PHARMACOKINETICS

DRUGS AND THE PHARMACEUTICAL SCIENCES

A Series of Textbooks and Monographs

Edited by

James Swarbrick
School of Pharmacy
University of North Carolina
Chapel Hill, North Carolina

Additional Volumes in Preparation

PHARMACOKINETICS

Regulatory • Industrial • Academic Perspectives

edited by

PETER G. WELLING
Warner-Lambert Company
Ann Arbor, Michigan

FRANCIS L. S. TSE
Sandoz Research Institute
East Hanover, New Jersey

MARCEL DEKKER, Inc.   New York and Basel

Library of Congress Cataloging-in-Publication Data

Pharmacokinetics : regulatory, industrial, academic
   perspectives.

   (Drugs and the pharmaceutical sciences ; v. 33)
   Bibliography: p.
   Includes index.
   1. Pharmacokinetics. I. Welling, Peter G. II. Tse,
Francis L. S. III. Series. [DNLM: 1. Pharmacokinetics.
W1 DR893B v. 33 / QV 38 P5327]
RM301.5.P485   1988   615'.7   88-10874
ISBN 0-8247-7945-2

MARCEL DEKKER, INC.
270 Madison Avenue, New York, New York 10016

Current printing (last digit):
10 9 8 7 6 5 4 3 2 1

PRINTED IN THE UNITED STATES OF AMERICA

To Christine, Clara, Graham, and Stephen

Preface

The subject of pharmacokinetics, at least as we understand it
today, is just over 50 years old. From its inception in 1937 with the
classical papers of Torsten Teorell, pharmacokinetics has evolved at
an incredible rate. Advances in pharmacokinetic concepts, together
with improved analytical methods to determine compounds in biological
fluids, have made it possible to completely characterize the nature
and kinetics of drug and metabolite disposition in the body. The huge
volume of published material and innumerable symposia on pharmacokinetics and drug metabolism bear testimony to their pivotal
importance in the study, and understanding, of drug action.

As an interdisciplinary science, progress in pharmacokinetics
has been aided by advances in our knowledge of the biology and
chemistry of the living organism as well as the physicochemical properties of drug entities. As technology improves, the study of pharmacokinetics and metabolism continues to expand and to achieve new
levels of sophistication. These factors, together with improved understanding of the mechanisms of drug disposition and drug action, will
continue to expand the role of pharmacokinetics and drug metabolism
in drug discovery and development.

With the golden jubilee year of pharmacokinetics behind us, it is
appropriate to pause and take stock of where we are and where we
are going in the future. The objective of this book is to present information and opinions from researchers who are recognized and active
in their respective areas of pharmacokinetics and drug metabolism.
Contributions were sought from leading scientists in the pharmaceutical
industry, academia, and regulatory agencies in order to accurately
reflect perspectives of each of these important sectors.

The book is organized to provide continuity across the broad spectrum of topics covered. The first chapter considers some of the past developments in pharmacokinetics, issues currently confronting us, and future challenges. Chapter 2 considers recent developments in analytical methods, particularly microcolumn methods, separation of chiral compounds, and robotics. Chapter 3 reviews dosage routes, including the advantages and disadvantages of buccal, intranasal, inhalation, and transdermal delivery. Chapters 4 and 5 address the role of pharmacokinetics in drug discovery and development, both clinical and nonclinical. The underlying philosophies are based on scientific, regulatory, and economic issues, some of which have hitherto received little attention in the pharmacokinetic literature. Chapters 6 and 7 address topics in drug absorption simulation and systems for drug organ targeting, respectively. Chapter 8 provides a regulatory perspective in the important and controversial area of oral controlled drug delivery. Chapter 9 provides critical comparison of classical and population pharmacokinetics. Chapters 10 and 11 are devoted to drug metabolism, advances in methodology, and the importance of metabolism in drug discovery and design. Chapters 12 and 13 deal, respectively, with saturable and dose-dependent kinetics and their importance in bioavailability determination and time-dependent pharmacokinetics.

Our intent in preparing this book has been to present the very latest concepts and developments in rapidly expanding or changing areas of pharmacokinetics and drug metabolism and to draw opinions from a variety of informed sources. We hope we have achieved our objective through the generous contributions of our colleagues in academia, industry, and the regulatory area. We wish to thank the contributing authors, who willingly took time off from busy schedules to keep us abreast of trends and developments in their areas of expertise. We thank also, on behalf of all contributing authors, the secretarial staff responsible for preparing the manuscripts. Without their help this book would not have been completed.

PETER G. WELLING

FRANCIS L. S. TSE

Contents

Contributors

Wallace P. Adams, Division of Bioequivalence, Center for Drug Evaluation, U.S. Food and Drug Administration, Rockville, Maryland

Gordan L. Amidon, College of Pharmacy, The University of Michigan, Ann Arbor, Michigan

C. R. Banfield, Department of Pharmaceutics, University of Washington, Seattle, Washington

Tsun Chang, Parke-Davis Pharmaceutical Research Division, Warner-Lambert Company, Ann Arbor, Michigan

Wayne A. Colburn, Parke-Davis Pharmaceutical Research Division, Warner-Lambert Company, Ann Arbor, Michigan

Shrikant V. Dighe, Division of Bioequivalence, Center for Drug Evaluation and Research, U.S. Food and Drug Administration, Rockville, Maryland

C. Anthony Hunt, Department of Pharmacy, University of California at San Francisco, San Francisco, California

James M. Jaffe, Department of Drug Metabolism, Sandoz Research Institute, East Hanover, New Jersey

Glen D. Leesman, College of Pharmacy, The University of Michigan, Ann Arbor, Michigan

Rene H. Levy, Department of Pharmaceutics, University of Washington, Seattle, Washington

Roderick D. MacGregor, Department of Pharmacy, University of California at San Francisco, San Francisco, California

Stephen C. Olson,   Parke-Davis Pharmaceutical Research Division,
Warner-Lambert Company, Ann Arbor, Michigan

Lawrence A. Pachla,   Parke-Davis Pharmaceutical Research Division,
Warner-Lambert Company, Ann Arbor, Michigan

K. Sandy Pang, Department of Pharmacology, University of
Toronto, Toronto, Ontario, Canada

Donald L. Reynolds,   Parke-Davis Pharmaceutical Research Division,
Warner-Lambert Company, Ann Arbor, Michigan

Gerald M. Rubin*,   Department of Pharmacy, University of California
at San Francisco, San Francisco, California

Horst F. Schran,   Department of Drug Metabolism, Sandoz Research
Institute, East Hanover, New Jersey

Ronald A. Siegel, Department of Pharmacy, University of California
at San Francisco, San Francisco, California

Patrick J. Sinko,   College of Pharmacy, The University of Michigan,
Ann Arbor, Michigan

Thomas N. Tozer,   Department of Pharmacy, University of California
at San Francisco, San Francisco, California

Francis L. S. Tse,   Sandoz Research Institute, East Hanover, New
Jersey

John G. Wagner, Department of Pharmacology, and Upjohn Center
for Clinical Pharmacology, The University of Michigan, Ann
Arbor, Michigan

Peter G. Welling,   Parke-Davis Pharmaceutical Research Division,
Warner-Lambert Company, Ann Arbor, Michigan

Thomas F. Woolf,   Parke-Davis Pharmaceutical Research Division,
Warner-Lambert Company, Ann Arbor, Michigan

D. Scott Wright,   Parke-Davis Pharmaceutical Research Division,
Warner-Lambert Company, Ann Arbor, Michigan

Xin Xu, Department of Pharmacology, University of Toronto, Toronto,
Ontario, Canada

Current affiliation: Drug Metabolism Department, Merrell Dow
Research Institute, Cincinnati, Ohio

PHARMACOKINETICS

1

Pharmacokinetics: Past Developments, Present Issues, Future Challenges

JOHN G. WAGNER   *The University of Michigan, Ann Arbor, Michigan*

I. PAST DEVELOPMENTS

A. Introduction

1. History of Pharmacokinetics

The history of pharmacokinetics has been covered well in a previous
review [1], published in 1981. Hence much of the expected content
of a chapter such as this has been omitted to avoid duplication. However, this chapter does attempt to indicate the present state of the
art of pharmacokinetics.

2. Other Specialties That Pharmacokinetics
Has Spawned

Figure 1 shows that pharmacokinetics is central to many other
specialties. Because of its earlier origins [1], pharmacokinetics
has spawned biopharmaceutics [2], pharmacogenetics [3,4], chronopharmacokinetics [5], toxicokinetics [6], and therapeutic monitoring
[7,8]. Pharmacokinetic principles are also involved in practical
therapeutics [9,10], in targeting of drugs [11], and in drug delivery research. In such a condensed review as this chapter, little
can be included about each of these subspecialities.

3. Pharmacokinetic Factors Involved in Producing
a Pharmacodynamic Effect

Figure 2 summarizes many of the factors involved in producing a
pharmacodynamic effect. There are hundreds of uncited articles
concerned with the factors in this figure.

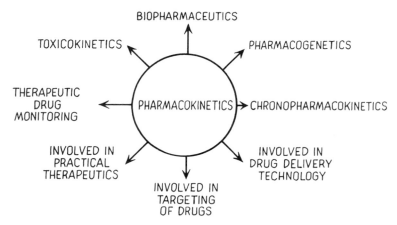

FIGURE 1 Pharmacokinetics is central to many other specialities.

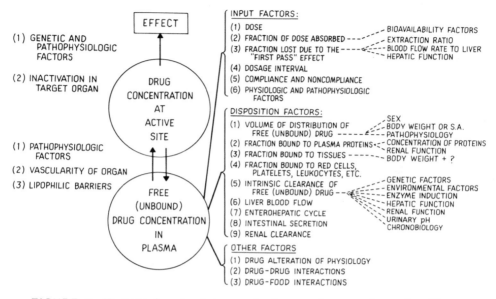

FIGURE 2 Factors involved in producing a pharmacodynamic effect.

B. Compartmental Models

1. Simple Classic Linear Compartmental Models

Compartmental models are utilized not only in pharmacokinetics but also in modeling metabolic systems (e.g., iodine or blood glucose) and by control engineers in designing feedback control systems. There have been three relatively recent reviews of linear compartment models [12–14].

Figure 3 shows schematically the most common compartmental models that have been used in pharmacokinetics. In the text that follows the equation for the concentration in the sampling compartment (i.e., the compartment containing V and C or V_p and C_p) is related to the schematic diagram of the compartment model in Figure 3. See Appendix for explanation of symbols.

a. One-Compartment Open Models

Model IA is the one-component open model with bolus intravenous administration:

$$C = \frac{D_{IV}}{V} e^{-k_e t}$$

(1)

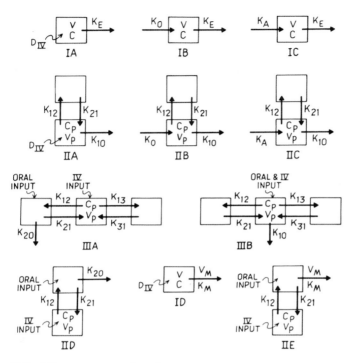

FIGURE 3 Schematic of the most common compartmental models that have been used in pharmacokinetics.

Model IB is the one-compartment open model with zero-order input:

$$C = \frac{k_0}{Vk_e}(1 - e^{-k_e t}) \tag{2}$$

Model IC is the one-compartment open model with first-order input:

$$C = \frac{FD}{V}\left(\frac{k_a}{k_a - k_e}\right)\left(e^{-k_e t} - e^{-k_a t}\right) \tag{3}$$

b. Two-Compartment Open Models

Model IIA is the classic two-compartment open model with bolus intravenous input:

$$C_p = \frac{D_{IV}}{V_p(\lambda_2 - \lambda_1)}[(k_{21} - \lambda_1)e^{-\lambda_1 t} - (k_{21} - \lambda_2)e^{-\lambda_2 t}] \quad (4)$$

Model IIB is the classic two-compartment open model with zero-order input:

$$C_p = \frac{k_0}{V_p}\left[\frac{(k_{21} - \lambda_1)(e^{+\lambda_1 t} - 1)e^{-\lambda_1 t}}{\lambda_1(\lambda_2 - \lambda_1)} + \frac{(k_{21} - \lambda_2)(e^{+\lambda_2 t} - 1)e^{-\lambda_2 t}}{\lambda_2(\lambda_1 - \lambda_2)}\right] \quad (5)$$

The postinput equation corresponding to Equation (5) is simply obtained by replacing $e^{+\lambda_1 t}$ by $e^{+\lambda_1 T}$ and $e^{+\lambda_2 t}$ by $e^{+\lambda_2 T}$, where T is the zero-order input time and t remains the time from the beginning of the zero-order input.

Model IIC is the classical two-compartment open model with first-order input:

$$C_p = \frac{FD}{V_p}k_a\left[\frac{(k_{21} - \lambda_1)e^{-\lambda_1 t}}{(\lambda_2 - \lambda_1)(k_a - \lambda_1)} + \frac{(k_{21} - \lambda_2)e^{-\lambda_2 t}}{(k_a - \lambda_2)(\lambda_1 - \lambda_2)}\right.$$
$$\left. + \frac{(k_{21} - k_a)e^{-k_a t}}{(\lambda_2 - k_a)(\lambda_1 - k_a)}\right] \quad (6)$$

In Equations (4) through (6), $\lambda_1 < \lambda_2$ and

$$\lambda_1 + \lambda_2 = k_{12} + k_{21} + k_{10} \quad (7)$$

$$\lambda_1\lambda_2 = k_{21}k_{10} \quad (8)$$

c. Three-Compartment Models

There are actually 21 three-compartment models for bolus intravenous administration, and models IIIA and IIIB are those most commonly used. Model IIIA has been called the "first-pass" three-compartment open model (Ref. 15, p. 114) and was first emphasized by Gibaldi and Feldman [16]. Equations for this model have been omitted here.

Model IIIB is the classical three-compartment open model in which sampling, input (both orally and intravenously), and elimination all occur in the central compartment. For intravenous bolus administration, the equations for this model are (Ref. 15, p. 117) [17].

$$C_p = \frac{D_{IV}}{V_p} \left[\frac{(k_{21} - \lambda_1)(k_{31} - \lambda_1)e^{-\lambda_1 t}}{(\lambda_2 - \lambda_1)(\lambda_3 - \lambda_1)} \right. $$

$$\left. + \frac{(k_{21} - \lambda_2)(k_{31} - \lambda_2)e^{-\lambda_2 t}}{(\lambda_1 - \lambda_2)(\lambda_3 - \lambda_2)} + \frac{(k_{21} - \lambda_3)(k_{31} - \lambda_3)e^{-\lambda_3 t}}{(\lambda_1 - \lambda_3)(\lambda_2 - \lambda_3)} \right]$$

$$\hspace{10cm} (9)$$

$$\lambda_1 + \lambda_2 + \lambda_3 = k_{10} + k_{12} + k_{13} + k_{21} + k_{31} \hspace{2cm} (10)$$

$$\lambda_1 \lambda_2 \lambda_3 = k_{10} k_{21} k_{31} \hspace{4cm} (11)$$

$$\lambda_1 \lambda_2 + \lambda_1 \lambda_3 + \lambda_2 \lambda_3 = k_{10} k_{21} + k_{13} k_{21} + k_{10} k_{31} + k_{21} k_{31} + k_{12} k_{31}$$

$$\hspace{10cm} (12)$$

2. Linear Two-Compartment Open Model with Peripheral Compartment Elimination

Models IA through IIC do not exhibit a first-pass effect and hence give erroneous parameter values for drugs that exhibit a first-pass effect. Model IIIA exhibits a first-pass effect, and Rowland et al. [18] showed that model IID also exhibits a first-pass effect and is much simpler. The equations applying to model IID for bolus intravenous input are

$$C_p = \frac{D_{IV}}{V_p(\lambda_2 - \lambda_1)} [(k_{20} + k_{21} - \lambda_1)e^{-\lambda_1 t} (k_{20} + k_{21} - \lambda_2)e^{-\lambda_2 t}]$$

$$\hspace{10cm} (13)$$

$$\lambda_1 + \lambda_2 = k_{12} + k_{21} + k_{20} \hspace{3cm} (14)$$

$$\lambda_1 \lambda_2 = k_{12} k_{20} \hspace{5cm} (15)$$

3. Physiologically Based and Circulatory Transport Models

Physiologically based pharmacokinetic models were introduced by Bischoff and Dedrick [19]. The models employ the lumped compartmental approach with the restriction that the volumes, flows, and other properties be physiologically meaningful and, usually, independently measured. The concept of flow-limited conditions is utilized for all body regions. In applying such a model one writes a differential mass balance equation for each body region. Chen and Gross

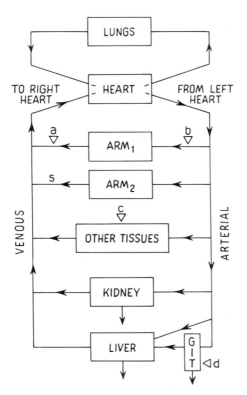

FIGURE 4 Model. (a) Intravenous. (b) Intra-arterial. (c) Subcut-aneous, buccol or intramuscular. (d) Oral.

[20] reviewed the applications of such models to anticancer drugs. Figure 4 is an illustration of such a model taken from Tozer [21]. The advantage of this particular example is that it shows the loca-tions of different input and sampling sites. Recently, Ball et al. [22] described a systematic approach to the design of this type of model and Gerlowski and Jain [23] discussed some of the principles and applications. The circulatory transport models studied by Vaughn and Hope [24] and Weiss and Föster [25] have properties similar to those of physiologically based models.

  Physiologically based pharmacokinetic models are utilized to *simulate* not to fit real data. However, the degree of closeness of the simulation to the real data may be quantitated by a statistical parameter, such as the coefficient of determination, r^2. This has not been done to the writer's knowledge. The author has not been too favorably impressed with the visual observations of the relation between the simulated and real data in the many literature applications of these models. In addition, the models simulate an "average" since the applications are based on average blood flows, average partition coefficients, and so on. Hence such models provide little or no information concerning intra- or interpatient variation.

4. One-Compartment Open Model with Michaelis-Menten Elimination

Model ID of Figure 3 is the one-compartment open model with Michaelis-Menten elimination and bolus intravenous input. Equation (16) is the differential equation, and Equation (17) is the integrated expression for this model:

$$- \frac{dC}{dt} = \frac{V'_m C}{K_m + C} \tag{16}$$

$$C_1 - C_2 + K_m \ln \frac{C_1}{C_2} = V'_m (t_1 - t_2) \tag{17}$$

where C_1 and C_2 are any two points on the C, t curve corresponding to times t_1 and t_2, respectively, and $V'_m = V_m/V$.

Other models (not shown) could be obtained by substituting Michaelis-Menten elimination for first-order elimination (rate constant k_e) in models IB and IC. The reader is referred to Wagner et al. [26] for many equations relating to these models and model ID.

Important consequences of Michaelis-Menten elimination kinetics are as follows:

1. AUC increases more than proportionally with increase in the size of single doses.
2. Steady-state blood concentrations increase more than proportionally with increase in the dose rate.
3. Drug clearance changes at every instant after a single dose, and in the elimination phase the clearance increases with decrease in the blood concentration.
4. The percentage of drug metabolized via a Michaelis-Menten pathway decreases with increase in the dose or dose rate.
5. The slower the rate of absorption or input, the smaller is the AUC for a given dose; conversely, the greater the rate of absorption or input, the larger is the AUC. Such effects occur if the ratio of the intrinsic clearance to liver blood flow is large enough.
6. The time required to reach steady state on multiple dosing increases with increase in the dose.

7. In the elimination phase, rectilinear plots of C versus t are pseudolinear for about two-thirds their length, but this does *not* indicate that zero-order kinetics are being obeyed.
8. The concept that there is a sudden jump from zero-order kinetics at high doses to first-order kinetics at low doses [27] is *not true*. In saturable metabolism the Michaelis-Menten equation explains the pharmacolinetics at all concentrations.

5. Two-Compartment Nonlinear Physiologic Pharmacokinetics Model with Michaelis-Menten Elimination

a. First-Pass Elimination

Use of the classic models IIA, IIB, and IIC became established before the first-pass effect became well recognized. Unfortunately, these models do not incorporate a first-pass effect, whereas models IID, IIE, IIIA, and IIIB do incorporate a first-pass effect. Hence the latter models are much more desirable for drugs exhibiting a first-pass effect. In these models, when drug is administered intraveneously into the "central compartment" 1, no elimination via metabolism occurs in that compartment but rather the drug must move to an adjacent compartment before it can be eliminated by metabolic processes. However, when the drug is administered orally it first enters the compartment from which elimination via metabolism occurs; hence the entire dose is exposed directly to the drug-metabolizing enzymes. The fraction that is bioavailable (i.e., reaches the central compartment unchanged) in models IID and IIIA on oral administration is $F = k_{21}/(k_{20} + k_{21})$, and the fraction extracted (metabolized eventually) is $E = k_{20}/(k_{20} + k_{21})$. With reference to the model of Figure 4, administration intraveneously, subcutaneously, intramuscularly, and buccally avoids this first pass effect. Model IIE also has a first-pass effect with the difference that the k_{20} of model IID is equivalent to V_m/V_2K_m of model IIE.

b. Arterial-Venous Concentration Differences

Intuitively and based on physiology, one would expect the arterial drug concentration to exceed the venous drug concentration shortly after a bolus intravenous dose or short infusion of drug. It is less obvious that at some later time the two concentrations become momentarily equal and from that time onward the venous concentration exceeds the arterial concentration. Simulations with such models as IID, IIE, and IIIA of Figure 3 and the model of Figure 4 confirm these expectations. Similar observations have been confirmed clinically or experimentally by several authors with a variety of drugs [28−31].

However, Chiou and Lau [30] made the following statement: "At the steady-state there is no A-V blood level difference during zero-order absorption, intravenous infusion, or net A-V blood level difference during a dosing interval following multiple dosing, provided that the compound is not eliminated from or formed in the sampling tissues or organ." Actually all first-pass drugs exhibit measurable arterial-venous concentration differences at steady state, and this was recently clearly shown to be the case for 5-fluorouracil [31]. We have also observed such steady-state A-V differences for the bromine analog of 5-fluorouracil in the rabbit and the dog. The simple model IIE of Figure 3 has been extensively studied by Wagner et al. [32], and the same model was used to explain the results in humans with 5-fluorouracil [31], propranolol [33], and verapamil [34]. Quantitative pooling of parallel Michaelis-Menten metabolite paths [35] greatly expands the usefulness of the simple model IIE in Figure 3. The chapter written by Tozer [21] clearly outlines the importance of A-V differences with anticancer drugs and provides many of the equations needed to apply such a model, as does the article of Wagner et al. [32].

c. *The Model and Equations*

Many of the equations may be considered noncompartmental and are treated as such and written in words rather than with symbols in Section I.D.2. However, the equations written in this section refer to a simple model. First we assume that the eliminating organ (e.g., the liver) has liver blood flow Q, that the arterial drug concentration at steady state c_{ss}^A is the concentration entering the organ, and that the venous drug concentration at steady state c_{ss}^V is the concentration leaving the organ. Drug is administered at a constant rate R_0 until a steady state is attained. The steady-state venous drug concentration is given by

$$c_{ss}^V = \frac{K_m R_0}{V_m - R_0} \tag{18}$$

The steady-state arterial drug concentration is given by Equation (19), and the flow parameter Q is given by Equation (20), which is Fick's law. Note that Equation (19) may be derived from Equations (18) and (20).

$$c_{ss}^A = \frac{R_0}{Q} + \frac{K_m R_0}{V_m - R_0} \tag{19}$$

$$Q = \frac{R_0}{c_{ss}^A - c_{ss}^V} \tag{20}$$

When we have collected such data experimentally we have measured across the eliminating organ, that is, by measuring drug in hepatic arterial blood and in hepatic venous blood. In such cases one would expect the flow parameter Q to average liver blood flow if the liver is the only eliminating organ. However, in the case of both 5-fluorouracil and nitroglycerin the flow parameter comes out equal to cardiac output, apparently because both these drugs are metabolized everywhere in the body.

It is not easy to obtain permission to take arterial blood samples from normal human volunteers. Fortunately, models IID and IIE may be used to involve venous blood only. One can consider that these models are akin to the isolated liver perfusion system in which compartment 1 is the reservoir and compartment 2 is the isolated organ. One can then consider that one always measures the drug in compartment 1. When drug is administered intraveneously it is infused into compartment 1, and when drug is administered either orally or into the hepatic artery one infuses the drug into compartment 2. Hence in the oral administration case an equation similar to Equation (18) holds where C_{ss}^{V} is replaced by C_{ss}^{PO}, meaning the concentration in compartment 1 when drug is infused into compartment 2. In intravenous administration, an equation similar to Equation (19) holds where C_{ss}^{A} is replaced by C_{ss}^{IV}, meaning the concentration in compartment 1 when drug is infused into compartment 1. This approach was taken by Wagner et al. [32].

If there is urinary excretion of unchanged drug as well as metabolism, such urinary excretion should be considered out of compartment 1 of the models IID and IIE since it is arterial blood-containing drug that goes to the kidney. In such cases Equations (18) and (19) must be modified [32].

6. Identifiability, Sensitivity Functions, and Optimization

The identifiability problem is concerned with determining whether the parameters of the model would be uniquely determined given a model of the system, specific input and output conditions, and error-free data. Hence identifiability is an a priori theoretical problem [36—47]. The identifiability problem was first introduced by Bellman and Aström [48].

For example, consider the models IIA and IID of Figure 3 and a third model that has elimination rate constants k_{10} and k_{20} from both compartments 1 and 2, respectively. It is easily shown [40] that the three models are structurally equivalent, if drug is introduced into compartment 1 and measurements are made in compartment 1 only and the three models are indistinguishable. However, Landaw et al. [41] presented an algorithm for computing all the uniquely identifiable sums and products of unidentifiable parameters of the general n-pool mammillary model when input and sampling occur in the central compartment. Chau [43] considered the case when input to the n-compartment mammillary model is into any arbitrary compartment and measurement is in the same arbitrary compartment and showed that a set of 2n elementary combinations of the model parameters can be determined. However, the model parameters themselves can only be localized each within an interval, and he showed how these intervals can be calculated.

The optimization problem can be formulated as follows. Given (1) an initial estimate of the parameter values, (2) that sampling is restricted to the time interval $0 < t \leqslant T$, (3) that the number of samples to be taken is n, and (4) the variance of the sampling errors, find the distribution of sampling times $(0, T)$ that optimizes the expected value of some function of the variances of the parameter estimates. The choice of the criterion function depends upon the error structure as well as on the goals of the experiment [44]. Bremermann [49] gave a method of unconstrained global optimization [49].

7. Mathematics of Other Compartmental Models

In the past decade or so many articles (e.g., see Refs. 50–79), other than those cited previously [12–79] have been published concerning compartmental model mathematics. Limited space in this chapter precludes discussion of most of them.

Suzuchi and Saitoh [50] discussed the use of a monoexponential equation, such as Equation (1), as an approximation to a biexponential equation, such as Equation (4), which may also be written as

$$C_p = C_1 e^{-\lambda_1 t} + C_2 e^{-\lambda_2 t} \tag{21}$$

Suzuchi and Saitoh [50] indicated that the critical ratios in such an approixmation were C_2/C_1 and λ_2/λ_1.

Later, MacKichan et al. [57] discussed the same problem and showed that the error in clearance (CL) when a monoexponential equation is assumed, when the descriptive equation is really a biexponential equation, is given by

$$\% \text{ error in CL} = 100 \frac{\lambda_1 C_2}{\lambda_2 C_1} \tag{22}$$

Estimates made with Equation (22) are most useful in clinical pharmacokinetics. If the disposition equation is triexponential, such as

$$C_p = C_1 e^{-\lambda_1 t} + C_2 e^{-\lambda_2 t} + C_3 e^{-\lambda_3 t} \qquad (23)$$

then the error in the clearance when a monoexponential equation is assumed is given by

$$\% \text{ error in CL} = 100 \left[\frac{\lambda_1}{C_1} \left(\frac{C_2}{\lambda_2} + \frac{C_3}{\lambda_3} \right) \right] \qquad (24)$$

where $\lambda_1 < \lambda_2 < \lambda_3$. The problem of vanishing exponential terms has been discussed and illustrated [52]. Another cause of a vanishing exponential term is a prolonged infusion time. The second term on the right-hand side of Equation (5) becomes less and less important as the infusion time increases, until, after a sufficiently long infusion time, the distribution phase vanishes completely and post-infusion data are described by a simple monoexponential equation.

Thron [55] presented a method to estimate the parameters V, k_a, and k_e for model IC of Figure 3 using only three pairs of C, t points.

An entire issue of *Arzneimittel-Forschung* [56] was devoted to pharmacokinetic model building. Kirby [58] discussed the matrix representation of compartment models and showed in a general way that the area under the curve (AUC) $0 - \tau$ at steady state was equal to AUC $0 - \infty$ after a single dose for constant doses at τ intervals, which supported the earlier statement of Wagner et al. [80].

The preceding discussion of compartment models is deterministic in nature, but there is a whole other world of stochastic models of compartmental systems [59, 61-64, 68-70]. The article of Matis and Wehrly [59] is a good introduction; they show that regression functions of stochastic models may be different from those of deterministic models.

Jacquez et al. [76] presented several papers on the kinetics of capillary exchange. Smith and Smith [81] described a new type of compartmental model, which they called the unsteady model, and illustrated its application. Wise [82] showed that many sets of pharmacokinetic data that were fit by polyexponential equations could also be fit by a γ curve:

$$C = at^{-\alpha} e^{-\beta t} \qquad (25)$$

C. Corollaries of Compartmental Model
    Pharmacokinetics

1. Absorption Kinetics

a. Wagner-Nelson Method

The Wagner-Nelson method [83–90] provides estimates of the amount
of drug absorbed in some specific time divided by the volume of
distribution and/or the fraction absorbed; it is based on the disposition model shown as model IA of Figure 3. The method may be
applied to single-dose data [83] or to multiple-dose data [85]. The
elimination rate constant used in application of the method should be
estimated from terminal blood concentration-time data of the same data
set as analyzed in the initial phase for absorption kinetics. This is
because of intrasubject variation of the elimination rate constant.
The method was incorrectly modified by Hendeles et al. [91] for
theophylline data since they recommended using the rate constant
and the asymptotic value derived from oral solution or intravenous
data to apply to absorption data from an oral sustained-release dosage
form. Experimental proof that this incorrect modification gives
erroneous results is given by Wagner [87–89,92]. There is a
modified Wagner-Nelson method when Michaelis-Menten elimiantion
kinetics are operative (Ref. 15, p. 200) [90]. In almost all cases
the Wagner-Nelson method provides the correct kinetics of absorption
when the method is applied to data from the two-compartment open
model with zero-order input [86], which is model IIB of Figure 3.
However, the method provides incorrect absorption kinetics when
applied to the analogous first-order input model, which is model IIC
of Figure 3 [84].

b. Loo-Riegelman Method and Exact Loo-
    Riegelman Method

Based on the disposition model IIA of Figure 3 and by assuming
the blood concentration-time curve consisted of piecewise linear segments, Loo and Riegelman [93] derived Equations (26) and (27):

$$\frac{(Aa)_{tn}}{V_p} = (C_p)_{t_n} + k_{10} \int_0^{t_n} C_p \, dt + (C_2)_{t_n} \tag{26}$$

$$(C_2)_{t_n} = (C_2)t_{n-1} \, e^{-k_{21}\Delta t} + \frac{k_{12}}{k_{21}} (C_p)_{t_{n-1}} (1 - e^{-k_{21}\Delta t})$$

$$+ \frac{k_{12}}{k_{21}} \Delta C_p - \frac{k_{12}}{k_{21}^2} \frac{\Delta C_p}{\Delta t} (1 - e^{-k_{21}\Delta t}) \tag{27}$$

where $(C_2)_{t_n} = (A_2)_{t_n}/V_p$ and A_a and A_2 are the amounts of drug absorbed and amount in the peripheral compartment, respectively. Wagner (Ref. 15, p. 433) [94] showed that improved results could be obtained with the Loo-Riegelman method [93] by fitting a smooth function through the data points and interpolating data between the observed data points. A FORTRAN computer program to do this was published (Ref. 15, p. 433). Wagner [94] also shows that the Loo-Riegelman method provided the correct absorption kinetics whether metabolism occurs in compartment 1 only, compartment 2 only or in both compartments of the two-compartment open model.

Wagner [95] derived a so-called exact Loo-Riegelman equation:

$$\frac{A_T}{V_p} = C_T + k_{10} \int_0^T C_p \, dt + k_{12} e^{-k_{21}T} \int_0^T C_p \, e^{+k_{21}t} \, dt$$

(28)

which is based on the disposition model IIA of Figure 3. The third term on the right-hand side of Equation (28) replaces Equation (27) of the Loo-Riegelman original method. Wagner et al. [96] showed that one could estimate the value of V_p from oral solution data and then fit the terminal C, t data of a solid oral dosage form and derive the parameters k_{12}, k_{21}, and k_{10} needed to apply Equation (28) to the early C, t solid oral dosage form data to obtain absorption kinetics. Thus intravenous data are not essential to apply the method. Proost [97] improved the accuracy of the exact Loo-Riegelman method [95] by choosing to use the linear or logarithmic trapezoidal rules on the basis of the sign of the second derivative. The exact Loo-Riegelman method, Equation (28), also gives the correct kinetics of absorption whether drug metabolism occurs only in compartment 1, only in compartment 2, or in both compartments 1 and 2 of the two-compartment open model.

c. *Other Absorption Methods Based on*
   Compartmental Models

The article of Wagner [95] also gives an equation to estimate absorption kinetics when disposition is triexponential. The method assumes that model IIIB of Figure 3 applies, and the needed constants are derived from Equations (9) through (12). This method also provides the correct kinetics of absorption independently of where metabolism occurs in the three-compartment system.

With the exception of the method proposed by Wagner et al. [96], application of Equations (26) through (28) usually requires prior administration of the drug intraveneously, fitting of the intravenous data to Equation (4), and estimation of the constants

k_{12}, k_{21}, and k_{10}. This procedure assumes no intrasubject variation of the pharmacokinetic parameters in going from the intravenous
to the oral experiments. Gerardin et al. [98] described a method in
which both the microscopic rate constants k_{12}, k_{21}, and k_{10} of model
IIA of Figure 3 and absorption kinetics are simultaneously estimated.
The writer has had no experience with this method.

2. *Rapidly Attaining Steady-State*

Based on model IIA of Figure 3, there have been various recommendations for attaining steady state rapidly. Krüger-Thiemer [99] rec-
comended administering a loading dose and then a continuous infusion, the rate of which decreases exponentially to the proper steady-
state rate. However, this technique is very difficult to initiate in a
given case. Boyes et al. [100] recommended intravenously administering a bolus loading dose equal to R_0/k_{10} and, at the same time,
starting a constant rate infusion at the rate R_0, where k_{10} is the
microscopic elimination rate constant of model IIA. Mitenko and
Ogilvie [101,102] made a similar recommendation but claimed that the
loading dose should be made equal to R_0/λ_1 [see Equations (7) and
(8)]. These recommendations have the disadvantage of producing
very high initial blood concentration values as a result of the bolus
loading dose and a relatively long period of time before a true plateau
blood concentration is produced.

Wagner [103] recommended a method of two consecutive infusions
based on model IIB, where the first infusion rate R_1 is given by
Equation [29] and continues for T hours:

$$R_1 = \frac{R_2}{1 - e^{-\lambda_1 T}} \qquad (29)$$

and the second infusion rate R_2 is given by

$$R_2 = \text{plasma clearance} \times C_{ss} \qquad (30)$$

where C_{ss} is the steady-state concentration desired and the λ_1 in
Euqation (29) is the apparent elimination rate constant. This solution to the problem is based on the concept that the fall of the
plasma level from the peak at time T to the steady-state concentration C_{ss} is rapid and based on λ_2 and not on λ_1. The method is
much safer since the peak blood concentration at T hours is never
nearly as high than if a loading dose equal to R_1T was given as a
bolus injection. Vaughan and Tucker [104] provided a generalized
derivation of Equation (29) that holds for any linear disposition
model.

Also independent of the disposition model, Vaughan and Tucker [105] showed how one could instantly attain and then maintain a constant blood level of a drug by combining an initial bolus loading dose, a constant rate intravenous infusion, and an exponential intravenous infusion; they then applied the method to lidocaine.

For oral therapy, a suitable loading dose D to aid in rapidly attaining steady state is given by

$$D_L = D_m \frac{\int_0^\tau C_{ss} \, dt}{\int_0^\tau C \, dt} = D_m \frac{\int_0^\infty C \, dt}{\int_0^\tau C \, dt} \tag{31}$$

where D_m is the maintenance dose administered every τ hours, C refers to blood concentration after a single dose or the first dose of a multiple-dose regimen, and C_{ss} refers to the steady-state concentration at time t after the dose D_m at steady state. Thus, $\int_0^\tau C_{ss} \, dt$ is the AUC in a dosage interval at steady state and is equal to $\int_0^\infty C \, dt$ for the single dose, and $\int_0^\tau C \, dt$ is the AUC up to τ hours after a single dose. Equation (31) is a consequence of the fact that $\int_0^\tau C \, dt / \int_0^\infty C \, dt$ is the fraction of the steady state attained at τ hours after the first dose of a multiple-dose regime [106].

3. Dosage Regimens and Prediction of Steady-State Levels

Much of the earlier literature on dosage regimen calculations is covered by Wagner (Ref. 15, pp. 129–172) and Gibaldi and Perrier [17] and is not repeated here. In pharmacokinetic studies, drugs are usually given at uniform time intervals so that only the area in one dosage interval (usually 4, 6, 8, or 12 hr) need be measured at steady state. However, in the treatment of disease, drugs are often prescribed to be taken at nonuniform time intervals. Several articles [107–113] are concerned with the mathematical prediction of steady-state concentrations under such conditions.

Wheeler and Sheiner [114] discussed a dosage regimen optimization method that is based on a compartmental model and minimization of a quadratic function of the differences between the compartmental drug levels.

Veng-Pedersen [115] a methodology for predicting steady-state drug concentrations for nonlinear systems in which, following an intravenous bolus dose, the derivatives of the drug concentration-time profile at arbitrary drug levels are independent of the dose given. Michaelis-Menten and parallel Michaelis-Menten and first-order elimination kinetics are included in such nonlinear systems.

An excellent review of dosage regimen design was recently published [116], as well as some other excellent articles [117—119], including one on computerized dosage regimens [118] and another [119] on a new method in cases of renal insufficiency. The Bayesian adjustment procedure was described by Sheiner et al. [120,121] and is most useful in therapeutic drug monitoring.

In dosing drugs that obey Michaelis-Menten elimination kinetics, dose changes must be conservative since a given change in dosage in one patient may make little difference in the steady-state drug concentrations but the same change in another patient may change the drug blood concentration from subtherapeutic to toxic. The writer believes that it is most important to know whether a drug obeys Michaelis-Menten kinetics in the therapeutic blood concentration range prior to introduction of the drug to the market and fails to understand the administration attitudes in some companies that such information should be hidden or downplayed.

4. Time-Dependent Pharmacokinetics

Time-dependent pharmacokinetics is distinguished from dose-dependent pharmacokinetics in that the former involves an actual physiological or biochemical alteration in the organ(s) of the body associated with the drug disposition parameters in question [122] but the latter does not. Levy [122] published an excellent review of time-dependent pharmacokinetics (see also Chap. 13).

5. Drug Metabolite Kinetics

There have been two excellent reviews of drug metabolite kinetics [123,124]; one of these [124] concerns only linear metabolite kinetics, and the other [123] is mainly concerned with linear kinetics. Chapter 10 in this book is concerned with drug metabolite kinetics. Unfortunately, nonlinear metabolite kinetics has been largely ignored in these reviews despite its great importance in practical therapeutics. Examples are aspirin and salicylic acid [125] whose pharmacokinetics are nonlinear and have been reviewed by Levy [126], who was largely responsible for working out the metabolite kinetics of these drugs.

6. Reversible Metabolism Models

Several examples of reversible drug metabolism have been reported [127—133], including cortisone-hydrocortisone, prednisone-prednisolone, sulfonamide-N_4-acetylsulfonamide, penicillamine-penicillamine disulfide and 3-hydroxydiazepam-3-hydroxydiazepam glucuronide. Several linear models [127,128] have been proposed in such cases, and one of these leads to two elimination clearances and two intercompartmental clearances, which introduces considerable complications in the pharmacokinetics in such cases. Even bioavailability in such cases must be estimated in a different way from the classic manner. Recently, the prednisone-prednisolone case has been studied in considerable detail [129,130]; it was shown that during infusion of prednisone in the rabbit the metabolite, prednisolone, is formed by first-order kinetics but the reverse reaction, namely the conversion of prednisolone to prednisone, becomes saturated and eventually proceeds at a zero-order rate over a certain range of concentrations. The same system was also studied in humans by the same authors, and results await publication. In the simplest linear case in reversible drug metabolism, the unchanged drug after bolus intravenous injection can produce a biexponential equation to describe the data, which is the result of the reversible metabolism, not drug distribution as is the usual case.

7. Mean Residence Time and Volume of Distribution Steady State

Wagner [134,135] summarized much of the literature concerning mean residence time (MRT) and volume of distribution steady state (V_{ss}) and concluded that these parameters are model dependent since both the site of administration and site(s) of elimination determine the magnitude of the MRT and V_{ss}. He also showed that, based on models IA, IC, IIA, IIC, and IID of Figure 3, the dosage interval τ could be chosen based on Equation (32) such that if τ was estimated with Equation (32) then

$$\tau = (a\ factor)(plasma\ compartment\ MRT + absorption\ site\ MRT)$$

$$(32)$$

$C_{ss}^{max}/C_{ss}^{min} \cong 2$. For example, for model IC, Equation (32) becomes

$$\tau = 1.35 \left(\frac{1}{k_e} + \frac{1}{k_a} \right) \tag{33}$$

and such a τ value provides a $C_{ss}^{max}/C_{ss}^{min}$ ratio averaging about 2 and a percentage variation at steady state of about ±33%.

8. Population Pharmacokinetics and Use of NONMEM

Population pharmacokinetics have been extensively studied [137−141], particularly by Sheiner and Beal [136−139,141−145]. Population pharmacokinetic parameter quantify population mean kinetics, interindividual variability, and residual variability, including intraindividual variability and measurement error [136]. A major quest of population kinetics is to discover which measurable pathophysiologic factors cause change in the dose-concentration relationship and to estimate the degree to which they do so [145]. Population pharmaco-

kinetic studies are usually carried out during routine clinical
use of a drug. Population kinetic studies add to, but cannot replace, thorough evaluation by classic pharmacokinetic and pharmacodynamic studies in humans. NONMEM is a user-unfriendly program
that has been used in deriving population pharmacokinetic parameters
[138]. Martin et al. [143] discussed the problems and pitfalls in
estimating average pharmacokinetic parameters. They concluded:

> NONMEM, Nonlinear Mixed Effect Model, a recently developed
> computer program for estimating population pharmacokinetics
> from routine patient data, simultaneously takes care of all the
> parameters of the model, including the variance parameters. It
> carefully analyzes the variances of the total error, i.e., the
> intra- and inter-individual variation, inadequate pharmacokinetic
> modelling, analytical error and residual error, using a method
> called extended least squares. This program seems to avoid
> the shortcomings of both "standard" methods, the naive pooled
> data approach and the two-stage approach. It provides ac-
> curate and precise estimates of all parameters and computes their
> confidence intervals.

Probably the best example of use of NONMEM is the report of
Grasela et al. [140], in which 780 steady-state phenytoin concentrations and associated dose rates from 322 patients were analyzed.
Recently, Sheiner and Benet [145] reported the pros and cons of
therapeutic drug monitoring of patients in phase III clinical trials
of new potential drug products and the information that might be
obtained from applying population pharmacokinetic principles to the
resulting data collected.

The author believes there are certain problems with population
pharmacokinetics.

1. A model must be specified for the population. In a study
of amobarbital given by bolus intravenous injection to 28 subjects
[146], the number of exponential terms needed to describe each data
set was chosen by sound statistical methods; 5 subjects (18%) required only one exponential term; 16 subjects (57%) required two
exponential terms; and 7 subjects (25%) required three exponential
terms. Thus, the model needed varies with the subject studied.
Szpunar [147] studied the pharmacokinetics of flurbiprofen in
humans following oral administration of three different doses in the
form of tablets and one dose as an aqueous solution. The absorption
of the drug administered in solution form in individual subjects and
the average plasma concentrations resulting from administration of
each of the tablet doses were shown to be explained well by first-
order kinetics, but in individual subjects the absorption following
administration of the drug in tablets was clearly not first order,
but about one-half exhibited zero-order kinetics; the other half gave

S-shaped plots of fraction absorbed versus time. Thus the absorption kinetics from individual subject data were different from that from mean or pooled data. Thus the author believes that the population pharmacokinetic parameter values may be considerably biased since the model used in the analysis may be inappropriate for many of the patients studied. Such effects could be studied by a simulation technique.

    2. Little accumulated experience: There have been several theoretical articles [136—139,141—145] on population pharmacokinetic methods, but very few applications like the study by Grasela et al. [140]; thus there are few data upon which to make a real judgment.

    3. Cost: If one wished to study 15 different factors, NONMEN requires two runs per factor, and on our mainframe computer the cost averages about $18 per run; hence such a study analysis would cost $540.

    4. Some administrators, naive about pharmacokinetic knowledge, appear to have been "oversold" on population pharmacokinetics and believe they can replace classic pharmacokinetic studies in new drug development procedures. Classic studies are the backbone of new drug applications and should remain so. Population pharmacokinetics has a place but it is restricted.

D. Noncompartmental Analysis

1. Introduction

"Noncompartmental" and "model-independent" have been used more frequently in the literature of the past 5 years or so, and some investigators appear to believe this makes their articles more in vogue. However, the author thinks that this is a misinterpretation and that such an idea is unwarranted.

    There are pharmacokinetic concepts and parameters that are truly noncompartmental and even model independent. Some of these are given here as word equations:

Bioavailability with respect to entire body

    = fraction of the administered dose that reaches circulation unchanged

$$(34)$$

Bioavailability with respect to eliminating organ

$$= \frac{\text{rate or presentation of drug to organ} - \text{rate of elimination of drug by organ}}{\text{rate of presentation of drug to organ}} \qquad (35)$$

Blood flow in eliminating organ

$$= \frac{\text{constant input rate of drug to organ}}{\substack{\text{concentration of drug in} \\ \text{arterial blood entering}} - \substack{\text{concentration of drug in} \\ \text{venous blood exiting}}} \qquad (36)$$

Extraction ratio of drug by eliminating organ

$$= \frac{\text{rate of elimination of drug by organ}}{\text{rate of presentation of drug to organ}} \qquad (37)$$

Metabolic clearance of drug by eliminating organ

$$= \frac{\text{rate of elimination of drug by organ}}{\text{concentration of drug in blood exiting from organ}}$$

$$= \frac{\text{constant rate of input of drug to organ}}{\text{concentration of drug in venous blood exiting}} \qquad (38)$$

Total body clearance

$$= \frac{\text{constant input rate of drug to body}}{\text{drug concentration in arterial blood}}$$

$$= \frac{\text{rate of elimination of drug from body}}{\text{drug concentration in arterial blood}} \qquad (39)$$

The following two mass balance equations appear to be truly "noncompartmental" when kinetics are linear:

$$D_{IV} = CL_{TB}(AUC)_{IV} \qquad (40)$$

$$FD_{PO} = CL_{TB}(AUC)_{PO} \qquad (41)$$

where D is the dose, F is bioavailability with respect to the entire body, AUC is area under the blood concentration-time curve, CL_{TB} is total body clearance, and subscripts IV and PO refer to intravenous and oral, respectively.

However, most ideas in pharmacokinetics that are referred to as noncompartmental and some that are referred to as model independent actually depend upon the structured model shown in Figure 5, which is a modification from Di Stefano [148]. Thus, most so-called noncompartmental items assume central compartment input, elimination, and sampling, and in essence this noncompartmental compartment concept is the same as the n-compartment open mammillary model except that the rate constants to peripheral compartments are not specified. It must be stressed a structure like that in Figure 4 is inappropriate to describe the pharmacokinetics of first-pass drugs [16,18,21,32] and that models IID and IIE of Figure 3 are the minimum models to do so.

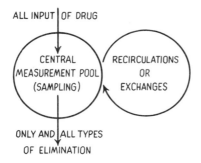

ALL INPUT OF DRUG

CENTRAL MEASUREMENT POOL (SAMPLING)

RECIRCULATIONS OR EXCHANGES

ONLY AND ALL TYPES OF ELIMINATION

FIGURE 5 Model IV. The basic physical model for most "noncompart-mental" analysis.

2. Deconvolution

Rescigno and Segré [149] introduced deconvolution to pharmacokinetics but called it "the inverse operation of convolution." Convolution and deconvolution may be explained as follows. Figure 6 shows a "black box", which is a physical system that transforms input into output. The input and output are given by continuous or sectionally con-tinuous linear functions. If X(t) is the input function (which is the rate of appearance of drug in the "black box") and Y(t) is the out-put function, then there is a weighting function G(t) such that

$$Y(t) = \int_0^t G(t - T)X(T) \, dT \qquad (42)$$

Hence it is said that Y(t) is given by the *convolution* between G(t) and X(t) where $0 \leqslant T \leqslant t$, and Equation (42) is called a con-volution integral. Transformation of Equation (42) into the Laplacian domain gives

$$y(s) = g(s)x(s) \qquad (43)$$

y(s), g(s), and x(s) are the Laplace transforms of Y(t), G(t), and X(t), respectively. Also g(s) is called the *transfer function* and its

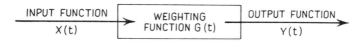

INPUT FUNCTION X(t) | WEIGHTING FUNCTION G(t) | OUTPUT FUNCTION Y(t)

FIGURE 6 "Black box."

matrix is called the transfer matrix of the black box. As applied
in pharmacokinetics, $Y(t)$ is usually the function describing the
plasma concentration-time curve following extravascular (usually oral)
administration, $G(t)$ is the function describing the plasma concentration-time curve following bolus intravenous (or impulse) administration, and $X(t)$ is the function describing the input.

It is instructive to indicate the functions for model IC of Figure
3. Related to Equation (42), for this model we have

$$Y(t) = \int_0^t \underbrace{e^{-k_e(t-T)}}_{G(t\ -\ T)}\underbrace{k_a\frac{D}{V}e^{-k_aT}}_{X(T)}\ dT = \frac{D}{V}\left(\frac{k_a}{k_a - k_e}\right)\left(e^{-k_et}\ -\ e^{-k_at}\right)$$

$$(44)$$

In the Laplacian domain for the same model we have

$$L[Y(t)] = L[G(t)]L[X(t)] \tag{45}$$

$$\underbrace{\frac{k_a(D/V)}{(S + k_a)(S + k_e)}}_{y(s)} = \underbrace{\frac{1}{S + k_e}}_{g(s)}\ \underbrace{\frac{k_a(D/V)}{S + k_a}}_{x(s)} \tag{46}$$

and $g(s)$ is the transfer function from the absorption site to the
blood and is given by

$$g(s) = \frac{y(s)}{x(s)} = \frac{\text{Laplace transform of the output function}}{\text{Laplace transform of the input function}} \tag{47}$$

Various methods have been proposed to deconvolute—that is,
obtain $X(t)$ when $Y(t)$ and $G(t)$ are known [149–161]. One of
these [159] described a computer program, DECONV, that required
that all the coefficients of the polyexponential equation describing
the impulse response $G(t)$ be positive. In such a case Wagner [95]
showed that the new model-dependent methods, such as the exact
Loo-Riegelman method, were exactly equal to the so-called model-
independent method of Veng-Pedersen [155]. Later, Gillespie and
Veng-Pedersen [160] gave a source listing for a new computer
program, DCON, in which the impulse response $G(t)$ could be a polyexponential function with one or more negative coefficients. They
illustrated the use of DCON by using C, t data obtained following
oral administration of an aqueous solution of ibuprofen to obtain
$X(t)$ data following oral administration of ibuprofen in tablet form.
They indicated that the $X(t)$ obtained with DCON "represents the

in vivo release rate from the (solid or oral) dosage form." However, this is untrue since such X(t) data also contain information about stomach emptying and are not simply a measure of in vivo release rate. It should also be noted that Wagner et al. [96] evaluated the same ibuprofen data by model-dependent methods [95,96], but their analysis provided data on the overall rate of appearance of ibuprofen in the blood, rather than the "apparent rate of appearance of ibuprofen at the absorption site," as was the case with use of DCON [160]. If the G(t) data used with DCON had been the impulse response from a bolus intravenous injection, then the X(t) results would also represent the rate of appearance of drug in blood. It should also be noted that deconvolution methods as described to date assume that there is no intrasubject variation in pharmacokinetics from the intravenous or aqueous solution trial in a given person to the trial with the solid oral dosage form. Such intrasubject variation is often considerable [162–166]. The model-dependent absorption method of Wagner et al. [96] takes care of intrasubject variation of the k_{12}, k_{21}, and k_{10} of model IIA of Figure 3 but requires the assumption of constant V_p and complete bioavailability and yields the data from which the kinetics of absorption may be obtained.

It should also be noted that, as usually applied, deconvolution assumes that the metabolism of a drug is exactly the same following intravenous and oral administrations—which often is not the case, as with quinidine and propranolol, for example.

3. Plasma Protein and Tissue Binding

The assumption of Behm and Wagner [167] and many other scientists prior to 1983 that no volume shift occurs during equilibrium dialysis was in error. A number of articles [168–173] published during 1983 and 1984 clearly showed that volume shifts occur during equilibrium dialysis and if binding is nonlinear or concentration dependent this must be taken into consideration or erroneous results are obtained. Several methods have been proposed to make the appropriate correction for the volume shift [168–173]. Behm and Wagner [167] also showed that in cases of nonlinear binding the bound versus free concentration data must be fit to the appropriate binding equation and then the free concentrations found from the total concentrations via a rearrangement of the appropriate binding equation. When the method of Tozer et al. [169] is used to correct for the volume shift it is their C_b'' values that are related to the C_f values, where C_b'' is the bound concentration of drug assuming no volume shift and C_f is the free concentration measured in the buffer at dialysis equilibration.

Gibaldi and Koup published a significant article in 1986 [174]. They showed that the apparent volume of distribution and drug clearance from the blood should be treated as independent pharmacokinetic parameters and that volume of distribution per se has no effect on clearance or on average steady-state blood levels. They also showed that although changes in tissue binding will affect partition coefficient and apparent volume of distribution, such changes will have no effect on average steady-state blood levels of either total or free drug. They suggested that rather than writing the clearance equation as Equation (48) it should be written as Equation (49):

$$CL = VK \qquad\qquad\qquad\qquad (48)$$

$$K = \frac{CL}{V} \qquad\qquad\qquad\qquad (49)$$

since the latter equation clearly indicates that K rather than CL is the dependent variable.

Wilkinson [175] reviewed plasma and tissue binding considerations in drug disposition. He discussed two extremes of behavior following intravenous drug administration when binding is linear. If clearance or extraction is high (i.e., the intrinsic clearance of unbound drug is much greater than liver blood flow), the total drug concentration is relatively independent of the degree of binding and the unbound concentration is simply related by the unbound fraction. On the other hand, if hepatic extraction is low (i.e., liver blood flow is much greater than the intrinsic clearance of unbound drug), the total drug concentration in blood is inversely proportional to the unbound fraction and binding has little effect on unbound drug concentrations. After oral administration, regardless of the magnitude of the drug's free intrinsic clearance, total drug concentration depends on binding, but the unbound levels are determined only by the metabolic parameter, although changes in the shape of the concentration-time curve may be present owing to alterations in systemic elimination.

Bachmann and Sullivan [176] showed that when model ID of Figure 3 holds and V_m and K_m are estimated from total drug concentrations, then the K_m estimated is really K'_m/f_m, where K'_m is the parameter in terms of unbound concentration and f_u is the fraction unbound. Similarly, Wagner [177] showed that when model IIE of Figure 3 holds then K_m estimated with Equation (18) from the total concentrations is K'_m/f_{u2}, where K'_m is the parameter in terms of unbound concentrations and f_{u2} is the unbound fraction in venous blood exiting from the liver.

4. Michaelis–Menten Kinetics

The differential and integrated Michaelis-Menten equations, which also apply to model ID of Figure 3, are Equations (16) and (17) in Section I.B.4 and the consequences of Michaelis-Menten elimination kinetics are listed in the same section. Some of the fundamental properties of the Michaelis-Menten equation were discussed formerly [178]. Veng-Pedersen [115] discussed the superimpossibility of data obeying Equation (17), and Wagner et al. [179] showed a practical application of this property using ethanol in humans. Data obeying Equation (17) have usually been obtained by numerical integration of Equation (16), but Beal [180,181] has given an explicit solution to Equation (50):

$$\frac{dC}{dt} = \frac{R_0}{V} - \frac{V'_m \, C}{K_m + C} \tag{50}$$

and Veng-Pedersen and Suaréz [183] have given an explicit solution to Equation (16). Wagner et al. [26] gave equations for time courses, areas under curves and clearances for model ID of Figure 3 with various types of input and for single doses and the steady state.

The minimum steady-state concentration, C_{ss}^{min} for model IA of Figure 3 when a maintenance dose D_m is administered every τ hours is given by

$$C_{ss}^{min} = \left(\frac{D_m}{V}\right)\left(\frac{e^{-k_e \tau}}{1 - e^{-k_e \tau}}\right) = \left(\frac{D_m}{V}\right)\left(\frac{1}{e^{+k_e \tau} - 1}\right) \tag{51}$$

Sawchuk and Rector [184] showed that for the nonlinear model ID of Figure 3 under the same conditions, $k_e \tau$ must be replaced by Q, where $Q = (V_m \tau - D_m)/VK_m$. It is also easily shown that for the nonlinear model ID Q is also equal to $(1 - D_m/V_m \tau)k_e \tau$ since $k_e = V_m/VK_m$. Hence when changing from first-order to Michaelis-Menten elimination kinetics, one must multiply the first-order exponent $k_e \tau$ by $(1 - D_m/V_m \tau)$.

Single-dose data derived from the Michaelis-Menten Equation (16) that obey Equation (17) have the shape of a hockey stick. The upper two-thirds of such data are pseudolinear, but his does not indicate zero-order kinetics. If one joints the two points corresponding to the initial concentration C_0 and a concentration C_0/e or $C_0/2.718$, the slope k_0 of such a line is given by

$$k_0 = \frac{V'_m(0.632C_0)}{K_m + (0.632C_0)} \tag{52}$$

and since $C_0 = D/V$ the slope depends upon all the parameters V_m, K_m, D, and V.

There are no "special cases" of the Michaelis-Menten equation. If we let $v = -dC/dt$ in Equation (16), then all cases may be changed to one curve by plotting relative velocity v/V_m versus relative concentration C/K_m so that Equation (16) becomes

$$\frac{v}{V_m} = \frac{C}{K_m + C} = \frac{C/K_m}{1 + C/K_m} \tag{53}$$

First-pass drugs usually obey Michaelis-Menten elimination kinetics as a result of high concentrations reaching the metabolism sites in the gut wall and the liver after oral administration. Hence the rate of input of drug given orally may significantly affect the bioavailability of the drug, and slow input, such as provided by sustained-release dosage forms, would provide lower bioavailabilities than immediate-release dosage forms. The extremes of input rate are bolus administration and zero-order input. Based on model ID of Figure 3 and these two extremes of input rate, Wagner [33] showed that the ratio of areas in a dosage interval at steady state is given by

$$\frac{(AUC\ 0 - \tau)_{zero\ order}}{(AUC\ 0 - \tau)_{bolus}} = \left(\frac{V_m}{V_m - R_0}\right)\left(\frac{1}{1 + D_m/VK_m[1/2 + 1/(e^Q - 1)]}\right) \tag{54}$$

A plot of the area ratio of Equation (54) versus the dose rate R_0 gives a U-shaped curve such that the area ratio is equal to unity at $R_0 = 0$ and at $R_0 \rightarrow V_m$ and becomes a minimum somewhere in the interval $0 < R_0 < V_m$. Equation (54) was applied to propranolol data and it explained why reported sustained-release forms had low bio-availabilities [33].

For model IIE of Figure 3, Equation (18) may also be written as

$$C_{ss}^V = \frac{R_0}{CL_i(1 - R_0/V_m)} \tag{55}$$

where CL_i is the intrinsic metabolic clearance and is equal to V_m/K_m and the bioavailability F for the same model for oral administration is given by

$$F = \frac{1}{1 + (CL_i/Q)(1 - R_0/V_m)} \qquad (56)$$

Equation (56) indicates that when $R_0 = 0$, the intrinsic bioavailability (corresponding to first-order kinetics) is given by $F = 1/(1 + CL_i/Q)$ and this is a minimum value. F then increases as the dose rate R_0 increases until bioavailability is complete ($F = 1$) when $R_0 = V_m$. It should be noted that Equation (56) depends upon the same input rate when drug is administered intraveneously and orally [32] or there is one input rate when drug is measured in arterial and venous blood on either side of the liver and $F = C_V/C_A$. Theoretically and practically the oral bioavailability can exceed 100% when Michaelis-Menten elimination kinetics are obeyed. This was shown recently for ethanol [185] since the administration rate when the alcohol was administered intravenously was less than that when it was administered orally.

Veng-Pedersen and Suaréz [186] expanded the superimpossibility phenomenon of nonlinear kinetics [115] and gave a model-independent method of estimating the peak, trough, and average steady-state concentrations of a drug obeying nonlinear elimination kinetics

Metzler and Tong [187] discussed "the ill-conditioning of the estimation of parameters of a differential equation that includes the so-called Michaelis-Menten output," in other words the estimation of V_m' and K_m of Equation (16) from downslope C, t data obeying Equation (17). However, Wagner [86] showed that when V_m' and K_m were estimated from downslope postinfusion ethanol concentration-time data, then the Wagner-Nelson method [83] was applied to the data obtained during infusion, that the known zero-order infusion rate constant was estimated almost exactly. This accuracy implies that the parameters V_m' and K_m that were estimated were most probably accurately determined and of course were useful pharamcokinetically.

5. Bioavailability and Use of Stable Isotopes

The usual objective in a comparative bioavailability trial is to show that the in vivo bioavailability characteristics of a new formulation of an active ingredient are essentially identical to those of an already approved, standard formulation. Classically this was done by hypothesis testing using such characteristics as plasma concentration at each sampling time, amount excreted in the urine at each sampling time, AUC, peak plasma concentration, and time of the peak plasma concentration. Westlake [188-190] proposed that symmetrical confidence intervals replace hypothesis testing, but the statisticians differ among themselves and several other methods [191-196] have been proposed as well as methods [197,198] for special conditions. The real problem in comparative bioavailability testing, however, does not appear to have been addressed to date. This is how to make an overall assessment of equivalence or inequivalence in bioavailability on the basis of all plasma and/or urinary data at once rather than a series of the same tests being performed on multiple sets of data obtained in the same bioavailability trial.

An important complicating factor in crossover comparative bioavailability trials is intrasubject variation in pharmacokinetics from one phase of the study to the next. This is true with respect to both the rate and efficiency of absorption of the drug involved in the trial. A suitable solution to the problem of intrasubject variation of pharmacokinetics is use of the drug labeled with a stable isotope along with the drug containing the usual isotope of the same element [199–202]. If the drug, such as phenobarbital [196], obeys linear kinetics, then the clearance CL_L may be estimated from the data resulting from the tracer dose of stable istopically labeled drug that accompanied the usual dose of drug in a bioavailability trial and this clearance used to estimate the bioavailability of the nonisotopically labeled drug F_U according to Equations (57) and (58):

$$CL_L = \frac{D_L}{(AUC)_L} \tag{57}$$

$$F_U = \frac{CL_L (AUC)_U}{D_U} \tag{58}$$

where L refers to labeled and U refers to unlabeled. If the drug, such as phenytoin [199,201], obeys Michaelis-Menten kinetics and the study is a steady-state study, then the clearance of isotopically labeled drug will be given by

$$CL_U = \frac{V_m}{K_m + C_U + C_L} \tag{59}$$

where C_U is the steady-state concentration of unlabeled drug. In the linear case one could also use the data collected from the single dose of isotopically labeled drug to estimate disposition parameters k_{12}, k_{21}, and k_{10} of model IIA of Figure 3 if applicable then use the exact Loo-Riegelman method of Wagner [95] to elucidate the kinetics of absorption of the nonisotopically labeled drug or use the isotope data as the impulse response to apply one of the deconvolution methods [150–161]. The author believes that the use of stable isotopically labeled drug will increase dramatically in the future as a result of their use obviating the intrasubject variation problem in pharmacokinetics.

Intestinal excretion of some drugs from blood to intestinal lumen [203] and biliary cycling [204,205] complicates pharmacokinetics, but Shepard et al. [204] showed that the comparison of AUC is still a valid procedure for estimation of bioavailability in cases of biliary cycling of a drug.

6. Variable V_d Model and Problems

Takada and Asada [206−208] presented a variable volume of distribution model to describe drug disposition curves after bolus intravenous administration. Their single-dose equation is shown as Equation (60):

$$C = \frac{De^{-kt}}{V_1 + (V_2)_{max}t/(K_d + t)} \tag{60}$$

and at steady state [207] the concentration-time curve is given by

$$C_{ss} = \frac{De^{-kt}}{V_1 + (V_2)_{max}} \tag{61}$$

The authors described this as a model-independent approach, but of course Equation (60) is a model itself; hence the method is obviously model dependent. Equation (60) indicates that the volume of distribution expands from its initial value of V_1 at time of dosing ($t = 0$) to the final value of $V_1 + (V_2)_{max}$.

There appear to be fundamental problems with this approach. First, the model indicates that the mass of drug in the body does not build up on multiple dosing (which it does), but rather it is a change in the volume of distribution that causes the concentration to change on multiple dosing or infusion of drug. Second, making a ratio of Equation (61) to Equation (60) for $t = 0$ (time of dosing of first does and time of dosing at steady state) yields $C_{ss}(0)/C(0) = V_1/[V_1 + (V_2)_{max}] < 1$, when of course the steady-state concentration has to be equal to or greater than $C(0)$. Colburn [209] described other similar models, and this author has similar problems with those equations.

II. PRESENT ISSUES

A. Estimation of Pharmacokinetic Parameters

Statistical aspects of estimating pharmacokinetic parameters have recently been reviewed [210] and hence are not covered in this chapter.

A present issue is the problem of choosing weights in nonlinear regression analysis [211], and extended least-squares nonlinear regression was offered as a possible solution to this problem [212]. This author believes the results are important, not necessarily the method by which they were obtained; by this $\underline{I}$ mean that the important thing is to obtain a minimum $\Sigma \, \text{dev}^2 = \Sigma(\hat{C} - C)^2$ (note that weighting is absent in the expression) for a given data set and that the method is best that produces this result.

Another present issue is that some scientists appear to think it is superior to say they calculated pharmacokinetic parameters by noncompartmental or model-independent methods. As stated previously, model IV is really the structured model assumed in so-called noncompartmental analysis. There are noncompartmental pharmacokinetic parameters, as indicated in Section D.1, but despite literature to the contrary [213–222] the system mean residence time and the volume of distribution steady state depend upon the site of input, the site of sampling, and the site of elimination. This is most important to understand since for classic models, such as models IIA, IIB, IIC, and IIIB, V_{ss} is independent of k_{10}, but such models are unsatisfactory for first-pass drugs. For nonclassic models, such as models IID and IIIA, which satisfactorily explain pharmacokinetics of first-pass drugs, V_{ss} is dependent upon k_{20}. There are really two types of system MRT—one type that I term the system moment MRT is given by Equation (62); the other type, which I term the system matrix MRT, is given by Equation (63):

$$\text{MRT} = \frac{\int_0^\infty tC \, dt}{\int_0^\infty C \, dt} \tag{62}$$

$$\text{MRT} = \frac{\int_0^\infty A_b \, dt}{D} \tag{63}$$

where A_b is the amount of drug in the body at time t after a single dose of size D. For the classic models IIA, IIB, IIC, and IIIB, the MRT given by Equations (62) and (63) are equal in each case, whereas for the nonclassic models IID and IIIA, the MRT given by Equation (62) and (63) are not the same for each model.

Physiologically oriented models based on circulatory drug transport have been proposed as alternatives to classic pharmacokinetic models and to better understand what various pharmacokinetic parameters depend upon [24,25,219–222]. Since these articles are more difficult to understand than the usual classic pharmacokinetic articles it may be some time before their content becomes widely used.

B. Modeling of Substrate Elimination by the Liver

Four principal types of models have been presented to explain substrate elimination by the liver. These are as follows: (1) venous equilibration (or well-stirred) model [223–225], (2) the sinusoidal perfusion (or parallel-tube) model [226–228], (3) the albumin receptor model [229–231], and (4) the dispersion model [232]. The pros and cons of the first three has been well treated by Morgan et al. [233].

Determinants of substrate elimination by the liver are hepatic blood flow Q, fraction of substrate unbound in the blood F_u, the intrinsic clearance of substrate ($CL_i = V_m/K_m$), and the rate of presentation of drug to the liver. The venous equilibration model views the liver as a single well-mixed compartment with the concentration of substrate in the effluent blood in equilibrium with that throughout the liver. In the first-order region intrinsic clearance is equal to the velocity of metabolism divided by the concentration of drug in the effluent blood. The sinusoidal perfusion model views the sinusoids as parallel cylindrical tubes and the substrate concentration declines exponentially along the sinusoid; the mean sinusoidal concentration is the logarithmic average $\bar{C}$ of the hepatic inflow C_i and outflow C_0 concentrations; that is, $\bar{C} = (C_i - C_0)/\ln (C_i/C_0)$; in the first-order region intrinsic clearance is equal to the velocity of metabolism divided by $\bar{C}$. The venous equilibration model indicates that oral bioavailability F in the first-order region is given by

$$F = \frac{1}{1 + CL_i/Q} \tag{64}$$

and the sinusoidal perfusion model indicates that bioavailability is given by

$$F = e^{-CL_i^*/Q} \tag{65}$$

where the asterisk indicates that the intrinsic clearances differ for the two models. The albumin receptor model proposes that the transfer of albumin-bound substrate to the hepatocyte surface is facilitated by a specific interaction of the albumin-substrate complex with a receptor in the hepatocyte plasma membrane. Although data that may be explained by the albumin receptor model cannot be explained by the sinusoidal perfusion model, most can be explained by the venous equilibration model [233]. Even if the albumin receptor model of the liver is later abandoned, albumin-bound testosterone is biologically active and can enter tissues [234]; this must be explained and the serum protein-mediated hepatic uptake of warfarin [235] must be explained in the future. The dispersion model [232] is based upon well-known mass transport phenomena and was stated to have one extreme limit equivalent to the venous equilibration model and another extreme limit equivalent to the sinusoidal perfusion model. The difficulty this author has with these conclusions is that the theory indicates these limits would have the same intrinsic clearance but two different bioavailabilities, when in reality there should be different intrinsic clearances and equal bioavailabilities [see Equations (64) and (65)].

C. Toxicokinetics

When toxicology in animals is carried out in pharmaceutical companies, the doses administered on a milligram per kilogram basis are usually many times those that are subsequently administered to humans to treat disease. The high doses often lead to nonlinear pharmacokinetics [6,236]. This author would like to recommend that the toxicokineticist seriously consider more steady-state studies than single-dose studies since the steady-state data are more amenable to pharmacokinetic analysis than single-dose data. When Michaelis-Menten kinetics are operative, one can readily estimate V_m and K_m values and flow parameters from steady-state data [31,32,33,34,90], but the appropriate parameters cannot be extracted from single-dose data in most cases. The concept that parallel Michaelis-Menten metabolite paths frequently pool to give a pooled V_m and pooled K_m, similar to the addition of parallel first-order paths, does not appear to be well known [35].

D. Intra-arterial Drug Administration

Considerable research has been and currently is being done in an attempt to show an advantage of intra-arterial over intravenous drug administration [237-242]. There are two possible types of advantages of intra-arterial administration: (1) a pharmacokinetic advantage that exists only for high-clearance first-pass drugs, which has been treated well by Collins [238]; and (2) a higher local concentration effect which that at present appears to be approachable by tissue biopsy experiments.

E. Parameter Redundancy

An excellent chapter in another book [243] treats parameter redundancy both qualitatively and quantitatively. Parameter redundancy arises when the proposed kinetic model is too detailed for the actual information content of the measurable data. For example, data generated with a higher number of exponential terms are often adequately fit by a lower number of exponential terms [52,244-246].

Parameter redundancy is a defect caused by the mathematical structure of the proposed model, not by experimental inaccuracy or by
using an inappropriate model. Parameter redundancy is usually
associated with computer fitting of data such that one and the
same curve can, with reasonable accuracy, be produced by totally
different parameter sets. Hence, parameter redundancy is also a
problem in data simulation as is done with physiologically based
pharmacokinetic models [19,20]. The author is not aware of any
detailed study of parameter redundancy in such physiologically based
models. Because of the problems of parameter redundancy, it is
important in the fitting of sums of exponential terms to apply an F
test [247] or the Akaike information criterion [248] to statistically
determine the optimum number of exponential terms for a given set
of data. In addition, the standard deviations of the estimated
parameters provide information about parameter redundancy. For
example, with data that are well fit by a biexponential equation one
usually finds the ratio of the standard deviation to the estimated
parameter value to be less than about 0.3 for each coefficient and
exponent. However, if the same data are fit with a triexponential
equation and parameter redundancy exists, then the same ratio for
the third coefficient and third exponent may be as high as $50-300$.
Such an example occurred in fitting lysergic acid diethylamide (LSD)
data $[244-246,249]$.

Surely parameter redundancy is an issue in application of the
program NONMEM [138]. To apply the program one pharmacokinetic
model must be specificed and examples have specified single-compart-
ment Michaelis-Menten kinetics [137], a linear monoexponential equation [141], and a linear biexponential equation [139]. However, in a
study of amobarbital pharmacogenetics with 28 subjects, the optimum
number of exponential terms needed to describe the disposition of
amobarbital determined by F test [247] was only one term in 18% of
the trials, two terms in 57% of the trials, and three terms in 25% of
the trials [146]. In a recent study in my own laboratory with
adinazolam, four of eight subjects exhibited linear kinetics and the
other four subjects exhibited Michaelis-Menten kinetics in the same
dose range. It appears that choice of a single model for all patients
for the application of NONMEM to a specific drug, for example,
presents many problems indicated by these two examples, and parameter redundancy would just be one of those problems.

F. Translation of Pharmacokinetics to Clinical Medicine

Dettli, himself a physician, wrote a chapter [250] entitled Translation
of Pharmacokinetics to Clinical Medicine. He indicated that the
translation of pharmacokinetics to practical medicine must meet one
condition of utmost importance: *simplicity*. As an example he illustrated that drug accumulation may be well defined mathematically by

a pharmacokineticist, but as a qualitative definition for the practicing physician it may be defined as "The amount of drug in the organism after repeated administration of the dose is higher than that after the administration of one dose." He also indicated that it is important to stress to the practicing physician that the extent of drug accumulation is not a property of the drug but rather a property of the dosage regimen of the drug. Dettli suggested two matters of importance: (1) even the most correct pharmacokinetic analysis is useless in clinical practice unless it can be adapted to the physician's background in mathematics; and (2) there is an urgent need for promoting mathematical thinking in medical education. It must be remembered that the application of almost any basic science information to the actual practice of medicine lags far behind the development of the basic science.

During most of my own career I have worked with a number of physicians in pursuit of common goals. I have been often very frustrated with the physicians' lack of mathematical knowledge. Undoubtedly they have been frustrated with me since I have often not succeeded in translating the mathematics into something they can understand. This is an important issue. Dettli's suggestions, indicated above, must be continually worked upon.

III. FUTURE CHALLENGES

In a departure from the format of this chapter, in this section, I merely list those areas I believe harbor future challenges. I do not discuss each of them beyond such listing except the last item.

1. Pharmacokinetics of peptides and proteins.
2. Stereoselective metabolism and transport
3. Chronopharmacokinetics and circadian timing of doses of drugs
4. Nonlinear toxicokinetics
5. Elucidation of molecular structure-pharmacokinetic correlations
6. Pharmacokinetics involving drugs labeled with stable isotopes
7. Elucidation of renal transport mechanism and the effect of protein binding and urinary flow rate
8. CD-ROM retrieval of pharmacokinetic data, including drug-drug interaction data
9. Determining relative magnitudes of intra- and intersubject variability of pharmacokinetic parameters
10. Estimation of bioavailability based upon overall profiles of blood concentrations and urinary excretion data
11. Production of user-friendly computer programs for extended least-squares and NONMEM
12. Improved modeling of pharmacokinetics and pharmacodynamics at the same time
13. Pharmacokinetic symbolism and terminology

There always has been a problem with symbolism and terminology in the field of pharmacokinetics since different authors differ considerably. However, the situation is becoming intolerable and in the near future we must do something about it. First, I believe the word *intrinsic* should be associated only with parameter values in the first-order region or those that are limits of nonlinear expressions as the dose or dose rate approaches zero. This is analogous to the intrinsic solubility of an organic acid, which is the solubility as the pH approaches zero. Hence if we assign total body clearance CL_{TB}^i and the limiting metabolic clearance CL_m^i as those values in the first-order region, then I propose CL_{TB} and CL_m be used for the clearances at dose rates R_0. We also should distinguish whether such clearances are determined from single doses or at steady state. There are many other examples of such gaps in our current systems, and we must tackle these problems in the near future.

APPENDIX: SYMBOLS USED IN THE TEXT

Symbol	Equation	Definition
$(A_a)t_n$	26	Amount of drug absorbed to time t_n
A_b	63	Amount of drug in the body at time t
A_T	28	Amount of drug absorbed to time T
$(AUC)_{IV}$, $(AUC)_{PO}$	40, 41	Areas under intravenous and oral concentration-time curves
C	1	Concentration of drug at time t
C_1, C_2	17	Concentration of drug at time t_1 and t_2
C_T	29	Concentration of drug at time T
C_{ss}^A	19	Steady-state concentration of drug in arterial blood
C_{ss}^V	18	Steady-state concentration of drug in venous blood
$(C_p)t_n$, $(C_p)t_{n-1}$	26, 27	Plasma concentration of drug at times t_n and t_{n-1}
C_0	52	Initial concentration of drug at time zero
CL	48	Systemic clearance

CL_i	55, 64	Intrinsic or metabolic clearance under first-order conditions for venous equilibration model
CL_i^*	65	Intrinsic or metabolic clearance under first-order conditions for sinusoidal perfusion model
C_U, C_L	59	Concentrations of unlabeled and labeled drug
C_{ss}^{min}, C_{ss}^{max}	Follows 32	Steady-state minimum and maximum drug concentrations
CL_{TB}	40	Total body (systemic) clearance
D	60, 61, 63	Dose of drug
D_{IV}	1	Intravenous dose of drug
D_L	31	Loading dose of drug
D_m	31	Maintenance dose of drug
F	3, 64, 65	Bioavailability of drug under first-order conditions
$G(t)$, $g(s)$	43	Weighting function and its Laplace transform
K	49	First-order rate constant obtained at a ratio of CL to V
k_a	3	First-order absorption rate constnat
k_e	1	First-order elimination rate constant
k_0	2	Zero-order input rate constant
k_{10}, k_{12}, k_{21}	4, 7	First-order rate constants of models IIA, IIB, IIC
k_{20}		First-order elimination rate constant of model IID
k_{10}, k_{12}, k_{21}, k_{13}, k_{31}	9–12	First-order rate constants of model IIIB
K_m	16	Michaelis constant
MRT	62, 63	System mean residence time

Q	19, 54, 56, 64, 65	In Equations (19), (56), (64), and (65) Q represents liver blood flow, but in Equation (54) $Q = (V_m \tau - D_m)/VK_m$
R_0	18	Zero-order input rate constant
R_1, R_2	29, 30	Initial and final zero-order infusion rates
t	1	Time after administration of drug
Δt	27	Time interval
V	1	Volume of distribution of drug in models IA, IB, and IC
V_m	16	Maximal velocity of metabolism (mass/time)
V'_m	16	$V'_m = V_m/V$
v	53	Velocity of metabolism
V_1	61	Initial volume of distribution
$(V_2)_{max}$	60	Maximum volume of distribution
V_p	4	Volume of central compartment of models IIA, IIB, and IIC
X(t), x(t)	42, 43	Input function and its Laplace transform
Y(t), y(t)	42, 43	Output function and its Laplace transform
λ_1, λ_2	4–7	Defined by Equations (7) and (8)
λ_1, λ_2, λ_3	9–12	Defined by Equations (10) to (12)
τ	31	Dosage interval

REFERENCES

1. J. G. Wagner. History of pharmacokinetics. Pharmacol. Ther. 12: 537–562, 1981.
2. J. G. Wagner. Biopharmaceutics: Absorption aspects. J. Pharm. Sci. 50: 359–387, 1961.
3. F. Vogel and A. G. Motulsky. Human Genetics. Springer-Verlag, Berlin, 1979.

4. W. Kalow. Pharmacogenetics, Heredity and the Response to Drugs. W. B. Saunders, Philadelphia, 1962.

5. A. Reinberg and F. Halzerg. Circadian pharmacology. Annu. Rev. Pharmacol. 11: 455–492, 1971.

6. F. DiCarlo. Metabolism, pharmacokinetics, and toxicokinetics defined. Drug Metab. Rev. 13: 1–4, 1982.

7. M. Sokolow and A. L. Edgar. Blood quinidine concentration as a guide in the treatment of cardiac arrhythmias. Circulation 1: 576–592, 1950.

8. B. B. Brodie. Physiological and biochemical aspects of pharmacology. JAMA 202: 600–604, 1967.

9. L. Z. Benet (ed.). The Effect of Disease States on Drug Pharmacokinetics. American Pharmaceutical Association, Academy of Pharmaceutical Sciences, Washington, D.C., 1976.

10. L. Z. Benet, N. Massoud, and J. G. Gambertologlio (eds.). Pharmacokinetic Basis for Drug Treatment. Raven Press, New York, 1984.

11. R. T. Borchardt, A. J. Repta, and V. J. Stella. Directed Drug Delivery. A Multidisciplinary Problem. Humana Press, Clifton, New Jersey, 1985.

12. R. F. Brown. Compartmental system analysis: State of the art. IEEE Trans. Biomed. Eng. BME-27: 1–11, 1980.

13. C. D. Thron. Linear pharmacokinetic systems. Fed. Proc. 39: 2442–2449, 1980.

14. G. Segré. Pharmacokinetics—compartmental representation. Pharmacol. Ther. 17: 111–127, 1982.

15. J. G. Wagner. Fundamentals of Clinical Pharmacokinetics. Drug Intelligence Publications, Inc., Hamilton, Illinois, 1975.

16. M. Gibaldi and S. Feldman. Pharmacokinetic basis for the influence of route of administration on the area under the plasma concentration-time curve. J. Pharm. Sci. 58: 1477–1480, 1969.

17. M. Gibaldi and D. Perrier. Pharmacokinetics. Marcel Dekker, New York, 1982, pp. 92–98.

18. M. Rowland, L. Z. Benet, and E. G. Graham. Clearance concepts in pharmacokinetics. J. Pharmacokinet. Biopharm. 1: 123–136, 1973.

19. K. B. Bischoff and R. L. Dedrick. Thiopental pharmacokinetics. J. Pharm. Sci. 57: 1347–1357, 1968.

20. H.-S. G. Chen and J. F. Gross. Physiologically based pharmacokinetic models for anticancer drugs. Cancer Chemother. Pharmacol. 2: 85–94, 1979.

21. T. N. Tozer. Pharmacokinetic concepts basic to cancer chemotherapy. In Pharmacokinetics of Anticancer Agents in Humans. Edited by M. M. Ames, G. Powis, and J. S. Kovack. Elsevier, New York, 1983, pp. 1–28.

22. R. Ball, O. Skliar, and S. L. Schwartz. A systematic approach to the design of physiological pharmacokinetic models (abstract 4157). Fed. Proc. 44(4): 1121, 1985.
23. L. E. Gerlowski and R. K. Jain. Physiologically based pharmacokinetic modeling: Principles and applications. J. Pharm. Sci. 72: 1103–1226, 1983.
24. D. P. Vaughan and I. Hope. Applications of a recirculatory stochastic pharmacokinetic model: Limitations of compartment models. J. Pharmacokinet. Biopharm. 7: 207–225, 1979.
25. M. Weiss and W. Förster. Pharmacokinetic model based on circulatory transport. Eur. J. Clin. Pharmacol. 16: 287–293, 1979.
26. J. G. Wagner, G. J. Szpunar, and J. J. Ferry. Michaelis-Menten elimination kinetics: Areas under curves, steady-state concentrations, and clearances for compartment models with different types of input. Biopharm. Drug Dispos. 6: 177–200, 1985.
27. J. L. Holtzman. Definition and implications of dose-dependent kinetics in clinical medicine. Drug Metab. Rev. 14: 1103–1117, 1983.
28. P. K. Wilkinson and J. L. Rheingold. Arterial-venous blood alcohol concentration gradients. J. Pharmacokinet. Biopharm. 9: 279–307, 1981.
29. S. Bøjholm, O. B. Paulson, and H. Flacks. Arterial and venous concentrations of phenobarbital, phenytoin, clonezepam, and diazepam after rapid intravenous injections. Clin. Pharmacol. Ther. 32: 478–483, 1982.
30. W. L. Chiou and G. Lam. The significance of the arterial-venous plasma concentration difference in clearance studies. Int. J. Clin. Pharmacol. 20: 197–203, 1982.
31. J. G. Wagner, J. W. Gyves, P. L. Stetson, S. C. Walker-Andrews, I. S. Wollner, M. K. Cochran, and W. D. Ensminger. Steady-state nonlinear pharmacokinetics of 5-fluorouracil during hepatic arterial and intravenous infusion in cancer patients. Cancer Res. 46: 1499–1506, 1986.
32. J. G. Wagner, G. J. Szpunar, and J. J. Ferry. A nonlinear physiologic pharmacokinetic model. I. Steady-state. J. Pharmacokinet. Biopharm. 13: 73–92, 1985.
33. J. G. Wagner. Propranolol: Pooled Michaelis-Menten parameters and the effect of input rate of bioavailability. Clin. Pharmacol. Ther. 37: 481–487, 1985.
34. J. G. Wagner. Commentary: Predictability of verapamil steady-state plasma levels from single-dose data explained. Clin. Pharmacol. Ther. 36: 1–4, 1984.
35. A. J. Sedman and J. G. Wagner. Quantitative pooling of Michaelis-Menten equations in models with parallel metabolite formation paths. J. Pharmacokinet. Biopharm. 2: 149–160, 1974.

36. S. Vajda. Identifiability of first order reaction systems. React. Kinet. Catal. Lett. 11: 39–43, 1979.

37. J. Delforge. New results on the problem of identifiability of a linear system. Math. Biosci. 52: 73–96, 1980.

38. S. Vajda. Identifiability classes in reaction kinetics. React. Kinet. Catal. Lett. 13: 191–196, 1980.

39. S. Vajda. Identifiability classes in reaction kinetics. React. In Advances in Physiological Science, Vol. 34, Mathematical and Computational Methods in Physiology. Edited by L. Fedina, B. Kanjar, B. Kocsis, and M. Kollai. Pergamon Press, Budapest, 1981, pp. 157–168.

40. S. Vajda. Structural equivalence of linear systems and compartmental models. Math. Biosci. 55: 39–64, 1981.

41. E. M. Landaw, B. C-M. Chen, and J. J. Distefano, III. An algorithm for the identifiable parameter combinations of the general mammillary compartmental model. Math. Biosci. 72: 199–212, 1984.

42. N. P. Chau. Linear n-compartment catenary models: Formulas to describe tracer amount in any compartment and identification of parameters from a concentration-time curve. Math. Biosci. 76: 185–206, 1985.

43. N. P. Chau. Parameter identification in n-compartment mammillary models. Math. Biosci. 74: 199–218, 1985.

44. J. A. Jacquez and P. Grief. Numerical parameter identifiability and estimability: Integrating identifiability, estimability, and optimal sampling design. Math. Biosci. 77: 201–277, 1985.

45. Y. Cherrault and V. B. Sarin. Identification of pharmacokinetic parameters of two compartment open model with first order absorption. Int. J. Biomed. Comput. 16: 127–133, 1985.

46. I. Gonda. Analytical approximations of sensitivities of steady-state predictions to errors in parameter estimation. J. Pharmacokinet. Biopharm. 10: 559–574, 1982.

47. S. L. Lehman and L. W. Stark. Three algorithms for interpreting models consisting of ordinary differential equations: Sensitivity coefficients, sensitivity functions, global optimization. Math. Biosci. 62: 107–122, 1982.

48. R. Bellman and K. J. Aström. On structure identifiability. Math. Biosci. 7: 329–339, 1970.

49. H. J. Bremermann. A method of unconstrained global optimization. Math. Biosci. 9: 1–15, 1970.

50. T. Suzuki and Y. Saitoh. Pharmacokinetic analysis of blood level data interpreted by a two compartment model. Chem. Pharm. Bull. 21: 1458–1469, 1973.

51. J. Radziuk. An integral equation approach to measuring turnover in nonsteady compartmental and distributed systems. Bull. Math. Biol. 38: 679–693, 1974.

52. J. G. Wagner. Linear pharmacokinetic models and vanishing exponential terms: Implications in pharmacokinetics. J. Pharmacokinet. Biopharm. 4: 395–425, 1976.

53. J. G. Wagner. Linear pharmacokinetic equations allowing direct calculation of many needed pharmacokinetic parameters from the coefficient and exponents of polyexponential equations which have been fitted to the data. J. Pharmacokinet. Biopharm. 4: 443–467, 1976.

54. J. P. Kehoczky. A diffusion-approximation analysis of a general n-compartment system. Math. Biosci. 36: 127–148, 1979.

55. C. D. Thron. Quick estimation of kinetic parameters for a compartment with exponential absorption rate and first-order elimination rate. J. Pharm. Sci. 66: 127–129, 1977.

56. Arzneimittel forsch. 27: 897–931, 1977.

57. MacKichan, M. R. Dubrinska, P. G. Welling, and J. G. Wagner. Error dependent on renal function when monoexponential equation assumed. Clin. Pharmacol. Ther. 22: 609–614, 1977.

58. M. R. Kirby. The matrix representaiton of pharmacokinetic models. J. Theor. Biol. 77: 333–348, 1979.

59. J. H. Matis and T. E. Wehrly. Stochastic models of compartmental systems. Biometrics 35: 199–220, 1979.

60. G. W. Harrison. Compartmental models with uncertain flow rates. Math. Biosci. 43: 131–139, 1979.

61. S. El-Asfovri, B. C. McInnis, and A. D. Kapadia. Stochastic compartmental modeling and parameter estimation with application to cancer treatment follow-up studies. Bull. Math. Biol. 41: 203–215, 1979.

62. V. Capasso and S. L. Paveri-Fontana. Some results on linear stochastic multicompartmental systems. Math. Biosci. 55: 7–26, 1981.

63. A. Rescigno and J. H. Matis. On the relevance of stochastic compartmental models to pharmacokinetic systems. Bull. Math. Biol. 43: 245–247, 1981.

64. G. K. Agrafiotis. On the stochastic theory of compartments: A semi-Markov approach for the analysis of the K-compartmental systems. Bull. Math. Biol. 44: 809, 1982.

65. D. H. Anderson. Structural properties of compartmental models. Math. Biosci. 58: 61–81, 1982.

66. M. Barzegar-Jalai and M. Toomanian. Theoretical consideration for the cases where absorption rate constant approaches elimination rate constant in the linear one-compartment open models. Int. J. Pharmaceutics, 12: 351–354, 1982.

67. P. Veng-Pedersen and R. Brashear. Kinetic interpretation of the microparameters in compartmental modeling when adjoining compartments are sampled. J. Pharm. Sci. 72: 576–577, 1983.

68. V. Capasso and S. L. Paveri-Fontana. Comments on statistical independence for linear stochastic multicompartmental systems. Bull. Math. Biol. 45: 431–435, 1983.

69. V. Capasso and S. L. Paveri-Fontana. Analysis of the correlations for stochastic multicompartmental systems. Bull. Math. Biol. 45: 555–569, 1983.

70. M. Witten. The diffusion process approach to one-compartmental stochastic models: A mathematical note. Bull. Math. Biol. 45: 425–430, 1983.

71. Y. Plusquellec and J.-L. Steimer. An analytical solution for a class of delay-differential equations in pharmacokinetic compartment modeling. Math. Biosci. 70: 39–56, 1984.

72. J. Eisenfeld and S. M. Grundy. Extension of compartmental parameters to blocks of compartments with application to lipoprotein kinetics. Math. Biosci. 68: 99–120, 1984.

73. J. Eisenfeld, W. F. Beltz, and S. M. Grundy. The role of nonreal eigenvalues in the identification of cycles in a compartmental system. Math. Biosci. 71: 41–55, 1984.

74. P. Macheras. Quick method for the calculation of the absorption rate constant of the linear one-compartment model using all available blood level data. Int. J. Pharmaceutics 19: 339–343, 1984.

75. D. H. Anderson. Properties of the transfer functions of compartmental models. Math. Biosci. 71: 105–119, 1984.

76. J. A. Jacquez et al. Kinetics of capillary exchange. Fed. Proc. 43: 147–184, 1984.

77. Y. Cherruault and V. B. Sarin. General treatment of linear mammillary models. Int. J. Biomed. Comput. 16: 119–126, 1985.

78. M. G. Leitnaker and P. Purdue. Non-linear compartmental systems: Extensions of S. R. Bernard's urn model. Bull. Math. Biol. 47: 193–204, 1983.

79. J. G. McWilliams and D. H. Anderson. Properties of the transfer functions of compartmental models II. Math. Biosci. 77: 287–303, 1985.

80. J. G. Wagner, J. I. Northam, C. D. Alway, and O. S. Carpenter. Blood levels of drug at the equilibrium state after multiple dosing. Nature 207: 1301–1302, 1965.

81. M. T. Smith and T. C. Smith. The unsteady model. An alternate approach to nonlinear pharmacokinetics. Eur. J. Clin. Pharmacol. 20: 387–398, 1981.

82. M. E. Wise. Negative power functions of time in pharmacokinetics and their implications. J. Pharmacokinet. Biopharm. 13: 309–346, 1985.

83. J. G. Wagner and E. Nelson. Per cent absorbed time plots derived from blood level and/or urinary excretion data. J. Pharm. Sci. 52: 610–611, 1963.

84. J. G. Wagner. Application of the Wagner-Nelson method to the two compartment open model. J. Pharmacokinet. Biopharm. 2: 469–486, 1974.

85. J. G. Wagner. Modified Wagner-Nelson absorption equations for multiple-dose regimens. J. Pharm. Sci. 72: 578—579, 1983.

86. J. G. Wagner. The Wagner-Nelson method applied to a multi-compartment model with zero order input. Biopharm. Drug Dispos. 4: 359—373, 1983.

87. J. G. Wagner. Effect of using an incorrect elimination rate constant in application of the Wagner-Nelson method to theophylline data in cases of zero order absorption. Biopharm. Drug Dispos. 5: 75—83, 1984.

88. J. G. Wagner. Estimation of drug absorption kinetics with emphasis on theophylline. In Sustained Release Theophylline in the Treatment of Chronic Reversible Airways Obstruction. International Workshop, Monte Ste. Marie, Canada. Edited by J. H. G. Jonkman, J. W. Jenne, and F. E. R. Simons. Excerpta Medica, Amsterdam, 1984, pp. 113—120.

89. J. G. Wagner. Unusual pharmacokinetics. Chapter 16 in Pharmacokientics. Edited by L. Z. Benet, G. Levy, and B. R. Ferraiolo. Plenum Publishing, New York, 1984, pp. 173—189.

90. J. G. Wagner. Theophylline. Pooled Michaelis-Menten parameters (V_{max} and K_m) and implications. Clin. Pharmacokinet. 10: 432—442, 1985.

91. L. Hendeles, R. P. Iafrate, and M. Weinberger. A clinical and pharmacokinetic basis for the selection and use of slow release theophylline products. Clin. Pharmacokinet. 9: 95—135, 1984.

92. J. G. Wagner. Estimation of theophylline absorption rate by means of the Wagner-Nelson equation. J. Allergy Clin. Immunol. 78: 681—688, 1986.

93. J. C. K. Loo and S. Riegelman. New method for calculating the intrinsic absorption rate of drugs. J. Pharm. Sci. 57: 918—928, 1968.

94. J. G. Wagner. Application of the Loo-Riegelman absorption method. J. Pharmacokinet. Biopharm. 3: 51—67, 1975.

95. J. G. Wagner. Pharmacokinetic absorption plots from oral data alone or oral/intravenous data and an exact Loo-Riegelman equation. J. Pharm. Sci. 72: 838—842, 1983.

96. J. G. Wagner, K. S. Albert, G. J. Szpunar, and G. F. Lockwood. Pharmacokinetics of ibuprofen in man. IV. Absorption and disposition. J. Pharmacokinet. Biopharm. 12: 381—399, 1984.

97. J. H. Proost. Wagner's exact Loo-Riegelman equation: The need for a criterion to choose between the linear and logarithmic trapezoidal rule. J. Pharm. Sci. 74: 793—794, 1985.

98. A. Gerardin, D Wantiez, and A. Jaouen. An incremental method for the study of the absorption of drugs whose kinetics are described by a two-compartment model: Estimation of the micro-

scopic rate constants. J. Pharmacokinet. Biopharm. 11: 401–424, 1983.

99. E. Krüger-Thiemer. Continuous infusion and multicompartment accumulation. Eur. J. Pharmacol. 4: 317–324, 1968.

100. R. H. Boyes, D. B. Scott, R. J. Jebson, M. J. Godman, and D. G. Julian. Pharmacokinetics of lidocaine in man. Clin. Pharmacol. Ther. 12: 105–115, 1971.

101. P. A. Mitenko and R. I. Ogilvie. Rapidly achieved plasma concentration plateaus, with observations on theophylline kinetics. Clin. Pharmacol. Ther. 13: 329–335, 1972.

102. P. A. Mitenko and R. I. Ogilvie. Pharmacokinetics of intravenous theophylline. Clin. Pharmacol. Ther. 14: 509–513, 1973.

103. J. G. Wagner. A safe method for rapidly achieving plasma concentration plateaus. Clin. Pharmacol. Ther. 16: 691–700, 1974.

104. D. P. Vaughan and G. T. Tucker. General theory for rapidly establishing steady state drug concentrations using two consecutive constant rate intravenous infusions. Eur. J. Clin. Pharmacol. 9: 235–238, 1975.

105. D. P. Vaughan and G. T. Tucker. General derivation of the ideal intravenous drug input required to achieve and maintain a constant plasma drug concentration. Theoretical application to lignocaine therapy. Eur. J. Clin. Pharmacol. 10: 433–440, 1976.

106. W. L. Chiou. Rpaid compartment- and model-independent estimation of times required to attain various fractions of steady-state plasma level during multiple dosing of drugs obeying superposition principle and having various absorption or infusion kinetics. J. Pharm. Sci. 68: 1546–1547, 1979.

107. H. Engberg-Pedersen, P. Mørch, and L. Tybring. Kinetics of serum aminosalicylic acid levels. Br. J. Pharmacol. 23: 1–13, 1964.

108. P. J. Niebergall, E. T. Sugita, and R. L. Schnaare. Calculation of plasma level versus time profiles for variable dosage regimens. J. Pharm. Sci. 63: 100–105, 1974.

109. J. R. Howell. Mathematical formulation for nonuniform multiple dosing. J. Pharm. Sci. 64: 464–466, 1975.

110. E. M. Faed. Model-independent linear pharmacokinetic equations for variable dosage regimens. Biopharm. Drug Dispos. 2: 299–302, 1981.

111. P. K. Ng. Prediction of multiple-dose blood level curves of drugs administered four times daily at non-uniform dosing intervals. Int. J. Biomed. Comput. 12: 217–226, 1981.

112. M. Weiss. Periodic dosage regimens with uneuqal dosing intervals. J. Pharm. Sci. 74: 1022, 1985.

113. H. Schwilden. A general method for calculating the dosage scheme in linear pharmacokinetics. Eur. J. Clin. Pharmacol. 20: 379–386, 1981.

114. L. A. Wheeler and L. B. Sheiner. A general method for optimal drug dose computation. J. Pharmacokinet. Biopharm. 4: 487–497, 1976.

115. P. Veng-Pedersen. Model-independent steady-state plasma level predictions in autonomic nonlinear pharmacokinetics. I. Derivation and theoretical analysis. J. Pharm. Sci. 73: 761–765, 1984.

116. C. L. DeVane and W. J. Jusko. Dosage regimen design. Pharmacol. Ther. 17: 143–163, 1982.

117. P. J. Niebergall, E. T. Sugita, and R. L. Schnaare. Potential dangers of common drug dosing regimens. Am. J. Hosp. Pharm. 31: 53–58, 1974.

118. F. J. Goicoechea and R. W. Jelliffe. Computerized dosage regimens for highly toxic drugs. Am. J. Hosp. Pharm. 31: 61–71, 1974.

119. R. Hori, K. Okumura, H. Nihira, H. Nakano, K. Akagi, and A. Kimiya. A new dosing regimen in renal insufficiency. Clin. Pharmacol. Ther. 38: 290–295, 1985.

120. L. B. Sheiner, S. Beal, B. Rosenberg, and V. Marathe. Forecasting individual pharmacokinetics. Clin. Pharmacol. Ther. 26: 294–305, 1979.

121. L. B. Sheiner, B. Rosenberg, and K. L. Melmon. Modelling individual pharmacokinetics for computer-aided drug dosage. Comp. Biomed. Res. 5: 441–459, 1972.

122. R. H. Levy. Time-dependent pharmacokinetics. Pharmacol. Ther. 17: 383–397, 1982.

123. J. B. Horeston. Drug metabolite kinetics. Pharmacol. Ther. 15: 521–552, 1982.

124. K. S. Pang. A review of drug metabolite kinetics. J. Pharmacokinet. Biopharm. 13: 633–662, 1985.

125. G. Levy. Clinical pharmacokinetics of salicylates: A reassessment. Br. J. CLin. Pharmacol. 10: 2855–2905, 1980.

126. G. Levy. Pharmacokinetics of salicylate in man. Drug Metab. Rev. 9: 3–19, 1979.

127. J. G. Wagner, A. R. DiSanto, W. R. Gillespie, and K. S. Albert. Reversible metabolism and pharmacokinetics: Application to prednisone-prednisolone. Res. Commun. Chem. Pathol. Pharmacol. 32: 387–405, 1981.

128. S. Hwang, K. C. Kwan, and K. S. Albert. A linear model of reversible metabolism and its application to bioavailability assessment. J. Pharmacokinet. Biopharm. 9: 693–709, 1981.

129. J. J. Ferry and J. G. Wagner. A pharmacokinetic model for prednisone after infusion to steady-state in the rabbit. Biopharm. Drug Dispos. 6: 335–339, 1985.

130. J. J. Ferry and J. G. Wagner. The non-linear pharmacokinetics of prednisone and prednisolone. I. Theoretical.
Biopharm. Drug Dispos. 7: 91–101, 1986.
131. C. E. Bourke, J. O. Miners, and D. J. Birkett. Reversible
metabolism of D-penicillamine in the rat. Drug Metab. Dispos. 12: 798–799, 1984.
132. T. B. Vree, C. A. Hekster, and E. van der Klein. Significance of apparent half-lives of a metabolite with a higher
elimination rate than its parent drug. Drug Intell. Clin.
Pharm. 16: 126–131, 1982.
133. G. J. Dutton and B. Burchell. Newer aspects of glucuronidation. In J. W. Bridges and L. F. Chasseaud. Progress in
Drug Metabolism. Edited by John Wiley, Bristol, England,
1977, pp. 1–70.
134. J. G. Wagner. Types of mean residence times. Biopharm.
Drug Dispos. submitted August 22, 1986.
135. J. G. Wagner. Dosage intervals based on mean residence
times. J. Pharm. Sci. 76: 35–38, 1987.
136. L. B. Sheiner, B. Rosenberg, and V. V. Marathe. Estimation
of population characteristics of pharmacokinetic parameters
from routine clinical data. J. Pharmacokinet. Biopharm. 5:
441–479, 1977.
137. L. B. Sheiner and S. L. Beal. Evaluation of methods for
estimating population pharmacokinetic parameters. I.
Michaelis-Menten model: Routine clinical pharmacokinetic
data. J. Pharmacokinet. Biopharm. 8: 553–571, 1980.
138. S. L. Beal and L. B. Sheiner. NONMEM Users Guide Part
I. Users Basic Guide. Division of Clinical Pharmacology,
University of California, San Francisco, 1979.
139. L. B. Sheiner and S. L. Beal. Evaluation of methods for
estimating population pharmacokinetic parameters. II. Biexponential mdoel and experimental pharmacokinetic data. J.
Pharmacokinet. Biopharm. 9: 635–665, 1981.
140. T. H. Grasela, L. B. Sheiner, B. Rambeck, H. E. Boenigk,
A. Dunlop, P. W. Mullen, J. Wadsworth, A. Richens, T.
Ishizaki, K. Chiba, H. Miura, K. Minagawa, P. G. Blain,
J. C. Mucklow, C. T. Bacon, and M. Rowlins. Steady-state
pharmacokinetics of phenytoin from routinely collected patient
data. Clin. Pharmacokinet. 8: 355–364, 1983.
141. L. B. Sheiner and S. L. Beal. Evaluation of methods for
estimating population pharmacokinetic parameters. III. Monoexponential model: Routine clinical pharmacokinetic data. J.
Pharmacokinet. Biopharm. 11: 303–319, 1983.
142. L. B. Sheiner. The population approach to pharmacokinetic
data analysis: Rationale and standard data analysis methods.
Drug Metab. Rev. 15: 153–171, 1984.

143. E. Martin, W. Moll, P. Schmid, and L. Dettli. Problems and pitfalls in estimating average pharmacokinetic parameters. Eur. J. Clin. Pharmacol. 26: 595–602, 1984.

144. S. L. Beal. Population pharmacokinetic data and parameter estimation based on their 1st 2 statistical moments. Drug Metab. Rev. 15: 173–193, 1984.

145. L. B. Sheiner and L. Z. Benet. Premarketing observational studies of population pharmacokinetics of new drugs. Clin. Pharmacol. Ther. 38: 481–487, 1985.

146. L. Endrenyi, T. Inabi, and W. Kalow. Genetic study of amobarbital elimination based on its kinetic in twins. Clin. Pharmacol. Ther. 20: 701–704, 1976.

147. G. J. Szpunar. The pharmacokinetics of flurbiprofen in man. Dissertation for Ph.D. in pharmaceutics, University of Michigan, 1984.

148. J. J. Di Stefano, III. Noncompartmental vs compartmental analysis: Some bases for choice. Am. J. Physiol. 243: R1–R6, 1982.

149. A. Rescigno and G. Segré. Drug and Tracer Kinetics. Blaisdell Publishing, Waltham, Massachusetts, 1966, p. 109.

150. L. Z. Benet and C.-W. Chiang. The use and application of deconvolution methods in pharmacokinetics. Abstracts of papers presented at the 13th National Meeting of the American Pharmaceutical Association Academy of Pharmaceutical Sciences, Chicago, November 5–9, 1972, Vol. 2, No. 2.

151. J. G. Wagner. Do you need a pharmacokinetic model, and, if so, which one? J. Pharmacokinet. Biophar. 3: 457–478, 1975.

152. H. Kiwada, K. Morita, M. Kayaski, S. Awaza, and M. Hanano. A numerical calculation method for deconvolution in linear compartment analysis of pharmacokinetics. Chem. Pharm. Bull. 25: 1312–1318, 1977.

153. D. J. Cutler. Numerical deconvolution by least squares: Use of prescribed input functions. J. Pharmacokinet. Biopharm. 6: 227–263, 1978.

154. D. P. Vaughan and M. Dennis. Mathematical basis of point-area deconvolution method for determining in vivo input functions. J. Pharm. Sci. 67: 663–665, 1978.

155. P. Veng-Pedersen. Model-independent method of analyzing input in linear pharmacokinetic systems having polyexponential impulse response. I. Theoretical analysis. J. Pharm. Sci. 69: 298–305, 1980.

156. P. Veng-Pedersen. Model-independent method of analyzing input in linear pharmacokinetic systems having poly-exponential impulse response. II. Numerical evaluation. J. Pharm. Sci. 69: 305–312, 1980.

157. P. Veng-Pedersen. Novel deconvolution method for linear pharmacokinetic systems with polyexponential impulse response. J. Pharm. Sci. 69: 312–318, 1980.

158. P. Veng-Pedersen. Novel approach to bioavailability testing: Statistical method for comparing drug input calculated by a least-squares deconvolution technique. J. Pharm. Sci. 69: 318–324, 1980.

159. P. Veng-Pedersen. An algorithm and computer program for deconvolution in linear pharmacokinetics. J. Pharmacokinet. Biopharm. 8: 463–481, 1980.

160. W. R. Gillespie and P. Veng-Pedersen. A polyexponential deconvolution method. Evaluation of the "gastrointestinal bioavailability" and mean in vivo dissolution time of some ibuprofen dosage forms. J. Pharmacokinet. Biopharm. 13: 289–309, 1985.

161. J. H. Proost. Application of a numerical deconvolution technique in the assessment of bioavailability. J. Pharm. Sci. 74: 1135–1136, 1985.

162. R. A. Upton, J. F. Thiercelin, T. M. Guentert, S. M. Wallace, J. R. Powell, L. Sanson, and S. Riegelman. Intraindividual variability in theophylline pharmacokinetics: Statistical verification in 39 of 60 healthy young adults. J. Pharmacokinet. Biopharm. 10: 123–134, 1982.

163. M. Miller, K. E. Upheim, V. A. Raisys, and A. G. Motolsky. Theophylline metabolism: Variation and genetics. Clin. Pharmacol. Ther. 35: 170–182, 1984.

164. A. Grahnen, M. Hammarlund, and T. Lundquist. Implications of intraindividual variability in bioavailability studies of furosemide. Eur. J. Clin. Pharmacol. 27: 595–602, 1984.

165. R. M. Nash, L. Stein, M. B. Penno, G. T. Passananti, and E. S. Vesell. Sources of interindividual variations in acetaminophen and antipyrine metabolism. Clin. Pharmacol. Ther. 36: 417–430, 1984.

166. M. Eichelbaum and A. Somogyi. Inter- and intra-subject variation in the first-pass elimiantion of highly cleared drugs during chronic dosing. Studies with deuterated verapamil. Eur. J. Clin. Pharmacol. 26: 47–53, 1984.

167. H. L. Behm and J. G. Wagner. Errors in interpretation of data from equilibrium dialysis protein binding experiments. Res. Comm. Chem. Path. Pharmacol. 26: 145–160, 1979.

168. J. J. Lima, J. J. MacKichan, N. Libertia, and J. Sabino. Influence of volume shifts on drug binding during equilibrium dialysis: Correction and attenuation. J. Pharmacokinet. Biopharm. 11: 483–498, 1983.

169. T. N. Tozer, J. G. Gambertoglio, D. E. Furst, D. S. Avery, and N. H. G. Holford. Volume shifts and protein binding estimates using equilibrium dialysis: Application to prednisolone binding in humans. J. Pharm. Sci. 72: 1442–1446, 1983.

170. G. F. Lockwood and J. G. Wagner. Plasma volume changes as a result of equilibrium dialysis. J. Pharm. Pharmacol. 35: 387—388, 1983.

171. J. Huang. Errors in estimating the unbound fraction of drug due to the volume shift in equilibrium dialysis. J. Pharm. Sci. 72: 1368—1369, 1983.

172. J. J. H. M. Lokman, P. M. Hooymans, M. T. Verhey, M. L. P. Koten, and F. W. H. M. Merhus. Influence of volume shifts in equilibrium dialysis to estimate plasma protein binding of drugs. Pharm. Res. 4: 187—188, 1984.

173. K. M. Giacomino, F. M. Wong, and T. N. Tozer. Correction for volume shift during equilibrium dialysis by measurement of protein concentration. Pharm. Res. 4: 179—180, 1984.

174. M. Gibaldi and J. R. Koup. Pharmacokinetic concepts—drug binding, apparent volume of distribution and clearance. Eur. J. Clin. Pharmacol. 20: 299—305, 1981.

175. G. R. Wilkinson. Plasma and tissue binding considerations in drug disposition. Drug Metab. Res. 14: 427—465, 1983.

176. K. Bachmann and T. J. Sullivan. Effect of plasma protein binding on clearance of drugs metabolized by Michaelis-Menten kinetics. J. Pharm. Sci. 71: 374—375, 1982.

177. J. G. Wagner. Effect of protein binding on steady-state equations. J. Pharmacokinet. Biopharm. 13: 559—560, 1985.

178. J. G. Wagner. Properties of the Michaelis-Menten equation and its integrated form which are useful in pharmacokinetics. J. Pharmacokinet. Biopharm. 1: 103—121, 1973.

179. J. G. Wagner, P. K. Wilkinson, A. J. Sedman, D. R. Kay, and P. J. Weidler. Elimination of alcohol from human blood. J. Pharm. Sci. 65: 152—154, 1976.

180. S. L. Beal. On the solution of the Michaelis-Menten equation. J. Pharmacokinet. Biopharm. 10: 109—113, 463, 1982.

181. S. L. Beal. Computation of the explicit solution to the Michaelis-Menten equation. J. Pharmacokinet. Biopharm. 11: 641—657, 1983.

182. J. G. Wagner. Effect of first-pass Michaelis-Menten metabolism on performance of controlled-release dosage forms. Presented at Drug Absorption from Sustained Release Formulations, A.Ph.A. Academy of Pharmaceutical Sciences Meeting, Minneapolis, October 21—24, 1985.

183. P. Veng-Pedersen and L. Suaréz. Practical solution to the Michaelis-Menten equation. J. Pharm. Sci. 72: 1483—1485, 1983.

184. R. J. Sawchuck and T. S. Rector. Steady-state plasma concentrations as a function of the absorption rate and dosing interval for drugs exhibiting concentration-dependent clearance: Consequences for phenytoin therapy. J. Pharmacokinet. Biopharm. 7: 543—555, 1979.

185. J. G. Wagner. Lack of first-pass metabolism of ethanol at blood concentrations in the social drinking range. Life Sci. 39: 407–414, 1986.

186. P. Veng-Pedersen and L. Suaréz. Model-independent method of predicting peak, trough, and mean steady-state levels in multiple intravenous bolus dosing in nonlinear pharmacokinetics. J. Pharm. Sci. 72: 1098–1100, 1983.

187. C. M. Metzler and D. D. M. Tong. Computational problems of compartment models with Michaelis-Menten type elimination. J. Pharm. Sci. 70: 733–737, 1981.

188. W. J. Westlake. Use of confidence intervals in analysis of comparative bioavailability trials. J. Pharm. Sci. 61: 1340–1341, 1972.

189. W. J. Westlake. Symmetrical confidence intervals for bio-equivalence trials. Biometrics 32: 741–744, 1976.

190. W. J. Westlake. Statistical aspects of comparative bioavailability trials. Biometrics 35: 273–280, 1979.

191. T. B. L. Kirkwood. Bioequivalence testing—a need to re-think. Biometrics 37: 589–594, 1981.

192. W. J. Westlate. Bioequivalence testing—a need to rethink: Reply. Biometrics 37: 591–594, 1981.

193. H. Fluehler, J. Hirtz, and H. A. Moser. An aid to decision-making is bioequivalence assessment. J. Pharmacokinet. Biopharm. 9: 235–243, 1981.

194. V. W. Steinijans and E. Diletti. Statistical analysis of bio-availability studies: Parametrix and nonparametric confidence intervals. Eur. J. Clin. Pharmacol. 24: 127–136, 1983.

195. H. Fluehler, A. P. Grieve, D. Mandallaz, J. Mau, and H. A. Moser. Bayesian approach to bioequivalence assessment: An example. J. Pharm. Sci. 72: 1178–1181, 1983.

196. W. W. Hauck and S. Anderson. A new statistical procedure for tesitng equivalence in two-group comparative bioavailability trials. J. Pharmacokinet. Biopharm. 12: 83–91, 1984.

197. R. Urso and L. Aarons. Bioavailability of drugs with long elimination half-lives. Eur. J. Clin. Pharmacol. 25: 689–693, 1983.

198. P. S. Collier and S. Riegelman. Estimation of absolute bio-availability assuming steady-state apparent volume of distribution remains constant. J. Pharmacokinet. Biopharm. 11: 205–214, 1983.

199. T. R. Browne, J. E. Evans, G. K. Szabo, B. A. Evans, D. J. Breenblatt, and G. E. Schumacher. Studies with stable isotopes. I. Changes in phenytoin pharmacokinetics and bio-transformation during monotherapy. J. Clin. Pharmacol. 25: 43–50, 1985.

200. T. R. Browne, J. E. Evans, G. K. Szabo, B. A. Evans, and D. J. Greenblatt. Studies with stable isotopes. II. Pheno-

barbital pharmacokinetics during monotherapy. J. Clin. Pharmacol. 25: 51—58, 1985.

201. T. R. Browne, D. J. Greenblatt, Harmatz, J. E. Evans, G. K. Szabo, B. A. Evans, and G. E. Schumacher. Studies with stable isotopes III. Pharmacokinetics of tracer doses of drug. J. Clin. Pharmacol. 25: 59—63, 1985.

202. M. Eichelbaum, G. E. von Unrush, and A. Somogyi. Application of stable labelled drugs in clinical pharmacokinetic investigations. Clin. Pharmacokinet. 7: 490—507, 1982.

203. P. G. Dayton, Z. N. Israili, and J. D. Henderson. Elimination of drugs by passive diffusion from blood to intestinal lumen: Factors influencing nonbiliary excretion by the intestinal tract. Drug Metab. Rev. 12: 1193—1206, 1983.

204. T. A. Shepard, R. H. Reuning, and L. J. Aarons. Interpretation of area under the curve measurements for drugs subject to enterohepatic cycling. J. Pharm. Sci. 74: 227—228, 1985.

205. W. A. Colburn. Pharmacokinetic analysis of concentration-time data obtained following administration of drugs that are recycled in bile. J. Pharm. Sci. 73: 313—320, 1984.

206. K. Takada and S. Asada. A model-independent approach to describe the blood disappearance profile of intraveneously administered drugs. Chem. Pharm. Bull. 29: 1462—1466, 1981.

207. K. Takada and S. Asada. Model-independent method to describe blood disappearance profile of drugs. J. Pharm. Dyn. 5: S-73, 1982.

208. K. Takada, S. Asada, and S. Meraniski. Statistical study of the model-independent method to describe the blood disappearance profile of instantaneously administered rugs. Chem. Pharm. Bull. 30: 2614—2617, 1982.

209. W. A. Golburn. A time-dependent volume of distribution term used to describe linear concentration-time profiles. J. Pharmacokinet. Biopharm. 11: 389—400, 1983.

210. C. M. Metzler. Estimation of pharmacokinetic parameters: Statistical considerations. Pharmacol. Ther. 13: 543—551, 1981.

211. C. C. Peck, L. B. Sheiner, and A. I. Michols. The problem of choosing weights in nonlinear regression analysis of pharmacokinetic data. Drug Metab. Rev. 15: 133—148, 1984.

212. C. C. Peck, S. L. Beal, L. B. Scheiner, and A. I. Nichols. Extended least squares nonlinear regression: A possible solution to the "choice of weights" problem in analysis of individual pharmacokientic data. J. Pharmacokinet. Biopharm. 12: 545—588, 1984.

213. D. P. Vaughan. Theorems on the apparent volume of distribution of a linear system. J. Pharm. Sci. 71: 793—795, 1982.

214. A. B. Straughn. Model-independent steady-state volume of distribution. J. Pharm. Sci. 71: 597–598, 1982.

215. W. L. Chiou. New physiologically based methods for calculating the apparent steady-state volume of distribution in pharmacokinetic studies. Int. J. Clin. Pharmacol. 20: 255–258, 1982.

216. L. Z. Benet and R. R. Galeazzi. Noncompartmental determination of steady-state volume of distribution. J. Pharm. Sci. 68: 1071–1074, 1979.

217. L. A. Bauer and M. Gibaldi. Computation of model-independent pharmacokinetic parameters during multiple dosing. J. Pharm. Sci. 72: 978–979, 1983.

218. M. Chung. Computation of model-independent pharmacokinetic parameters during multiple dosing. J. Pharm. Sci. 73: 570–571, 1984.

219. M. Weiss. Definition of pharmacokinetic parameters: Influence of the samplng site. J. Pharmacokinet. Biopharm. 12: 167–175, 1984.

220. M. Weiss. Steady-state distribution volume in physiologic multiorgan systems. Biopharm. Drug Dispos. 4: 141–156, 1983.

221. M. Weiss. Modelling of initial distribution of drugs following intravenous bolus injection. Eur. J. Clin. Pharmacol. 24: 121–126, 1983.

222. D. J. Culter. A linear recirculation model for drug disposition. J. Pharmacokinet. Biopharm. 7: 101–116, 1979.

223. J. R. Gillette. Factors affecting drug metabolism. Ann. N.Y. Acad. Sci. 174: 43–66, 1971.

224. M. Rowland, L. Z. Benet, and G. G. Graham. Clearance concepts in pharmacokinetics. J. Pharmacokinet. Biopharm. 1: 123–136, 1973.

225. K. S. Pang and M. Rowland. Hepatic clearance of drugs. I. Theoretical considerations of a "well-stirred" model and "parallel-tube" model. Influence of hepatic blood flow, plasma and blood cell binding, and the hepatocellular enzymatic activity on hepatic drug clearance. J. Pharmacokinet. Biopharm. 5: 625–653, 1977.

226. L. Bass, S. Keiding, K. Winkler, and N. Tygstrup. Enzymatic elimination of substrates flowing through the intact liver. J. Theor. Biol. 61: 393–409, 1976.

227. L. Bass, P. Robinson, and A. J. Brackan. Hepatic elimination of flowing substrates: The distributed model. J. Theor. Biol. 72: 161–184, 1978.

228. S. Johansen and S. Keiding. A family of models for the elimination of substrate in the liver. J. Theor. Biol. 89: 549–556, 1981.

229. R. Weisiger, J. Gollan, and R. Ockner. Receptor for albumin on the liver surface may mediate uptake of fatty acids and other albumin-bound substances. Science 211: 1048—1051, 1981.

230. E. L. Forker and B. A. Luxon. Albumin helps mediate removal of taurocholate by rat liver. J. Clin. Invest. 67: 1517—1522, 1981.

231. R. K. Ockner, R. A. Weisiger, and J. L. Gollan. Hepatic uptake of albumin-bound substances: Albumin receptor concept. Am. J. Physiol. 245: G13—G18, 1983.

232. M. S. Roberts and M. Rowland. Hepatic elimination-dispersion model. J. Pharm. Sci. 74: 585—587, 1985.

233. D. J. Morgan, D. B. Jones, and R. A. Smallwood. Modeling of substrate elimiantion by the liver: Has the albumin receptor model superseded the well-stirred model? Hepatology 5: 1231—1235, 1985.

234. A. Manni, W. M. Pardridge, W. Cefalu, B. C. Nisula, C. W. Baradin, S. J. Santner, and R. J. Santen. Bioavailability of albumin-bound testosterone. J. Clin. Endocr. Metab. 61: 705—710, 1985.

235. Y. Sugiyama, Y. Sawada, S. C. Tsao, T. Iga, M. Hanano, and S. Nagase. Serum protein-mediated uptake of drugs: Analysis by indicator dilution method, presented at The Third Japanese-American Conference on Pharmacokinetics and Biopharmaceutics, Kyoto, Japan, July 22—24, 1985.

236. A. Yacobi and H. Barry, III. Experimental and Clinical Toxicokinetics. Academy of Pharmaceutical Sciences, American Pharmaceutical Association, Washington, D.C., 1984.

237. W. D. Ensminger, A. Rosowsky, V. Raso, D. C. Levin, M. Glode, S Corne, G. Steele, and E. Frei. A clinical pharmacological evaluation of hepatic arterial infusions of 5-fluoro-2'-deoxyuridine and 5-fluorouracil. Cancer Res. 38: 3784—3792, 1978.

238. J. M. Collins. Pharmacologic rationale for regional drug delivery. J. Clin. Oncol. 2: 498—504, 1984.

239. W. D. Ensminger and E. Frei. High-dose intravenous and hepatic artery infusions of thymidine. Clin. Pharmacol. Ther. 24: 610—615, 1978.

240. A. J. Swistel, J. R. Bading, and J. H. Raof. Intraarterial versus intravenous adriamycin in the rabbit Vx-2 tumor system. Cancer 53: 1397—1404, 1984.

241. A. G. Bledin, E. E. Kim, V. P. Chuang, S. Wallace, and T. T. P. Haynie. Changes of arterial blood flow patterns during infusion chemotherapy as monitored by intraarterially injected $^{99}Tc^{m}$ macroaggregated albumin. Br. J. Radiol. 57: 197, 1984.

242. G. Milano, J. R. Boublil, J. N. Bruneton, J. Bourry, N. Renee, A. Thyss, P. Roux, and M. Namer. Systemic blood levels after intra-arterial administration of microencapsulated mitomycin C in cancer patients. Eur. J. Drug Metab. Pharmacokinet. 10: 197−201, 1985.

243. J. G. Reich. On parameter redundancy in curve fitting of kinetic data. In Kinetic Data Analysis, Design and Analysis of Enzyme and Pharmacokinetic Experiments. Edited by L. Endrenyi. Plenum Press, New York, 1981, pp. 39−50.

244. J. G. Wagner, G. K. Aghajanian, and O. H. L. Bing. Correlation of performance test scores with tissue concentrations of lysergic acid diethylamide in human subjects. Clin. Pharmacol. Ther. 9: 635−838, 1968.

245. C. M. Metzler. A mathematical model for the pharmacokinetics of LSD effect. Clin. Pharmacol. Ther. 10: 737−739, 1969.

246. G. Levy, M. Gibaldi, and W. J. Jusko. Multicompartment pharmacokinetic models and pharmacologic effects. J. Pharm. Sci. 58: 422−424, 1969.

247. H. G. Boxenbaum, S. Riegelman, and R. M. Flashoff. Statistical estimations in pharmacokinetics. J. Pharmacokinet. Biopharm. 2: 123−148, 1974.

248. H. Akaike. An information criterion (AIC). Math. Sci. 14: 5−9, 1976.

249. J. G. Wagner. Pharmacokinetics and bioavailability. Triangle 14: 101−108, 1975.

250. L. Dettli. Translation of pharmacokinetics to clinical medicine. In Pharmacology and Pharmacokinetics. Edited by T. Teorell, R. R. Dedrick, and P. G. Condliffe. Plenum Press, New York, 1974, pp. 69−85.

2

Recent Advances in Analytical Chemistry

LAWRENCE A. PACHLA, DONALD L. REYNOLDS, and D. SCOTT
WRIGHT *Parke-Davis Pharmaceutical Research Division, Warner-Lambert Company, Ann Arbor, Michigan*

I. INTRODUCTION

Advances in analytical chemistry have kept pace with the application
of principles from physics and chemistry. For example, gas chromatography (GC) (late 1950s to early 1960s) and gas chromatography-
mass spectrometry (GC-MS) (late 1960s) were developed from the
application of physical principles. All these technqiues have been
applied to understanding the pharmacokinetics of both old and new
drugs. Usually after several years of use, research associated with
new technology evolves into applying chemical principles or creating
new subtechniques in order to more adequately address analytical
problems. This chapter discusses the broadening application of
liquid chromatography and introduces a potentially new useful technology. The application of subtechniques—microcolumn liquid chromatography (MLC) and achiral separations—and the introduction
of robotics are discussed.

Microcolumn LC separations may never dominate the LC chromatography field. However, we view this technique as analogous
to capillary-gas chromatography. Microcolumn liquid chromatography
has its limitations and will not be universally used until advances in
instrumentation are implemented. In order to facilitate the rational
use of this technique in pharmacokinetic studies, we have included
not only theoretical considerations but also applications. Perhaps
the most exciting new technological development deals with the introduction of laboratory robotics. Although the technique may not
substantially improve detection limits, it should in principle improve
accuracy, precision, and sample throughput. Its eventual application
to pharmacokinetic studies should greatly facilitate the understanding
of drug pharmacokinetics. We envision that this technology will play
a dominant role in analytical chemistry during the next decade.

The final section of this chapter deals with the separation of
chiral drugs. Researchers are becoming increasingly aware of not
only the pharmacokinetic but also the toxicological differences associated with chiral drugs.

Because of the voluminous material that has recently been published, we have included only a representative sampling of the
available material on microcolumn and chiral separations. Only 100
manuscripts have been published concerning robotics, because of
the infancy of the field. The major intent of this chapter is to in-
troduce these new techniques and generate interest in the valuable
pharmacokinetic information that can be derived from their deploy-
ment.

II. MICROCOLUMN LIQUID CHROMATOGRAPHY

Microcolumn liquid chromatography (MLC), which involves the use of
miniature columns (15 μm to 2 mm internal diameter, i.d.), has been

applied to inorganic, biochemical, environmental, and pharmaceutical analysis. The potential of MLC has not yet been fully realized for biopharmaceutical studies. This section discusses microcolumn history, nomenclature, advantages, and disadvantages. Theoretical aspects governing the microcolumn, detector, injector, and other ancillary hardware are also considered. Recent applications and future directions are discussed.

Horvath et al. [1] were reported [2] to be the first to use microcolumn liquid chromatography. A 1 mm bore pellicular ion-exchange column was used for nucleotide separations. A decade passed before Scott and Kucera [3] revived interest in microcolumns by using 1 mm bore columns, 2 or 10 m in length for size exclusion. Recently, three excellent texts [4—6] appeared describing the theory and practice of MLC, and many excellent papers detail microcolumn fundamentals [2,7—15], compare microcolumns to conventional 4.6 mm bore columns [16—18], and consider instrumentation requirements [19].

Microcolumns can be classified into three major types: packed small-bore, packed capillary, and open-tubular capillary [20]. Small-bore packed columns are similar to conventional LC columns and are fabricated of stainless steel or plastic tubing using slurry packing procedures. Typically they have an internal diameter of 0.2—1 mm, a volumetric flow rate of 1—20 μl/min, and a sample capacity of 1—10 μg. Packed capillary columns are generally heavy-walled glass tubes packed with alumina or silica gel microparticles. Their internal diameter, volumetric flow rate, and sample capacity range from 40 to 80 μm, 0.5 to 2 μl/min, and 100 ng to 1 μg, respectively. Open-tubular capillary columns are similar to capillary gas chromatography columns but have an internal diamter of 15—50 μm, a volumetric flow rate of less than 1 μl/min, and a sample capacity of less than 100 ng [7,20].

Many advantages and some disadvantages have been ascribed to microcolumn liquid chromatography. At present, small-bore packed microcolumns are most practical for drug analysis. Packed capillary and open-tubular capillary columns place far too much demand on miniaturizing detection and injection volumes to be practical. Recently, several papers [16—18] have considered the advantages of small-bore packed microcolumns (1—2 mm i.d.) over conventional columns (4.6 mm i.d.). First, microcolumns allow a significant decrease in solvent consumption. The annual reduction in solvent consumption would result in a cost savings of 81 and 95% for 2 and 1 mm bore columns, respectively, when compared with conventional LC [11]. Second, less packing material is required, thus allowing the use of novel and expensive stationary phase (e.g., diamond dust and noble metals) [11]. A third advantage includes lower detection limits for concentration sensitive detectors [13]. The lower detection limit is a result of the higher solute concentration in the effluent [21].

In principle, the 1 mm bore microcolumn should allow a 21-fold improvement in detection limit compared with a 4.6 mm bore column. However, such practical problems as reduced detector sensitivity impede this level of improvement. The 1 mm bore columns can be coupled together to increase the number of theoretical plates for difficult separations [18]. This increase is proportional to overall column length but is less than that obtainable from conventional columns [22]. Since these columns can be operated at high linear flow velocities and low volumetric flow rates, they are very effective for high-speed separations and offer reduced solvent consumption when compared with conventional technology [11]. Perhaps the most exciting attribute is the allowance of new detection schemes in liquid chromatography [16—18]. Direct-coupled mass spectrometers and flame-based gas chromatographic detectors have been implemented, along with nanoliter volume amperometric detectors.

MLC is not without disadvantages. Small microcolumn volumes place miniaturization demands on associated instrumentation (i.e., pump, injector, and detector). Consequently, modification of conventional instrumentation is usually necessary to supply microliter per minute flow rates and submicroliter injection and detection volumes. However, commercial MLC instrumentation is being introduced that will alleviate the need to modify equipment. In addition, 1 mm bore columns are more difficult to pack than conventional columns [18].

A. Theory and Instrumentation

The underlying theoretical principles are identical for both MLC and conventional LC [23]. In MLC, all volumes and dimensions (except column length) must be reduced by a factor of (microcolumn diameter/ conventional diameter)^2 if the performance of a microcolumn is to be similar to conventional columns [24]. This subsection focuses on the dispersion (i.e., band broadening) resulting from each of the components of a chromatography system (column, detector, injector, pumping system, and connecting tubing). A number of key relationships are presented to allow the analyst to appropriately match microcolumn system components while minimizing dispersion.

Total solute dispersion resulting from all the components of a liquid chromatographic system can be represented by the total variance of the chromatographic solute peak σ_T^2. This total variance can be further subdivided into peak variance due to column dispersion σ_C^2 and peak variance resulting from extracolumn dispersion σ_{ext}^2; therefore,

$$\sigma_T^2 = \sigma_C^2 + \sigma_{ext}^2$$

TABLE 1 Some of the Commercially Available 1 mm Bore Microcolumns

Manufacturer	Bonded phase	Dimensions	
		dp (μm)	Length (cm)
Whatman Micro-B (Partisil)	C-18, C-8, Si	10	25
Alltech Microbore columns	C-18, C-8, Si	5, 10	25, 50
Chromega μChromega	All Chromega packings	3, 5, 10	10, 15, 25, 30, 50
EM Microbore (Lichrosorb)	C-18, C-8, Si	10	50
HRSM	C-18, C-8, Si	10	50
Varian MicroBore-1	C-18	4, 5	30
Brownlee 1 mm ID Microbore Column	C-18, C-8, Si, CN	5	25

Extracolumn variance is equal to the sum of variances of the detection, injection, and connecting tube systems. To attain maximal
column efficiency, dispersion from extracolumn components must be
minimized [19].

1. Column

Linear and coiled 1 mm bore microcolumns have been fabricated [25].
Glass-lined columns have a superior inner wall finish compared with
that of conventional small-diameter stainless steel tubing [26].
However, glass-lined columns are limited to the linear design. Stainless steel microcolumns are usually coiled when their length exceeds
1 m for ease of handling and thermostatting. Columns exceeding
1 m in length are used for very high resolution applications and are
usually fabricated in 1 m sections and then connected. Efficiency
loss is minimal when the coil radius is greater than 12 cm [26]. A
partial list of commercially available 1 mm bore microcolumns is given
in Table 1.

Realistically, microcolumns do not give higher efficiencies than
conventional columns if both are identically packed and operated
under the same conditions [23] since solute peak dispersion in the
column is independent of the column diameter [23,27]. The van
Deemter equation describes column peak dispersion as a sum of three
dispersion processes: multipath effects, longitudinal diffusion, and
the resistance to mass transfer of the solute between the stationary

and the mobile phases. In general terms, the solute dispersion in the column $\sigma_C{}^2$ can be calculated by the equation [19]

$$\sigma_C{}^2 = \frac{V_R{}^2}{N}$$

where N = the number of theoretical plates and V_R = the solute elution volume.

2. Detector

Although chromatographic detectors can be classified in a variety of ways, one scheme divides them into concentration-sensitive or mass-sensitivie detectors [28]. Concentration-sensitive detectors produce a signal proportional to the solute concentration in the detector. Mass-sensitive detectors generate a signal proprotional to the mass of solute entering the detector per unit time (i.e., mass flux). Ogan [28] has stated there are few "true" LC mass-sensitive detectors and that none are acceptable for MLC. He has provided a list of commercially available low-volume concentration-sensitive detectors.

Three terms that cause some confusion are detector response, detector sensitivity (minimum detectability), and limit of detection. Detector response is the slope of the detector signal versus solute concentration plot. Detector sensitivity is defined as the ratio of twice the detector noise to the detector response [28]. The limit of detection is classically defined as the analyte mass injected on the column that produces a response twice the noise level of the system [18].

Scott has shown [23] that the limit of detection is directly proportional to the square of the column radius. The following equation compares the relative limits of detection for two chromatographic systems with differing column bore sizes:

$$\frac{LOD_A}{LOD_B} = \frac{r_A{}^2}{r_B{}^2}$$

where

    LOD = limit of detection
    r = column radius
    A, B = columns with differing bore sizes

Thus a 1 mm bore column will have a 21-fold limit of detection advantage over a conventional 4.6 mm bore column. This equation is valid only when (1) both columns have the same total porosity, length, and plate number, (2) both systems are operated at the same linear flow velocity, and (3) the detector sensitivity for the two systems is constant [18]. Unfortunately, this last condition has proved to be a nemesis in allowing MLC to achieve its theoretical advantage for improving detection limits.

A major problem with spectrophotometric detectors is that when the flow cell volume is reduced to minimize dispersion and maximize microcolumn compatibility, the signal is reduced (due to shorter path length) and/or noise is increased (due to a reduction in the aperture) [11]. Scott and Kucera [29] reported that by judiciously reducing both the path length and aperture of the flow cell, they were able to retain approximately the same detector sensitivity as before modification. In addition, the use of optimal system components can improve detection limits. Cooke et al. [17] demonstrated the attainable decrease in detection limits when comparing 1.0 mm and 2.0 mm bore microcolumns to a conventional column (Fig. 1). In this example, the ultraviolet detection flow cells and flow rates were matched for each of the three systems to validate the detection limit comparison. Variable injections of a solution containing caffeine and 8-chlorotheophylline were made into each column to produce a caffeine peak height five times the baseline noise (peak-to-peak at 0.001 absorbance units full scale (AUFS)). The amounts injected indicate the detection limits of these three systems. A 0.42 ng caffeine injection onto a 4.6 mm bore column was comparable to 0.23 and 0.05 ng injections on 2.0 and 1.0 mm bore microcolumns, respectively.

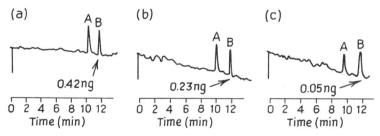

FIGURE 1 Limits of detection of the 4.6, 2.0, and 1.0 mm columns. (a) The standard 20 µl flow cell was used with the 4.6 mm column, and the 5 µl microflow cell was used with the (b) 2.0 mm and (c) 1.0 mm columns. Mobile phase: acetonitrile:water (10:90); flow rate: (a) 1.0 ml/min, (b) 0.2 ml/min, and (c) 0.55 ml/min; detection: UV 254 nm, 0.001 AUFS, 0.5 sec time constant. Peaks: A = 8-chlorotheophylline, B = caffeine. (From Ref. 17, reprinted with permission from N. H. C. Cooke, K. Olsen, and B. G. Archer. LC Mag. 2: 514, 1984. Copyright 1984 Aster Publishing Corporation.)

Therefore, the 1.0 mm bore system gave an approximately eightfold improvement in detection limit over the conventional system.

Another term often used in describing a liquid chromatographic system is concentration sensitivity, which is a function of the limit of detection. Concentration sensitivity is the smallest solute concentration that can be detected and can be equated to the minimum detectable mass dissolved in the maximum permissible sample volume [23]. Theoretically, microcolumns require less sample volume to achieve the same sensitivity as conventional columns [23].

A large detector flow cell volume or a large detector time constant can result in excessive solute zone dispersion. Dispersion is minimized in spectrophotometric flow cells by adjusting the flow cell volume to approximately one-half the injected volume. Katz [30] derived the following equation relating the maximum detector cell radius (and therefore volume) that can be used without causing significant dispersion (i.e., dispersion from detector <3% of dispersion from the column):

$$r = \left[\frac{0.72 D_M V_0^{\,2}}{\pi^2 N u L} \right]^{1/6}$$

where

r = cell radius
D_M = solute diffusivity in the mobile phase
V_0 = void volume
N = theoretical plate number
u = mobile-phase linear velocity
L = cell path length

This equation was used [30] to demonstrate the effects of the detector cell flow volume on column efficiency. The effect of V_0 on the geometry (r and L) of the flow cell for a column of 25,000 theoretical plates was also evaluated in terms of minimal dispersion. If the microcolumn is operated in a high-speed mode, the detector time constant and recorder response time become critical elements in minimizing dispersion. Kucera [25] indicates that the maximum permitted detector time constant t_D that produces a nominal 5% increase in dispersion is given by

$$t_D = 0.32 \frac{t_R}{(N)^{1/2}}$$

where t_R is the retention time.

3. Injector

Cooke and coworkers [17] emphasize that the best detection limits
for MLC are obtained when injecting the maximum sample volume
that does not significantly decrease efficiency. They assert that
MLC is useful in lowering detection limits only when the available
sample volume is too small to inject the maximal volume onto a conventional column.

For example, if a separation requires 5000 theoretical plates,
the maximal injection volumes for a 1 mm bore column and a conventional column of equivalent characteristics (except for internal diameter) are 14 and 320 μl, respectively [17]. Separations requiring
higher plate numbers have smaller maximal injection volumes. If
the maximal injection volumes of a 100 ng/ml sample are injected onto
each column and the solute band volume at the microcolumn exit is
0.1 ml and the solute band volume at the conventional column exit
is 2.12 ml [0.1 ml/2.12 ml is proportional to $(1 \text{ mm})^2/(4.6 \text{ mm})^2$],
solute concentration for each column is approximately 15 ng/ml.
Therefore, when maximal injection volumes are permissible, microcolumns offer no advantages. Conditions in which MLC is more advantageous are illustrated in Table 2. These data suggest that as
the permissible injection volume decreases the usefulness of conventional columns decreases. These data assume identical detector sensitivity. Realistically, these ratios are reduced for spectrophotometric detectors owing to the reasons previously outlined. However,
future technological advances may allow MLC to achieve its theoretical
advantage.

Dispersion of the solute zone resulting from sample injection
σ_i^2 can be described as [21]

$$\sigma_i^2 = \frac{V_i^2}{4}$$

where V_i is the sample injection volume and the constant 4 accounts
for the injection method and conditions. If the solute dispersion resulting from the injection process is only 5% of the column dispersion,
then the maximum injection volume is given by the equation [21]

$$V_{max} = \frac{0.24 d_c^2 (1 + k')L}{(N)^{1/2}}$$

where

d_c = column diameter
k' = capacity factor
L = column length
N = theoretical plate number

TABLE 2   Comparison of the Solute Concentration at Conventional and Microbore Column Exits for Various Sample and Injection Volumes

Sample volume (ml)[a]	Injection volume (ml)[b]		Solute concentration at column exit (ng/ml)		Concentration ratio of microbore to conventional
	Conventional	Microbore	Conventional	Microbore	
1	0.32	0.014	15	14	0.93
0.5	0.245	0.014	12	14	1.2
0.25	0.120	0.014	5.7	14	2.5
0.100	0.045	0.014	2.1	14	6.7
0.050	0.020	0.014	0.94	14	15
0.040	0.014	0.014	0.66	14	21

[a]Volume after sample preparation, solute concentration is constant at 100 ng/ml.
[b]Volume that allows two injections.

Therefore, the maximum injection volume is proportional to the column length and capacity factor and to the square of the column diameter and inversely to the square root of the theoretical plate number.

Ogan [31] has prepared a list of commercially available micro-column sample injectors. In general, 1 mm bore microcolumns require an injection volume ranging from 0.2 to 2.0 µl. If greater sample masses are required than can be supplied by these injection volumes, sample preconcentration methods (on-column or off-column) should be used [11,17].

4.   Pump and Connecting Tubing

Dispersion of the solute zone resulting from connecting tubing σ_t^2 can be represented as [21]

$$\sigma_t^2 = \frac{\pi r^4 lF}{24D_m}$$

where

r = connecting tube radius
l = connecting tube length

F = volumetric flow rate
D_m = solvent diffusion coefficient

This equation can be incorporated into an expression that yields tubing dimensions r and l when the variance contribution of the tubing is 1% of the column variance [21]:

$$r^4 l = \frac{0.06 D_m E(1 + k')d_c^2 Lt_R}{N}$$

where

E, d_c, L = column porosity, diameter, and length
k' = capacity factor
t_R = solute retention time
N = theoretical plate number

Tubing specifications resulting from this equation can be easily met. Katz [30] indicated that a common length and bore of connecting tube are 10 cm and 0.006 in., respectively. Minimal solute dispersion is as follows: serpentine-shaped tubes < coiled tubes < straight connecting tubes.

Recently, a list of microcolumn components and complete manufactured systems has appeared [19]. Typically, microcolumns require pumps that can deliver solvent flow rates of 10–100 μl/min. Both reciprocating piston and syringe pumps have been used. Ogan [31] has provided a list of commercially available microcolumn system solvent pumps and describes the approaches and concepts for gradient formation.

B. Applications

Microcolumns of 1 mm and 2.1 mm bore are most commonly used for drug analysis because of solvent economy and detection limits. This section describes several recent microcolumn applications and is subdivided into spectroscopic and electrochemical detection.

1. Spectroscopic Detection

The majority of microcolumn drug analysis applications have involved ultraviolet (UV) absorbance detection. Dickinson and coworkers [32] developed a sensitive method for pentamidine in blood serum using a 2.1 mm bore microcolumn (15.0 cm length). Pentamidine and internal standard (hexamidine) were ion-pair extracted from serum and separated by ion-pair chromatography. This method was more precise than a fluorimetric method and more sensitive than a bioassay.

Eckers et al. [33] used 1 mm bore microcolumns and ultraviolet detection at 254 nm to analyze reserpine in equine plasma and trichlormethiazide in equine urine. Reserpine was isolated from equinine plasma samples by liquid-liquid extraction and chromatographed using a Whatman ODS-3 microcolumn (30 cm × 1 mm). Detection limits in the high picograms per milliliter of plasma range should be attainable. Their method for trichlormethiazide in equine urine used hydrochlormethiazide as an internal standard along with an extraction step, prior to chromatographic analysis of the drug and internal standard. An Alltech C-18 microcolumn (50 cm × 1 mm) was used for separation. A quantitation limit of 10 ng/ml urine is reported.

Shipe and coworkers [34] developed a sensitive and selective microcolumn method for bethanidine in plasma using UV detection (210 nm) that was found to be more suitable then an available fluorometric or gas-liquid chromatographic (GLC) method. The MLC method involved liquid-liquid extraction of plasma and a 50 μl injection of the reconstituted volume into the 2.1 mm bore C-18 microcolumn (25 cm). The recovery and within-run precision for a 1.25 mg/liter bethanidine plasma sample were 99 and 4% RSD, respectively. Calibration curves were linear (r = 0.9996) from 0.7 to 5.0 mg/liter, with a detection limit of 0.02 mg/liter. When compared with a conventional column system (25 cm × 4.6 mm C-18 and a 5 μm particle size), the microcolumn system reduced the solvent consumption by 90% and produced a fivefold increase in peak area along with a decrease in noise.

Nielen et al. [35] introduced an automated column switching method for the analysis of clobazam and desmethylclobazam in plasma. The microcolumn was constructed by drilling through the axis of a Valco six-port switching valve to give a cavity of 4.5 × 1 mm, which was then packed with 40 μm C-8 particles. Plasma samples were diluted 1:1 with water, and 100 μl of the final volume was loaded onto the microprecolumn for trace enrichment. Following a water wash step, the drug and metabolite were transferred to a 1 mm bore analytical microcolumn (20 cm length, 3 μm C-18). Quantitation was performed at 254 nm (1 μl flow cell volume). Detection limits and precision (%RSD) were 2.5 ng/ml and 1.7% for desmethylclobazam, and 5 ng/ml and 1.1% for clobazam. This method of online trace enrichment in a microprecolumn can result in a two-order of magnitude decrease in detection limit when compared to an equivalent loop injection.

Kamperman and Kraak [36] devised a fluorimetric method for epinephrine and norepinephrine in plasma. The method involved liquid-liquid extraction followed by on-column concentration of the aqueous layer and ion-pair analysis using a C-18 microcolumn. Excitation and emission wavelengths were 278 and 317 nm, respectively. Epinephrine and norepinephrine calibration plots were linear (0.9998) over the range 20−16,000 pg/ml. The microcolumn method was claimed to be more stable and more sensitive than a conventional column system. The feasibility of attaining femtogram per milliliter sensitivities using a laser excitation source was also noted.

The remaining applications [24,37—39] involve methods for drugs in nonbiologic fluids using 1 mm bore microcolumns and UV detection. Gill [37] demonstrated the advantage of coupling three 1 mm bore silica microcolumns (30 cm length per column) to produce a high plate count, which was equal to the sum of the individual microcolumn plate counts. This column combination was used to separate a mixture of 10 basic drugs. The author states that this system could be very useful for drug screening.

Tsuji and Binns [38] have demonstrated individual normal-phase separations (silica, 1 mm × 50 cm) of seven steroids, tolbutamide and tolazamide, novobicin from its impurities, and neomycin B and C. Reversed-phase separations (C-8, 1 mm × 25 cm) were illustrated for ibuprofen and valerophenone (internal standard), and for ampicillin and its decomposition products. The authors claim their microcolumn systems to be practical and advantageous over conventional column systems. Solvent consumption savings ranged from 90 to 99%. Decreases in mass detection limits for trace analyses were from 10- to 16-fold. High-speed chromatography was practical with these systems, and only small sample volumes were required.

High-speed microcolumn separations of drugs also appeared [24, 39]. Kucera [39] developed a 30 sec separation of diazepam and its metabolites using a 15 cm × 1 mm bore C-18 microcolumn and a flow rate of 1.5 ml/min. Hartwick and Dezaro [24] reported a rapid separation of four analgesics in 20 sec using an ion-pairing microcolumn system (15 cm × 1 mm C-18).

2. Electrochemical Detection

Only microcolumn applications using amperometric detection are described here. Most of these involve 1 mm bore C-18 microcolumn systems for the analysis of biogenic amines in biologic fluids. Carlsson and coworkers [40] introduced a method for analyzing dopamine and its metabolites in small volumes (2 μl) of rat brain microinfusion dialysates. An ion-pair microcolumn (1 × 250 mm, C-18) system was used for separation. Amperometric detection was accomplished using a glassy carbon working electrode at 0.65 V versus Ag/AgCl. The detector cell volume was 1 μl. This microcolumn system was critically compared with an equivalent conventional amperometric system and significant advantages were found. The microcolumn system had a 50-fold smaller detection limit (0.06 pg), and the higher mass sensitivity of MLC allowed the use of very small sample volumes, enabling more frequent sample collections. Thus, more rapid measurements of dopamine release and metabolism were possible. The small volumes also permitted slower brain perfusion speeds, which facili-

tated perfusate detection in brain regions containing minuscule
amounts of biogenic amines.

Durkin et al. [41] developed an amperometric microcolumn system for analyzing catecholamines in tissue, blood plasma, and cerebrospinal fluid. After sample extraction, which afforded cleanup and
preconcentration, analytes were determined using a C-18 microcolumn
(1.2 mm × 10 cm) with an ion-pairing mobile phase. Detection was
accomplished using a glassy carbon working electrode at 0.60 V
versus Ag/AgCl, with a flow cell volume of 1 μl. Detection limits
for norepinephrine, epinephrine, and dopamine were 280, 400, and
800 fg, respectively, which are 10-fold less than detection limits
of conventional amperometric systems. Intra- and interassay precision were 5% for catecholamine levels in the range 50—200 pg/ml. The
microcolumn system was reported to have many advantages over conventional systems: greatly reduced column cost as the foremost,
lower solvent consumption, and lower detection limits.

Caliguri and Mefford [42] have described detection limits of 50—
100 fg for biogenic amines using a C-18 microcolumn system (1 mm
× 25 cm) with amperometric detection. Rat brain tissue samples
of less than 1 μg were processed before injecting 1 μl of the supernatant into the chromatograph. Detection was accomplished using a
carbon paste working electrode at 0.600 V versus Ag/AgCl. Precision
was better than 8.1% RSD at the 1—5 pg level. A 50-fold detection
limit improvement over conventional column systems was reported.

Krejci and coworkers [43] have described trace analysis and enrichment techniques using amperometric microcolumn systems for
phenothiazines, sulfonamides, tetracyclines, catecholamines, and
dipeptides. Microcolumns (0.7 mm × 15 cm) were prepared from
capillary glass columns packed with either C-18 or silica materials,
and injection volumes varied from 0.2 to 100 μl. Amperometric detector selectivity was varied by adjusting the working electrode potential and/or working electrode material.

C. Future Directions

A brief overview of microcolumn liquid chromatographic theory has
been given, along with representative microcolumn applications to
drug analysis. By and large, spectroscopic and electrochemical
detection schemes have been predominant. Future directions in MLC
for drug analysis will center around novel detection types, such as
flame-based and laser-based detectors. Technological refinements
in the pump and injector, along with further miniaturization of the
detector flow cell volume, will make packed capillary and open-tubular
capillary columns practical for drug analysis.

A relatively new detection type in the microliquid chromatographic
domain is the mass spectrometer. Liquid chromatography with mass
spectrometric (LC-MS) detection is gaining popularity in the field of

drug analysis. Recent publications have reviewed the general principles of LC-MS [44], micro-LC-MS with direct liquid introduction [45], and micro-LC-MS applied to drug analysis [18,37].

III. ROBOTICS

Robotics is a recent technological innovation that will dramatically impact future pharmacokinetic and drug metabolism research. This technology, introduced in the spring of 1982, allows total sample preparation and analysis. Before this time, sample preparation and handling was the weak link that prevented complete automation of analytical procedures. Recently there has been a dramatic increase in the utilization of laboratory robots [46,47]. This increase is a direct result of improved robotic module design and the ingenuity of laboratory personnel. A recent publication has described the anatomic function of a robot [48].

Laboratory robotics was met with the same skepticism and glee that was originally directed toward chromatographic autoinjectors and integrators in the 1970s. Most laboratory workers were pleased that they no longer had to be enslaved to chromatographic instrumentation but were initially skeptical of the accuracy and precision of the devices or worried about job security or a mandated increase in work load. These concerns are dissipating. Laboratory personnel will find that they can process a greater number of samples per day and also devote more time to career-building projects (e.g., pharmacokinetic or metabolic interpretations and report writing). At present, the number of robotic publications devoted to sample preparation and sample handling does not exceed 100 reports, and most papers are published either in *Proceedings of the International Robotics Symposia* [46,47] or in the September 1986 issue of the *Journal of Liquid Chromatography*. A section of this latter issue was devoted to product descriptions and comments from robot suppliers and manufacturers [49—54]. In addition, manuscripts have appeared pertaining to the use of robotics in synthesis [55], blood banking [56], dissolution testing [57], tablet uniformity analysis [58], and automated Simplex experimental design [59].

A. Advantages and Disadvantages

Many research managers view laboratory robotics as a means to improve productivity and reduce costs. This section discusses several scientific and managerial advantages and disadvantages of using laboratory robotics. Examples of improving productivity and reducing costs [60,61], advantages and disadvantages of laboratory robotics [62,63], and the philosophy of robotic design [64] have been documented.

1. Improved Precision and Accuracy

One of the most cited scientific reasons for using robotics is to improve assay precision and accuracy. These numerous citations can
be attributed to the ability of the robot to simulate human sample
manipulations identically for all samples. Nevertheless, improvements
in accuracy and precision may not be realized for all robotized
methods. Improvements are normally seen in procedures in which
accuracy or precision is time dependent. For example, if the analyte
degrades during actual work-up or a derivatization reaction produces several time-dependent products, then serial robotic sample
processing will result in assay improvement. However, if assay conditions were rigorously defined, no time-dependent factors were
found, or a rigorous proven chemistry has been utilized, improvement may not be realized. In this case, the accuracy and precision
of the robotic sample preparation may only equal that attained from
a competent analyst. An excellent review has appeared comparing
the precision of manual versus robotic sample analysis procedures
for pharmaceutical, foodstuff, polymer, and biologic samples [65].

2. Improved Morale and Career Enhancement of Laboratory Personnel

Improvements in laboratory worker morale is another reason for
considering laboratory robotics. Most scientifically trained personnel
obtain their educational degree because of a desire to solve scientific
problems. Personnel morale may be negatively affected when faced
with monotonous repetitive analyses. Fortunately, robotic analyses
can generate equivalent or improved data. Total automation of a
monotonous procedure can free laboratory personnel and allow them
to enhance their careers by performing duties previously associated
with their superiors (e.g., report writing and pharmacokinetic
analysis). This enhancement of professional responsibilities ultimately benefits the technical personnel and may also accelerate scientific
and corporate goals.

3. System Setup

Several years ago, robotic system setup required dedicating a bench
chemist for application programming. The initial application was
usually functional within the first several months. Although programming was simple, one's creativity was often tested when attempting
to exactly duplicate manual manipulations. For example, the attach-
ing of a pipette tip to a robotic hand required an electronic switch
contact closure to ensure that this function was successfully completed. At present, the Zymark Corporation has greatly simplified
this process via the introduction of PyTechnology. This technology
involves preprogrammed modules, which absolves the individual from

assuring that the program replicates a particular sample manipulation. Preprogrammed modules for pipetting, vortexing, extraction, and diluting are readily available. The robotic application chemist can invoke these "subroutines" from a master program and create a functional robotic procedure within a single day. Preassembled units for performing "routine" procedures, such as radioimmunoassay (RIA), enzyme-linked immunosorbent assay (ELISA), Karl Fisher, and dissolution testing, are now commercially available and can be implemented within a day.

Ideally, the robotic expert should be dismissed from everyday laboratory responsibilities if the major objective is to fully explore robotic capabilities. As in all newly developed technology, many more improvements in productivity and ease of use await the eager scientist. Reports have appeared that reaffirm the hypothesis that total dedication of a robotic applications scientist will ultimately yield a durable and intelligent system. Several investigators have interfaced a microprocessor with a robotic sample preparation system, allowing the system to determine whether the results were acceptable [66]. The microprocessor monitored system pressure, availability of mobile phase, and chromatographic resolution. Whenever any parameter is determined unacceptable, the microcomputer instructed the robot to complete sample preparation but not inject the samples. Finally, the ideal robotic application person should be an expert analyst with mechanical and electronic experience if state-of-the-art procedure adaptions are expected.

4. Increased Data Output

A natural result of robotic assay procedures is increased data output, which allows more rapid interpretation of the pharmacokinetic results. Although robotic assays may be slower than manual assays, the robot can function 24 hr/day.

5. Improved Laboratory Safety

Robotic assay procedures can minimize human exposure to hazardous chemicals and conditions and provide an alternative to redevelopment of a potentially hazardous assay. For example, Hurni et al. [67] utilized a robot to radioiodinate antibody proteins for an RIA procedure. Brodack and coworkers [68] utilized a robot to prepare positron-emitting pharmaceuticals. Robotic implementation of these procedures reduced radioactive exposure to laboratory personnel and allowed the final products to be available in a timely fashion. Another paper described the fabrication and special material constraints for successfully completing Los Alamos radioactive studies [69].

Perhaps the most wasteful utilization of resources concerns the redevelopment of assay procedures that uses a chemical that may have been recently placed on the "suspected carcinogen" list. A prime example would be the use of benzene as an extraction solvent in the plasma analysis of codeine. During the 1970s, many investigators wasted precious time finding a suitable selective extraction solvent that met OSHA standards. Perhaps this lengthy redevelopment time could have been avoided if a liquid-liquid robotic extraction system had been available.

B. Interfacing with Chromatographic Instrumentation

Ideally, robotics allows total automation of laboratory procedures, thus obviating the need for constant surveillance by laboratory personnel. Total automation should include sample identification, sample preparation, quantitation of analytes, and data reduction. Fortunately, robotic sample preparation units are modular in design. Therefore a single robot can be used for many different procedures. Flexible system design should be extended not only to the sample preparation module but also to the design of auxiliary functional components. A modular approach to system design should be incorporated into each implementation phase. Modular design of the overall system ensures flexibility and timely use of completed modules. The highest priority should be assigned to the sample preparation robotic module, since sample preparation is the weak link. Once this module has been thoroughly tested for the analysis of a variety of different "similar" assays, then the robot is ready to interface sample preparation with the detection system (e.g., analysis of processed samples). Finally, the last step should be interfacing sample identification and data reduction modules (e.g., LIMS) laboratory inventory management system with the other tested modules. Careful system design and phased implementation of modules will provide maximum benefit and ease of system validation.

Examples of optimal system design for interfacing robots to chromatographic systems follow. Two recent publications by Johnson [70,71] illustrate sample preparation module optimization to accommodate the analysis of several drugs. In these reports, a solid-phase isolation procedure was developed for the "worst-case scenario." A generic program utilizing two wash steps and four solvent cleanup steps followed by the final elution step was included in the initialization program. Other drugs could be assayed using the same program provided that the new application required the equivalent or fewer wash or cleanup steps. For example, if a new application required only two cleanup washes, the operator would simply enter a volume of zero for the last two cleanup steps. These authors are at present incorporating the injection and analysis of samples in their application.

Van Antwerp and Venteicher [72] introduced a creative solution for assaying on a given day a variety of pharmaceutical dosage forms that required vastly different chromatographic separations. A robotic event controller was used to drive a column switching valve for analytical column selection. The event controller was also utilized as a contact closure device for selecting the appropriate wavelength, for selecting a UV fluorescence detector, or for selecting the flow rate from a programmable LC pump. Another application incorporated "artificial intelligence" into the system design. Halloran and Franze [66] designed a content uniformity analysis of multiple dosage forms. Their system not only prepared samples and injected the processsed samples into a liquid chromatograph but also monitored the integrity of the analysis. Their artificial intelligence system monitored the assay to ensure that (1) the detector was functioning properly, (2) there were not drastic shifts in retention times, and (3) the proper response for standards was obtained. This on-line monitoring of chromatographic data assured successful analysis on a day-to-day basis. These authors indicated that future designs would optimize integrator and attentuation settings and increase flow rate, column, and wavelength selection.

C. Applications

One of the first practical assays was published by Schoenhard and coworkers [73] for the plasma analysis of a synthetic analog of prostaglandin E_1. This robotic LC-RIA procedure involved addition of an ion suppressant reagent, isolation of the drug on a C-18 solid-phase isolation column, and elution of interferences followed by selective elution of the drug into a carousel for evaporation and high-performance liquid chromatographic (HPLC) injection. The prostaglandin E_1 analog HPLC fraction was then automatically isolated and quantified by an RIA procedure. Precision associated with the sample handling, sample preparation, and LC interface was 1.45% RSD, the corresponding manual precision was 10 times greater. Overall assay precision was 5.6% RSD at 751 pg/ml and 18.4% RSD at 70.1 pg/ml. This system performed exceedingly better than its manual version and required minimal human intervention. These authors have also adapted their robotic unit to survey optimal analytical isolation conditions for other drugs. A variety of solid-phase cartridges are used by the robot to prepare various cleanup and elution conditions.

An excellent report on the use of robotics to support safety evaluation studies has been reported by Lewis and coworkers [74]. Their application involved liquid-liquid extraction of drugs from small-volume plasma samples followed by liquid chromatographic analysis. Their motivation for automating their procedures was not only to improve accuracy, precision, and productivity but also to redirect resources to concentrate on method development and drug

metabolism studies. Innovative system designs include a variable
nitrogen evaporation flow rate to assist in complete sample evaporation, electronically monitoring the flow rate to ensure that flow has
not been interrupted, and weighing the evaporation vessel to ensure
complete evaporation. Overall method precision was 8.8% RSD for
the manual and 4.2% RSD for the robotic methods. These authors
reported that total system development time and validation using an
early version of the Zymark robot required 2.5 months for the first
drug candidate, 3 weeks for the second, and 1 week for the third
candidate. The reduced time required for subsequent assay valida-
tions was attributed to using variables for operational procedures
and generic programming enhancements.

Recently, Myers et al. [75] and Kramer and coworkers [76]
introduced robotic assays for the determination of tolazamide and
theophylline, and tolazamide, respectively. Both investigators
utilized a liquid-solid phase cleanup procedure and identical robotic
sample preparation schemes for tolazamide. However, Myers et al.
employed a batch sample preparation sequence whereas Kramer et al.
relied on a serial operation mode. Both methods produced similar
precision and accuracies when compared with a manual procedure
but required minimal operator intervention. A solid-phase robotic
extraction procedure for quantifying the cardiotonic enoxamine and
its sulfoxide metabolite has appeared [77]. This report describes
improvements that can be attained using robotic sample preparation.
The authors have also described an interactive microcomputer
module that verifies the integrity of the sample analysis segment of
the program. This module allows sample preparation to proceed but
prevents HPLC analysis if the chromatography deteriorates [78].

IV.   CHROMATOGRAPHIC TECHNIQUES FOR
CHIRAL RESOLUTION

Stereoisomers have identical molecular formulas but differ in their
three-dimensional orientation. Enantiomers are stereoisomers that
are nonsuperimposable mirror images (Fig. 2). In achiral media,
enantiomers possess identical physical and chemical properties (except for the direction in which they rotate plane polarized light)
and cannot be resolved using conventional separation techniques.
Diastereomers (Fig. 2), however, differ in physical and chemical
properties and can theoretically be resolved using normal separation
techniques.

Enantiomers may possess different physiological properties,
arising from steric interactions at chiral receptor sites. Toxicological
properties may also differ; for example, the (S)-(−) isomer of
thalidomide was responsible for its observed teratogenicity [79].
Metabolism of enantiomers may be different owing to enzyme stereo-

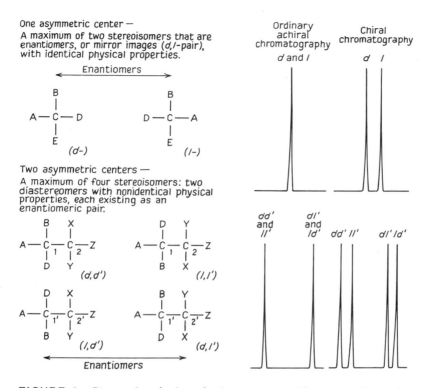

FIGURE 2 Stereochemical and chromatographic properties of optically active molecules. (From Ref. 88, reprinted with permission from I. W. Wainer. Chromatogr. Forum 1: 55, 1986. Copyright 1986, Cahners Publishing Company.)

selectivity [80] and thus impact on pharmacokinetic profiles. Consequently, rapid, inexpensive, and sensitive methods to separate and quantitate enantiomers were sought for many years.

Enantiomeric resolution is performed by interaction with an optically active reagent. Enantiomers are often converted to diastereomers or diastereomeric complexes and resolved using physical and chemical differences. Over the last several years, research efforts were directed toward understanding and designing gas and liquid chromatographic chiral separation techniques. These techniques offer high sensitivity and selectivity and are ideal for trace analysis.

Indirect and direct approaches have been utilized for separating enantiomers. Indirect approaches involve derivatization with an optically pure reagent and separation of the diastereomers by traditional achiral chromatography. Direct chromatographic resolution involves the use of a chiral stationary-phase or a chiral mobile-phase additive to resolve underivatized enantiomers. Numerous applications and reviews of these approaches have appeared [81-89]. A brief summary of indirect and direct approaches for GC and LC chiral separations is presented here.

A. Indirect Resolution

Indirect resolution techniques have been used for many years to resolve enantiomers. Specialized equipment is not required, and derivatization may be used to enhance detectability. However, derivatization is time consuming and requires the analyte to have a reactive functional group. Chiral derivatization reagents must be optically pure and stable toward racemization and have equal reactivity with both enantiomers.

1. Gas Chromatography

Numerous applications of indirect GC resolution have appeared. Wall-coated capillary columns have been frequently used to maximize separation and increase efficiency [90]. A major limitation of indirect GC resolution lies in obtaining optically pure reagents that give volatile derivatives. GC resolution techniques [90,91] and derivatization reagents [92,93] have been the subject of several reviews. Examples of indirect GC resolution of stereoisomers include derivatization of enantiomeric amines with (S,S)-N-trifluoroacetylproline anhydride [94], isopropyl isocyanate [95], or N-trifluoroacetyl-L-alanine [96]. Propranolol was resolved after derivatizing with S-$(-)$-1-phenylethyl isocyanate [97].

2. Liquid Chromatography

LC offers a wide range of stationary and mobile phases for the optimal selective separation of stereoisomers. Amines and alcohols are typically converted to diastereomeric amides and esters. Tocanide was derivatized with R-$(-)$-O-methyl mandelic acid chloride [98], and proxyphylline was derivatized with $(-)$-camphanoyl chloride [99] prior to achiral separation. Chiral acids can be resolved after esterifying, but stability considerations limit this approach. An example is ibuprofen, which was separated after esterification with S-$(+)$-2-octanol [100]. Optically active isothiocyanates have been used to form substituted thiourea diastereomers of racemic amines. Ephedrine, norephedrine, and pseudoephedrine were derivatized with 1-phenylethyl isothiocyanate [101], and amines including ephedrine and propranolol were derivatized with R-α-methylbenzyl isothiocyanate [102] before separation. Novel derivatization reagents include 1-((4-nitrophenyl)sulfonyl)-prolyl chloride [103] and $S(-)N$-1-(2-naphthylsulfonyl)-2-pyrrolidine carbonyl chloride [104].

B. Direct Resolution

Recent efforts have been focused on designing and optimizing direct separation methods. Direct resolution involves enantiomeric separation using a chiral stationary-phase or an LC chiral mobile-phase additive. Since derivatization is not required, chiral separation of compounds lacking a reactive functional group is possible. Chiral mobile-phase modifiers have been successfully used for LC resolution. A continuing source of reagent is necessary for this approach and may increase cost. Many inexpensive and stable chiral GC and LC stationary phases have become commercially available over the last few years.

1. Gas Chromatography

Although derivatization is not required for GC enantiomeric resolution, polar analytes must be derivatized to improve volatility. Achiral reagents are normally used to maintain the enantiomeric qualities of the analytes. Peptide, diamide, ureide, and metal complex GC phases have been used to achieve chiral separations. Resolution on these phases arises from steric interactions. One enantiomer will always be in a more favorable conformation to interact with the stationary phase, thereby facilitating resolution. Hydrogen bonding, dipole-dipole interactions, and van der Waals forces are also involved in obtaining resolution [91].

In 1966, Gil-Av et al. [105,106] reported the first peptide phases and resolved N-trifluoroacetyl (N-TFA) amino acid derivatives using capillary columns. A list of the numerous synthetic peptide phases has appeared [90]. These phases were predominantly used for separating N-TFA amino acids. Peptide phases should contain a N-TFA group, bulky side groups, and a large ester group to maximize resolution [90]. Recent efforts have been geared toward increasing stationary-phase stability.

Diamide phases have been most widely used for chiral GC resolution. N-t-butyl-L-valinamide-polysiloxane has been coated on borosilicate capillary columns (Chirasil Val) and has high thermal stability and low volatility. Wedlund et al. [107] resolved mephenytoin and its metabolite; McErlane and Pillai [108] investigated the stereoselective disposition of tocainide using this column. A similar phase, XE-60-L-valine-S-α-phenylethylamide, was used to resolve carbohydrates. A critical review of enantiomeric separation on amide phases has been reported [109].

Ureides are carbonyl(bis)amino acid esters capable of resolving racemic amine derivatives [90]. Ureides exist in solid, mesophase, and liquid states depending on column temperature. Resolution can vary depending on the state. GC metal complexation was first reported by Schurig [110] to resolve 3-methyl cyclopentene on a rhodium (I) chelate phase. Separation was achieved through π complexation. Other metal complex phases employ Ni(II) and Mn(II) [111–113].

2. Liquid Chromatography

Understanding and optimizing direct LC chiral separation techniques has received the major research emphasis over the last few years. Advantages of LC resolution include a wide choice of stationary phases, and polar enantiomers can be separated without derivatization. Chiral recognition occurs via interactions between enantiomers and the chiral stationary phase. Resolution results from differences in the conformation stability of the diastereomers. A minimum of three interactions is necessary for resolution, with at least one being stereochemically dependent. Interactions may be hydrogen bonding, dipole-dipole, charge transfer, hydrophobic, or repulsion forces. This concept was first reported by Dalgleish [114]. Pirkle and co-workers [115] have used this approach to rationally design new chiral stationary phases.

a. Chiral Mobile-Phase Additives

Enantiomers can be resolved on conventional LC columns using chiral mobile-phase additives. An obvious advantage is that both the chiral additive and the conventional stationary phase can be easily modified to optimize separations. A major limitation is that a continuing source of additive is required which may be expensive. Overall, resolution is the result of several interactions: the relative stability of the diasteriomeric complexes in the mobile phase, adsorption of additive on the stationary phase, and differential partitioning of the complex onto the stationary phase. Proteins, ion pairing, hydrogen bonding, metal chelates, and inclusion complexation reagents have been used.

α_1-Acid-glycoprotein and albumin have been used as chiral modifiers to resolve phenothiazines [116] and carboxylic acid derivatives [117], respectively. Factors influencing the observed retention models for predicting retention in these sytems were presented. Chiral ion-pair reagents have been used primarily in normal-phase LC to promote ion-pair formation. Pettersson [118] resolved naproxyn and derivatized amino acids using quinine and related amines. βBlockers have been resolved using (+) 10-camphor sulfonate [119]. Chiral hydrogen bonding agents derived from N-acetyl-L-valine have been used to separate N-acetyl-O-t-butyl amino acid derivatives [120]. Metal chelate complexes of transition metals and suitable ligands have been used as mobile-phase additives to resolve certain enantiomers. This approach is limited to solutes that can form tertiary complexes. Free amino acids have been resolved using mobile phases containing L-proline-Cu(II) [121,122], N,N-di-n-propyl-L-alanine-Cu(II) [123], or aspartame-Zn(II) [124] complexes. Gelber and Neumeyer [125]

used L-phenylalanine-Cu(II) complexes to resolve levodopa, methyldopa, and carbidopa. Karger et al. [126] reported the use of chiral
triamines, such as L-2-isopropyl-4-octyldiethylenetriamine-Zn(II), to
resolve dansylated amino acids.

Cyclodextrins are chiral cyclic glucose oligosaccharides containing
six to eight glucose monomers that are shaped like hollow truncated
cones. Inclusion complexes can form between solutes of the right
size and shape and the hydrophobic cyclodextrin cavity. Tightly
bound inclusion complexes must be formed to achieve resolution.
Sybilska et al. [127] resolved mephenytoin and several barbiturates
using an aqueous β-cyclodextrin mobile phase. A recent report
[128] describes the microbore LC separation of 12 dansyl amino racemates using β-cyclodextrin. Various hydantoin and barbiturate
enantiomers have been resolved using α-, β-, and heptakis (2,6-di-
O-methyl)-β-cyclodextrins [129].

b. Chiral Stationary Phases

Naturally occurring chiral substances, such as quartz, wool, lactose,
potato starch, and cellulose, have been used as stationary phases.
As early as 1944, Prelog and Wieland [130] reported separating
Troger's base on a lactose column and chiral separation on cellulose
was reported. Triacetylated cellulose offers increased resolution over
native cellulose.

Protein phases derived from bovine serum albumin (BSA) and
α_1-acid glycoprotein (α_1-AGP, orosomucoid) have been reported.
Allenmark et al. [131,132] bonded BSA to silica gel and separated
racemic sulfoxides and derivatized amino acids. Columns were stable,
but efficiencies were lower than with other bonded phases [132].
Hermansson et al. bonded α_1-AGP to silica gel and resolved several
racemic drugs and metabolites, including ketamine, disopyramide, and
pentazocine [133—135]. These phases have been applied to a wide
range of solutes and can be used with aqueous media.

Schill et al. [136,137] investigated the factors influencing chiral
resolution of cationic and anionic drugs on α_1-AGP columns. The
retention behavior of various solutes on BSA columns was reported
by Allenmark [138]. Hydrophobic, electrostatic, and steric effects
are important for resolution, but hydrogen bonding and charge
transfer interactions may also play an important role [138,139].

Synthetic chiral stationary phases are prepared either by bonding
a series of groups to a support, which forms a matrix capable of
achieving chiral recognition (cooperative), or by bonding individual
chiral molecules to a support (independent). Cooperative phases are
prepared by polymerization in the presence of a nonreactive chiral
template, leaving a chiral cavity. Polyacrylamide, polymethyl-acryl-
amide, and polytriphenylmethyl methacrylate supports are examples
of cooperative phases [140,141].

Recent efforts have been directed at designing and optimizing separations using independent phases. The four main types of independent phases include: π complex-charge transfer, fluorocarbon, ligand exchange, and inclusion complexation phases. The relative advantages, limitations, mechanisms, and utility of each are discussed here.

π Complex and Charge-Transfer Phases. Pirkle and coworkers have been leaders in designing chiral π-complex phases. The first commercially available phase was (R)-N-(3,5-dinitrobenzoyl)phenylglycine. Numerous applications have appeared, including the separation of ephedrine [142], propranolol [143], and amphetamine [144]. Chiral resolution results from π interactions, hydrogen bonding, dipole stacking, and/or steric effects and is shown in Figure 3. The advantages of these stationary phases include commercial availability, excellent peak shape, and efficiency [85]. However, limitations include the requirement that analytes have a π-donor group that can interact with the π-accepting dinitrobenzoyl stationary phase and that the phase is unstable with aqueous mobile phases. Highly polar analytes may require derivatization with achiral reagents (to maintain enantiomeric properties) to increase separation efficiency [145]. For example, methamphetamine and pseudophedrine were derivatized with β-naphthychloroformate prior to chiral separation [146].

Oi and coworkers [147] synthesized π-donor stationary phases using 1-(1-naphthyl)ethylamines. These phases are similar to Pirkle phases but are used for resolving π-acceptor solutes (e.g., DNB derivatives). A variety of π-donor phases were synthesized and evaluated for the separation of amines, alcohols, acids, and amino acids [148]. The best separation was achieved for solutes with strong π-acceptor properties. Charge transfer phases, such as 2-(2,3,5,7-tetranitro-9-fluorenylidineaminoxy)propionic amide, N-(2,4-dinitrophenyl)alanine amide, and bi-β-naphtholdiphosphate amide phases, have been reported [81].

Fluoroalcohol Phases. Fluoroalcohols can form two-point adducts with basic groups through interaction of the hydroxyl and carbinyl hydrogens [87]. Introduction of a π-donating group on the stationary phase and a π-accepting group on the analyte molecule provide the necessary three-point interaction. Pirkle and coworkers [149] used the chiral recognition model to rationally design a (R)-$(-)$-2,2,2-trifluoro-(9-(10-α-bromomethyl)anthranyl)ethanol phase. Resolution of 2,4-dinitrophenyl sulfoxides and 3,5-dinitrobenzyl alcohols, amines, and amino acids were reported.

Ligand Exchange. Ligand exchange involves formation of multidentate complexes between certain enantiomers and transition metals bound to chiral ligands. Aqueous mobile phases are used, thus allowing bio-

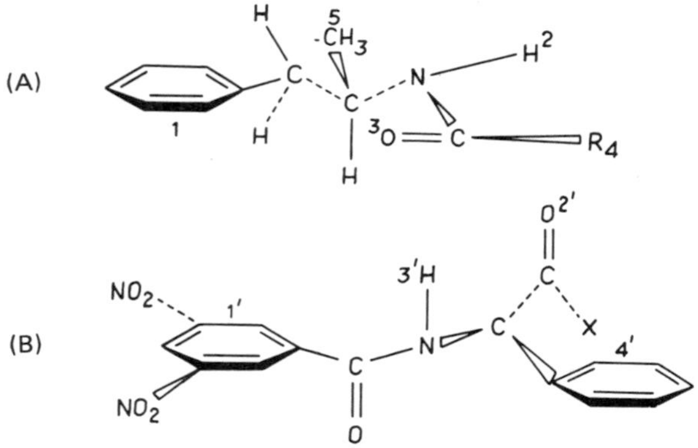

FIGURE 3 Bonding interaction between (S)-1-phenyl-2-aminopropane amide (A) and a Pirkle-type chiral stationary phase (B). X = $NH(CH_2)_3$, covalently bonded column; X = 0^-, ionically bonded column. Four possible sites for interaction between the solute and stationary phase are illustrated. (From Ref. 144, reprinted with permission from I. W. Wainer and T. D. Doyle. J. Chromatogr. 259: 465, 1983. Copyright 1983, Elsevier Science Publishers.)

fluid analysis. However, its use is limited to solutes capable of forming multidentate complexes. A proposed ligand-exchange interaction mechanism based on the stability of diastereomeric complexes is shown in Figure 4. In this example, the N-benzyl group of the chiral ligand blocks one axial position of the Cu(II) ion coordination sphere, and a water molecule occupying the other axial position stabilizes the overall complex [87]. Solutes in the less sterically hindered conformation form more stable complexes and are retained longer than the other enantiomer. A recent paper [150] indicates that hydrophobic and ionic interactions influence resolution. An approach to optimize ligand-exchange separations was proposed. This topic has also been reviewed [87].

These phases are highly stereoselective and widely used to resolve amino acids. Davankov et al. [151,152] introduced this approach for separating amino acids using an amino acid-polystyrene-divinylbenzene copolymer loaded with Cu(II), Ni(II), Zn(II), or Cd(II) ions. Although the amino acids were resolved, nonspecific interactions with the polymeric support resulted in poor peak shape. Gubitz et al. [153] prepared a more efficient phase by bonding L-proline and L-valine to silica gel. Selectivity can be modified by varying temperature, mobile-phase pH, organic modifier, ionic strength, and nature of metal ion used. Selectivity for amino acids decreases in the order Cu >> Ni > Zn > Cd [86]. Although ligand

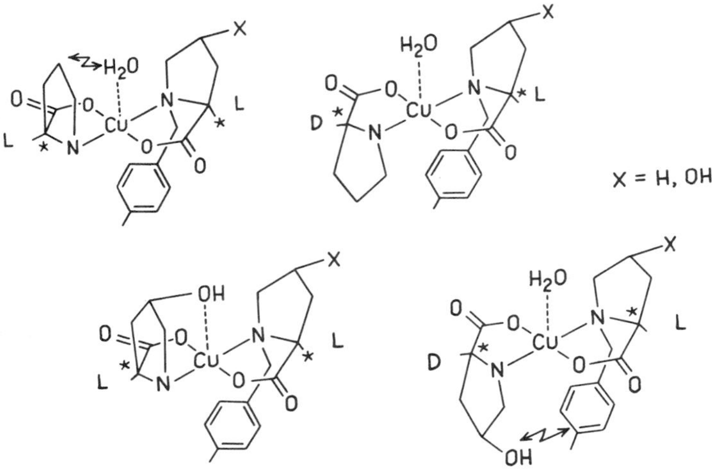

FIGURE 4 Binding of bidentate and tridentate ligands to L-proline-
and L-hydroxyproline-Cu(II) phases. The bidentate D isomer and
tridentate L isomer form the more sterically favorable complexes and
are retained to a greater extent than their respective enantiomers.
(From Ref. 87, reprinted with permission from V. A. Davankov,
A. A. Karganov, and A. S. Bochkov. Adv. Chromatogr. 22: 71,
1983. Copyright 1983, Chromatography Symposium Dept. Chemistry,
University of Houston.)

exchange phases are primarily used for resolving α-amino acids,
they have been applied to ephedrine and valinamide [154].

Inclusion Complexation Phases. The internal cavity of cyclodextrins
is hydrophobic, with secondary hydroxyl groups at the surface of
the large rim and primary hydroxyls around the smaller rim. The
resolution mechanism is based on enantiomer inclusion within the
cyclodextrin cavity. Solutes must have an aromatic group at or
near the chiral center with additional substituents near the cavity
rim and must tightly complex within the cavity in order to achieve
chiral resolution [155]. A three-point interaction is possible through
hydrophobic interaction within the cavity and with two interactions
at the rim.

    Hinze et al. [155] covalently bonded cyclodextrins to silica
gel to form a chiral stationary phase. The α, β, and γ cyclodextrin
columns are commercially available and capable of resolving enantiomers of various sizes. Cyclodextrin phases arc extremely stable
and are normally used with mixed aqueous solvents. Derivatization

is not normally necessary to achieve resolution. Preparation and use of these phases has been recently reviewed [84]. Cyclodextrin columns have been used to resolve a wide variety of solutes. A few examples include various dansyl- and β-naphthyl-amino acid derivatives, barbiturates, dansyl sulfonamides [155], and propranolol [85]. Structural isomers and epimers have also been resolved [84].

REFERENCES

1. C. G. Horvath, B. A. Preiss, and S. R. Lipsky. Fast liquid chromatography: An investigation of operating parameters and the separation of nucleotides on pellicular ion exhcangers. Anal. Chem. 39: 1422–1428, 1967.

2. R. P. W. Scott. An introduction to small-bore columns. J. Chromatogr. Sci. 23: 233–237, 1985.

3. R. P. W. Scott and P. Kucera. The exclusion properties of some commercially available silica gels. J. Chromatogr. 125: 251–263, 1976.

4. R. P. W. Scott et al. (eds.). Small Bore Liquid Chromatography Columns: Their Properties and Uses. Chemical Analysis. Edited by P. J. Elving, J. D. Winefordner, and I. M. Kolthoff. Vol. 72, John Wiley and Sons, New York, 1984.

5. P. Kucera (ed.). Microcolumn High-Performance Liquid Chromatography. Journal of Chromatography Library, Vol. 28. Elsevier, New York, 1984.

6. M. V. Novotny and D. Ishii (eds.). Microcolumn Separations. Journal of Chromatography Library, Vol. 30. Elsevier, New York, 1985.

7. J. H. Knox. Theoretical aspects of LC with packed and open small-bore columns. J. Chromatogr. Sci. 18: 453–461, 1980.

8. M. Novotny. Microcolumns in liquid chromatography. Anal. Chem. 53: 1294A–1308A, 1981.

9. F. J. Yang. Microbore column HPLC. J. High Resol. Chromatogr. Chromatogr. Commun. 6: 348–358, 1983.

10. D. Ishii, M. Goto, and T. Takeuchi. The efficient use of microcolumns in chromatographic systems. J. Pharm. Biomed. Anal. 2: 223–231, 1984.

11. D. Dezaro and R. A. Hartwick. Microbore columns. Chromatogr. Sci. (HPLC Nucleic Acid Res.) 28: 113–137, 1984.

12. N. Sagliano, Jr., H. Shih-Hsien, T. R. Floyd, T. V. Raglione, and R. A. Hartwick. Aspects of small-bore column technology. J. Chromatogr. Sci. 23: 238–246, 1985.

13. S. Van der Wal. Optimization of microbore HPLC separations for minimum detectable quantity and separation time. J. Chromatogr. Sci. 23: 341–347, 1985.

14. P. Gareil.   Recent advances in microbore high-performance liquid chromatography practice.   Biochem. Soc. Trans. 13: 1052—1055, 1985.

15. J. Bowermaster and H. M. McNair.   Sensitivity in microbore HPLC.   LC Mag. 1:   362—364, 1983.

16. R. Majors.   Micro-versus conventional HPLC.   LC Mag. 1: 80—81, 1983.

17. N. H. C. Cooke, K. Olsen, and B. G. Archer.   Microbore versus standard HPLC.   LC Mag. 2:   514—524, 1984.

18. R. Gill and B. Law.   Appraisal of narrow-bore (1 mm I.D.) high-performance liquid chromatography columns with view to the requirements of routine drug analysis.   J. Chromatogr. 354:   185—202, 1986.

19. F. M. Rabel.   Instrumentation for small-bore liquid chromatography.   J. Chromatogr. Sci. 23:   247—252, 1985.

20. M. Novotny.   In Microcolumn High-Performance Liquid Chromatography.   Edited by P. Kucera.   Journal of Chromatography Library, Vol. 28.   Elsevier, New York, 1984, Chap. 7.

21. G. Guiochon and H. Colin.   In Microcolumn High-Performance Liquid Chromatography.   Edited by P. Kucera.   Journal of Chromatography Library, Vol. 28.   Elsevier, New York, 1984, Chap. 1.

22. P. Kucera and G. Manius.   In Microcolumn High-Performance Liquid Chromatography.   Edited by P. Kucera.   Journal of Chromatography Library, Vol. 28,   Elsevier, New York, 1984, Chap. 4.

23. R. P. W. Scott (ed.).   In Small Bore Liquid Chromatography Columns: Their Properties and Uses.   Chemical Analysis, Vol. 72.   John Wiley and Sons, New York, 1984, Chap. 1.

24. R. A. Hartwick and D. D. Dezaro.   In Microcolumn High-Performance Liquid Chromatography.   Edited by P. Kucera. Journal of Chromatography Library, Vol. 28.   Elsevier, New York, 1984, Chap. 3.

25. P. Kucera (ed.).   In Microcolumn High-Performance Liquid Chromatography.   Journal of Chromatography Library, Vol. 28.   Elsevier, New York, 1984, Chap. 2.

26. C. Lochmuller.   In Small Bore Liquid Chromatography Columns: Their Properties and Uses.   Edited by R. P. W. Scott.   Chemical Analysis, Vol. 72.   John Wiley and Sons, New York, 1984, Chap. 5.

27. E. Katz, K. L. Ogan, and R. P. W. Scott.   Peak dispersion and mobile phase velocity in liquid chromatography: The pertinent relationship for porous silica.   J. Chromatogr. 270:   51—75, 1983.

28. K. Ogan.   In Small Bore Liquid Chromatography Columns: Their Properties and Uses.   Edited by R. P. W. Scott.   Chemical Analysis, Vol. 72.   John Wiley and Sons, New York, 1984, Chap. 4.

29. R. P. W. Scott and P. Kucera. Mode of operation and performance characteristics of microbore columns for use in liquid chromatography. J. Chromatogr. 169: 51–72, 1979.

30. E. D. Katz. In Small Bore Liquid Chromatography Columns: Their Properties and Uses. Edited by R. P. W. Scott. Chemical Analysis, Vol. 72. John Wiley and Sons, New York, 1984, Chap. 2.

31. K. Ogan. In Small Bore Liquid Chromatography Columns: Their Properties and Uses. Edited by R. P. W. Scott. Chemical Analysis, Vol. 72. John Wiley and Sons, New York, 1984, Chap. 3.

32. C. M. Dickinson, T. R. Navin, and F. C. Churchill. High-performance liquid chromatographic method for quantitation of pentamidine in blood serum. J. Chromatogr. 345: 91–97, 1985.

33. C. Eckers, K. K. Cuddy, and J. D. Henion. Practical microbore column HPLC: System development and drug applications. J. Liquid Chromatogr. 6: 2383–2409, 1983.

34. J. R. Shipe, A. F. Arlinghaus, J. Savory, M. R. Wills, and J. P. DiMarco. Determination of bethanidine in plasma by liquid chromatography with a microbore reversed-phase column. Clin. Chem. 29: 1793–1795, 1983.

35. M. W. F. Nielen, R. C. A. Koordes, R. W. Frei, and U. A. Th. Brinkman. Automated pre-column system for trace enrichment and clean-up of plasma samples in narrow-bore liquid chromatography. J. Chromatogr. 330: 113–119, 1985.

36. G. Kamperman and J. E. Kraak. Simple and fast analysis of adrenaline and noradrenaline in plasma on microbore high-performance liquid chromatography columns using fluorimetric detection. J. Chromatogr. 337: 384–390, 1985.

37. R. Gill. Application of narrow-bore high-performance liquid chromatography to the analysis of drugs. Anal. Proc. 21: 436–440, 1984.

38. K. Tsuji and B. Binns. Micro-bore high-performance liquid chromatography for the analysis of pharmaceutical compounds. J. Chromatogr. 253: 227–236, 1982.

39. P. Kucera. Design and use of short microbore columns in liquid chromatography. J. Chromatogr. 198: 93–109, 1980.

40. A. Carlsson, T. Sharp, T. Zetterstrom, and U. Ungerstedt. Determination of dopamine and its metabolites in small volumes of rat brain dialysates using small-bore liquid chromatography with electrochemical detection. J. Chromatogr. 368: 299–308, 1986.

41. T. A. Durkin, E. J. Caliguri, I. N. Mefford, D. M. Lake, I. A. Macdonald, E. Sundstrom, and G. Jonsson. Determination of catecholamines in tissue and body fluids using microbore HPLC with amperometric detection. Life Sci. 37: 1803–1810, 1985.

42. E. J. Caliguri and I. N. Mefford. Femtogram detection limits for biogenic amines using microbore HPLC with electrochemical detection. Brain Res. 296: 156−159, 1984.

43. M. Krejci, K. Slais, D. Kourilova, and M. Vespalcova. Enrichment techniques and trace analysis with microbore columns in liquid chromatography. J. Pharm. Biomed. Anal. 2: 197−205, 1984.

44. T. R. Covey, E. D. Lee, A. P. Bruins, and J. D. Henion. Liquid chromatography/mass spectrometry. Anal. Chem. 58: 1451A−1461A, 1986.

45. E. D. Lee and J. D. Henion. Micro-liquid chromatography/mass spectrometry with direct liquid introduction. J. Chromatogr. Sci. 23: 253−264, 1985.

46. G. L. Hawks and J. R. Strimatis (eds.). Advances in Laboratory Automation Robotics 1984. Zymark Corporation, Hopkinton, Massachusetts, 1984.

47. G. L. Hawks and J. R. Strimatis (eds.). Advances in Laboratory Automation Robotics 1985. Zymark Corporation, Hopkinton, Massachusetts, 1985.

48. K. R. Lung, C. H. Lochmuller, and P. M. Gross. The anatomy and function of the laboratory robot. J. Liquid Chromatogr. 9: 2995−3031, 1986.

49. D. L. Greene. Laboratory robots: Partners in productivity. J. Liquid Chromatogr. 9: 3159−3167, 1986.

50. W. W. Johnson. Laboratory robotics—an overview. J. Liquid Chromatogr. 9: 3168−3175, 1986.

51. L. G. Randall. An example of information exchange between a liquid chromatographic system and a robotic sample preparation system. J. Liquid Chromatogr. 9: 3177−3183, 1986.

52. M. G. Cirillo. The Perkin Elmer Masterlab system. J. Liquid Chromatogr. 9: 3185−3190, 1986.

53. T. H. Hight. Implementation of robotic workcells in the laboratory. J. Liquid Chromatogr. 9: 3191−3196, 1986.

54. J. N. Little. The Zymate laboratory automation system. J. Liquid Chromatogr. 9: 3197−3201, 1986.

55. A. R. Frisbee, M. H. Nantz, G. W. Kramer, and P. L. Fuchs. Robotic orchestration of organic reactions: Yield optimization via an automated system with operator-specified reaction sequences. J. Am. Chem. Soc. 106: 7143−7145, 1984.

56. L. I. Friedman and M. L. Severns. Application of robotics in blood banking. Vox Sang. 51: 57−62, 1986.

57. R. J. Eckstein, G. D. Owens, M. A. Baim, and D. A. Hudson. Unattended robotic drug release testing of enterically coated aspirin. Anal. Chem. 58: 2316−2320, 1986.

58. P. Walsh, H. Abdou, R. Barnes, and Cohen. Laboratory robotics for testing tablet content uniformity. Pharm. Technol. 10: 48−53, 1986.

59. C. H. Lochmuller and K. R. Lung. Applications of laboratory robotics in spectrophotometric sample preparations and experimental optimization. Anal. Chim. Acta 183: 257—262, 1986.

60. J. Curley. Robotics from a laboratory manager's view. In Advances in Laboratory Automation Robotics 1984. Edited by G. L. Hawks and J. R. Strimatis. Zymark Corporation, Hopkinton, Massachusetts, 1984, pp. 299—309.

61. F. E. Gainer. Robotics in the analytical laboratory—a management viewpoint. In Advances in Laboratory Automation Robotics 1985. Edited by G. L. Hawks and J. R. Strimatis. Zymark Corporation, Hopkinton, Massachusetts, 1985, pp. 1—14.

62. F. H. Zenie. Trends in laboratory automation—Technology and economics. In Advances in Laboratory Automation Robotics 1984. Edited by G. L. Hawks and J. R. Strimatis. Zymark Corporation, Hopkinton, Massachusetts, 1984, pp. 1—16.

63. F. H. Zenie. Strategic trends in laboratory automation—1985. In Advances in Laboratory Automation Robotics 1985. Edited by G. L. Hawks and J. R. Strimatis. Zymark Corporation, Hopkinton, Massachusetts, 1985, pp. 43—59.

64. P. Kool and Y. Michotte. Robotics in flexible analysis systems. Trends Anal. Chem. 4: 44—50, 1985.

65. J. N. Little. Precision in laboratory robotic-HPLC systems. J. Liquid Chromatogr. 9: 3033—3062, 1986.

66. K. J. Halloran and H. Franze. Interactions between a robotic system and liquid chromatograph—HPLC control, communication and response. LC-GC 4: 1020—1025, 1986.

67. W. M. Hurni, W. J. Miller, E. H. Wasmuth, and W. J. McAleer. A robot for performing radioiodinations. In Advances in Laboratory Automation Robotics 1985. Edited by G. L. Hawks and J. R. Strimatis. Zymark Corporation, Hopkinton, Massachusetts, 1985, pp. 497—507.

68. J. W. Brodack, M. R. Kilbourn, M. J. Welch, and J. A. Katzenellenbogen. Application of robotics to radiopharmaceutical preparations: Controlled synthesis of fluorine-18, 16α-fluoroestradiol-17β. J. Nucl. Med. 27: 714—721, 1986.

69. T. J. Beugelsdijk and D. W. Knobeloch. J. Liquid. Chromatogr. 9: 3093—3131, 1986.

70. E. L. Johnson, L. A. Pachla, and D. L. Reynolds. Robotic analysis of 3,7-dimethoxy-4-phenyl-N-$1H$-tetrazol-5yl-$4H$-furo-{3,2-b}-indole-2-carboxamide in human plasma. J. Pharm. Sci. 75: 1003—1005, 1986.

71. E. L. Johnson and L. A. Pachla. Generic robotic sample preparation of drugs from biological fluids using disposable cartridges. In Advances in Laboratory Automation Robotics 1986. Edited by G. L. Hawks and J. R. Strimatis. Zymark Corporation, Hopkinton, Massachusetts, 1986, pp. 23—36.

72. J. Van Antwerp and R. F. Venteicher. Improving the flexibility of an analytical robot system. LC-GC Mag. 4: 458–460, 1986.

73. G. Schoenhard, R. Schmidt, L. Kosobud, and K. Smykowski. Robotic assays for drugs in animal and human plasma. In Advances in Laboratory Automation Robotics 1984. Edited by G. L. Hawks and J. R. Strimatis. Zymark Corporation, Hopkinton, Massachusetts, 1984, pp. 61–70.

74. E. C. Lewis, D. R. Santarelli, and J. O. Malbica. Laboratory robotics for automated determinations of drugs in physiological samples. In Advances in Laboratory Automation Robotics 1984. Edited by G. L. Hawks and J. R. Strimatis. Zymark Corporation, Hopkinton, Massachusetts, 1984, pp. 237–255.

75. D. J. Myers, N. Szuminsky, and M. J. Levitt. Automating drug metabolism studies through laboratory robotics. In Advances in Laboratory Automation Robotics 1984. Edited by G. L. Hawks and J. R. Strimatis. Zymark Corporation, Hopkinton, Massachusetts, 1984, pp. 71–82.

76. S. F. Kramer, M. J. Levitt, and M. M. Passarello. Comparison of automated and manual extraction of drugs from biological fluids at trace levels. In Advances in Laboratory Automation Robotics 1985. Edited by G. L. Hawks and J. R. Strimatis. Zymark Corporation, Hopkinton, Massachusetts, 1985, pp. 465–479.

77. S. M. Walters, K. Y. Chan, and J. E. Coutant. An automated method for the determination of enoximone and its major sulfoxide metabolite in plasma using robotic technology—high performance liquid chromatography. J. Liquid Chromatogr. 9: 3133–3155, 1986.

78. S. M. Walters, personal communication.

79. G. von Blaschke, H. P. Kraft, K. Fickentscher, and F. Kohler. Chromatographic racemic separation of thalidomide and teratogenic activity of its enantiomers. Arzneimittel Forsch. 29: 1640–1642, 1979.

80. B. Testa and P. Jenner. Stereochemical methodology. In Drug Fate and Metabolism, Vol. 2. Edited by E. R. Garrett and J. L. Hirtz. Marcel Dekker, New York, 1978, pp. 143–193.

81. W. H. Pirkle and J. Finn. Separation of enantiomers by liquid chromatographic methods. In Asymmetric Synthesis, Vol. 1. Edited by J. D. Morrison. Academic Press, New York, 1983, pp. 87–124.

82. B. Testa. The chromatographic analysis of enantiomers in drug metabolism studies. Xenobiotica 16: 265–279, 1986.

83. R. Dappen, H. Arm, and V. R. Meyer. Applications and limitations of commercially available stationary phases for high-performance liquid chromatography. J. Chromatogr. 373: 1–20, 1986.

84. T. J. Ward and D. W. Armstrong. Improved cyclodextrin chiral phases: A comparison and review. J. Liquid Chromatogr. 9: 407–423, 1986.

85. D. W. Armstrong. Chiral stationary phases for high performance liquid chromatographic separation of enantiomers: A mini-review, J. Liquid Chromatogr. 7: 353–376, 1984.

86. S. Allenmark. Recent advances in methods of direct optical resolution. J. Biochem. Biophys. Methods 9: 1–25, 1984.

87. V. A. Davankov, A. A. Kurganov, and A. S. Bochkov. Resolution of racemates by high-performance liquid chromatography. Adv. Chromatogr. 22: 71–116, 1983.

88. I. W. Wainer. Comparison of the liquid chromatographic approaches to the resolution of enantiomeric compounds. Chromatogr. Forum 1: 55–61, 1986.

89. D. W. Armstrong. Optical isomer separation by liquid chromatography. Anal. Chem. 59: 84A–88A, 90A–91A, 1986.

90. R. H. Liu and R. H. Ku. Chiral stationary phases for the gas-liquid chromatographic separation of enantiomers. J. Chromatogr. 271: 309–323, 1983.

91. W. A. Koenig. Separation of enantiomers by capillary gas chromatography with chiral stationary phases. J. HRC & CC 5: 588–595, 1982.

92. J. H. Liu and W. W. Ku. Determination of enantiomeric N-trifluoroacetyl-L-prolyl chloride amphetamine derivatives by capillary gas chromatography/mass spectrometry with chiral and achiral stationary phases. Anal. Chem. 53: 2180–2184, 1981.

93. A. Hulshoff and H. Lingeman. Derivatization reactions in the gas-liquid chromatographic analysis of drugs in biological fluids. J. Pharm. Biomed. Anal. 2: 337–380, 1984.

94. J. D. Adams, T. F. Woolf, A. J. Trevor, L. R. Williams, and N. Castagnoli, Jr. Derivatization of chiral amines with (S,S)-N-trifluoroacetylproline anhydride for GC estimation of enantiomeric composition. J. Pharm. Sci. 71: 658–660, 1982.

95. W. A. Konig, I. Benecke, and S. Sievers. New procedure for gas chromatographic enantiomer separation. Application to chiral amines and hydroxy acids. J. Chromatogr. 238: 427–432, 1982.

96. K. Kruse, W. Francke, and W. A. Konig. Gas chromatographic separation of chiral alcohols, amino alcohols and amines. J. Chromatogr. 170: 423–429, 1979.

97. J. A. Thompson, J. L. Holtzman, M. Tsuru, C. L. Lerman, and J. L. Holtzman. Procedure for the chiral derivatization and chromatographic resolution of R-(+)- and S-(−)-propranolol. J. Chromatogr. 238: 470–475, 1982.

98. K.-J. Hoffmann, L. Renberg and C. Baarnhielm. Stereoselective disposition of RS-tocainide in man. Eur. J. Drug. Metab. Pharmacokin. 9: 215–222, 1984.

99.   M. Ruud-Christensen and B. Salvesen. Separation of (R)-
      and (S)-proxyphylline as diastereoisomeric camphanates by
      reversed-phase liquid chromatography. J. Chromatogr. 303:
      433−435, 1984.
100. E. J. D. Lee, K. M. Williams, G. G. Graham, R. O. Day,
      and G. D. Champion. Liquid chromatographic determination
      and plasma concentration profile of optical isomers of ibuprofen
      in humans. J. Pharm. Sci. 73: 1542−1544, 1984.
101. J. Gal. Resolution of the enantiomers of ephedrine, norephed-
      rine and pseudoephedrine by high-performance liquid chro-
      matography. J. Chromatogr. 307: 220−223, 1984.
102. J. Gal and A. J. Sedman. R-α-Methylbenzyl isothiocyanate,
      a new and convenient chiral derivatizing reagent for the
      separation of enantiomeric amino compounds by high-performance
      liquid chromatography. J. Chromatogr. 314: 275−281, 1984.
103. C. R. Clark and J. M. Barksdale. Synthesis and liquid chro-
      matographic evaluation of some chiral derivatizing agents for
      resolution of amine enantiomers. Anal. Chem. 56: 958−962,
      1984.
104. R. Shimizu, T. Kakimoto, K. Ishii, Y. Fujimoto, H. Nishi,
      and N. Tsumagari. New derivatization reagent for the resolu-
      tion of optical isomers in diltiazem hydrochloride by high-
      performance liquid chromatography. J. Chromatogr. 357: 119−
      125, 1986.
105. E. Gil-Av, B. Feibush, and R. Charles-Sigler. Separation of
      enantiomers by gas liquid chromatography with an optically
      active stationary phase. Tetrahedron Lett. 1009−1015, 1966.
106. E. Gil-Av, B. Feibush, and R. Charles-Sigler. Separation of
      enantiomers by gas-liquid chromatography with an optically
      active stationary phase. In Gas Chromatography 1966. Edited
      by A. B. Littlewood. Institute of Petroleum, London, 1967,
      pp. 227−239.
107. P. J. Wedlund, B. J. Sweetman, C. B. McAllister, R. A.
      Branch, and G. R. Wilkinson. Direct enantiomeric resolution
      of mephenytoin and its N-demethylated metabolite in plasma
      and blood using chiral capillary gas chromatography. J.
      Chromatogr. 307: 121−127, 1984.
108. K. M. McErlane and G. K. Pillai. Gas-liquid chromatographic
      resolution and assay of tocainide enantiomers using a chiral
      capillary column and study of their selective disposition in
      man. J. Chromatogr. 274: 129−138, 1983.
109. B. Koppenhoefer and E. Bayer. Chiral recognition in gas
      chromatographic analysis and enantiomers on chiral polysilox-
      anes. J. Chromatogr. Libr. 32: 1−42, 1985.
110. V. Schurig. Resolution of a chiral olefin by complexation
      chromatography on an optically active rhodium(I) complex.
      Angew. Chem. 89: 113−114, 1977.

111. V. Schurig and W. Burkle. Quantitative resolution of enantio- mers of trans-2,3-epoxybutane by complexation chromatography on an optically active nickel(II) complex. Angew. Chem. 90: 132—133, 1978.

112. V. Schurig, B. Koppenhoefer, and W. Burkle. Preparation and determination of configurationally pure trans-(2*S*,3*S*)-2,3- epoxybutane. J. Org. Chem. 45: 538—541, 1980.

113. V. Schurig and R. Weber. Manganese(II)-bis(3-heptafluoro- butyryl-1*R*-camphorate): A versatile agent for the resolution of racemic cyclic ethers by complexation gas chromatography. J. Chromatogr. 217: 51—70, 1981.

114. C. E. Dalgleish. The optical resolution of aromatic amino- acids on paper chromatograms. J. Chem. Soc. 3940—3942, 1952.

115. W. H. Pirkle, M. H. Hyun, and B. Bank. A rational ap- proach to the design of highly-effective chiral stationary phases. J. Chromatogr. 316: 585—604, 1984.

116. J. Hermansson. Direct liquid chromatographic resolution of racemic drugs by means of α_1-acid glycoprotein as the chiral complexing agent in the mobile phase. J. Chromatogr. 316: 537—546, 1984.

117. C. Pettersson, T. Arvidsson, A. L. Karlsson, and I. Marle. Chromatographic resolution of enantiomers using albumin as complexing agent in the mobile phase. J. Pharm. Biomed. Anal. 4: 221—235, 1986.

118. C. Pettersson. Chromatographic separation of enantiomers of acids with quinine as chiral counter ion. J. Chromatogr. 316: 553—567, 1984.

119. C. Pettersson and G. Schill. Separation of enantiomeric amines by ion-pair chromatography. J. Chromatogr. 204: 179—183, 1981.

120. A. Dobashi and S. Hara. Chiral recognition mechanisms in the enantioselectivity of chiral hydrogen bonding additives in liquid-solid chromatography. J. Chromatogr. 349: 143—154, 1986.

121. P. E. Hare and E. Gil-Av. Separation of D and L amino acids by liquid chromatography: Use of chiral eluants. Science 204: 1226—1228, 1979.

122. E. Gil-Av, A. Tishbee, and P. E. Hare. Resolution of un- derivatized amino acids by reversed-phase chromatography. J. Am. Chem. Soc. 102: 5115—5117, 1980.

123. S. Weinstein, M. H. Engel, and P. E. Hare. The enantiomeric analysis of a mixture of all common protein amino acids by high-performance liquid chromatography using a new chiral mobile phase. Anal. BIochem. 121: 370—377, 1982.

124. C. Gilon, R. Leshem, Y. Tapuhi, and E. Grushka. Reversed phase chromatographic resolution of amino acid enantiomers

with metal-aspartame eluants. J. Am. Chem. Soc. 101: 7612–7613, 1979.

125. L. R. Gelber and J. L. Neumeyer. Determination of the enantiomeric purity of levodopa, methyldopa, carbidopa and tryptophan by use of chiral mobile phase high-performance liquid chromatography. J. Chromatogr. 257: 317–326, 1983.

126. J. N. LePage, W. Lindner, G. Davies, D. E. Seitz, and B. L. Karger. Resolution of the optical isomers of dansyl amino acids by reversed phase liquid chromatography with optically active metal chelate additives. Anal. Chem. 51: 433–435, 1979.

127. D. Sybilska, J. Zukowski and J. Bojarski. Resolution of mephenytoin and some chiral barbiturates into enantiomers by reversed phase high performance liquid chromatography via β-cyclodextrin inclusion complexes. J. Liquid Chromatogr. 9: 591–606, 1986.

128. T. Takeuchi, H. Isai, and D. Ishii. Enantiomeric resolution of dansyl amino acids by micro high-performance liquid chromatography with β-cyclodextrin inclusion complexes. J. Chromatogr. 357: 409–415, 1986.

129. J. Zukowski, D. Sybilska, and J. Bojarski. Application of α- and β-cyclodextrin and heptakis(2,6-di-O-methyl)-β-cyclodextrin as mobile phase components for the sepration of some chiral barbiturates into enantiomers by reversed-phase high-performance liquid chromatography. J. Chromatogr. 364: 225–232, 1986.

130. V. Prelog and P. Wieland. Uber die spaltung der Troger'schen base in optische antipoden, ein beitrag zur stereochemie des dreiwertigen stickstoffs. Helv. Chim. Acta 27: 1127–1134, 1944.

131. S. Allenmark, B. Bomgren, and H. Boren. Direct liquid chromatographic separation of enantiomers on immobilized protein stationary phases. III. Optical resolution of a series of N-aroyl D,L-amino acids by high-performance liquid chromatography on bovine serum albumin covalently bound to silica. J. Chromatogr. 264: 63–68, 1983.

132. S. Allenmark, B. Bomgren, H. Boren, and P.-O. Lagerstrom. Direct optical resolution of a series of pharmacologically active racemic sulfoxides by high-performance liquid affinity chromatography. Anal. Biochem. 136: 293–297, 1984.

133. J. Hermansson, M. Eriksson, and O. Nyquist. Determination of (R)- and (S)-disopyramide in human plasma using a chiral α_1-acid glycoprotein column. J. Chromatogr. 336: 321–328, 1984.

134. J. Hermansson. Direct liquid chromatographic resolution of racemic drugs using α_1-acid glycoprotein as the chiral stationary phase. J. Chromatogr. 269: 71–80, 1983.

135. J. Hermansson. Liquid chromatographic resolution of racemic drugs using a chiral α_1-acid glycoprotein column. J. Chromatogr. 298: 67–78, 1984.

136. G. Schill, I. W. Wainer, and S. A. Barkan. Chiral separation of cationic drugs on an α_1-acid glycoprotein bonded stationary phase. J. Liquid Chromatogr. 9: 641–666, 1986.

137. G. Schill, I. W. Wainer, and S. A. Barkan. Chiral separations of cationic and anionic drugs on an α_1-acid glycoprotein-bonded stationary phase (Enantiopac). II. Influence of mobile phase additives and pH on chiral resolution and retention. J. Chromatogr. 365: 73–88, 1986.

138. S. Allenmark. Optical resolution by liquid chromatography on immobilized bovine serum albumin. J. Liquid Chromatogr. 9: 425–442, 1986.

139. S. Allenmark, B. Bomgren, and H. Boren. Direct liquid chromatographic separation of enantiomers on immobilized protein stationary phases. IV. Molecular interaction forces and retention behavior in chromatography on bovine serum albumin as a stationary phase. J. Chromatogr. 316: 617–624, 1984.

140. A.-D. Schwanghart, W. Backmann, and G. Blaschke. Untersuchung chromatographischer racemattrennungen. VII. Praparative trennversuche an optisch aktiven polyamiden. Chem. Ber. 110: 778–787, 1977.

141. H. Yuki, Y. Okamoto, and I. Okamoto. Resolution of racemic compounds by optically active poly(triphenylmethyl methacrylate). J. Am. Chem. Soc. 102: 6356–6358, 1980.

142. I. W. Wainer, T. D. Doyle, Z. Hamidzadeh, and M. Aldridge. Application of high-performance liquid chromatographic chiral stationary phases to pharmaceutical analysis. Resolution of ephedrine. J. Chromatogr. 261: 123–126, 1983.

143. I. W. Wainer, T. D. Doyle, K. H. Donn, and J. R. Powell. The direct enantiomeric determination of (−) and (+)-propranolol in human serum by high-performance liquid chromatography on a chiral stationary phase. J. Chromatogr. 306: 405–411, 1984.

144. I. W. Wainer and T. D. Doyle. Application of high-performance liquid chromatographic chiral stationary phases to pharmaceutical analysis. Direct enantiomeric resolution of amide derivatives of 1- phenyl-2-aminopropane. J. Chromatogr. 259: 465–472, 1983.

145. T. D. Doyle and I. W. Wainer. The resolution of enantiomeric drugs using HPLC chiral stationary phases. Pharm. Technol. 28, 30, 31–2 (February 1985).

146. T. D. Doyle, W. M. Adams, F. S. Fry, Jr., and I. W. Wainer. The application of HPLC chiral stationary phases to stereochemical problems of pharmaceutical interest: A general method for the resolution of enantiomeric amines as β-naphthyl-carbamate derivatives. J. Liquid Chromatogr. 9: 455–471, 1986.

147. N. Oi, M. Nagase, and T. Doi. High-performance liquid chromatographic separation of enantiomers on (S)-1-(α-naphthyl)-ethylamine bonded to silica gel. J. Chromatogr. 257: 111–117, 1983.

148. R. Dappen, V. R. Meyer, and H. Arm. New chiral covalently bonded pi-donor stationary phases for high-performance liquid chromatography, based on derivatives of optically active 1-(α-naphthyl)ethylamine. J. Chromatogr. 361: 93–105, 1986.

149. W. H. Pirkle and D. W. House. Chiral high-pressure liquid chromatographic stationary phases. I. Separation of the enantiomers of sulfoxides, amines, amino acids, alcohols, hydroxy acids, lactones, and mercaptans. J. Org. Chem. 44: 1957–1960, 1979.

150. H. Englehardt, Th. Koenig, and Sk. Kromidas. Optimization of enantiomeric separations with chiral bonded phases. Chromatographia 21: 205–213, 1986.

151. V. A. Davankov, S. V. Rogozhin, A. V. Semechkin, and T. P. Sachkova. Ligand-exchange chromatography of racemates. Influence of the degree of saturation of the asymmetric resin by metal ions on ligand exchange. J. Chromatogr. 82: 359–365, 1973.

152. V. A. Davankov. Resolution of racemates by ligand-exchange chromatography. Adv. Chromatogr. 18: 139–195, 1980.

153. G. Gubitz, W. Jellenz, and W. Santi. Resolution of the optical isomers of underivatized amino acids on chemically bonded chiral phases by ligand-exchange chromatography. J. Liquid Chromatogr. 4: 701–712, 1981.

154. V. A. Davankov, Yu. A. Zolotarev, and A. A. Kurganov. Ligand-exchange chromatography of racemates. XI. Complete resolution of some chelating racemic compounds and nature of sorption enantioselectivity. J. Liquid Chromatogr., 2: 1191–1204, 1979.

155. W. L. Hinze, T. E. Riehl, D. W. Armstrong, W. DeMond, A. Alak, and T. Ward. Liquid chromatographic separation of enantiomers using a chiral β-cyclodextrin-bonded stationary phase and conventional aqueous-organic mobile phases. Anal. Chem. 57: 237–242, 1985.

3

Dosage Routes, Bioavailability, and Clinical Efficacy

PETER G. WELLING   *Parke-Davis Pharmaceutical Research Division, Warner-Lambert Company, Ann Arbor, Michigan*

The last decade has witnessed a major shift in the focus of the pharmaceutical industry to the dosage form. This has resulted from a greater appreciation of the importance of drug absorption, the characteristics of circulating drug levels required to exert desired therapeutic effects, and the ability of new drug delivery systems to improve drug absorption from various dosage sites into the bloodstream.

Attention has naturally focused on conventional oral and parenteral dosage. With the oral route in particular, tremendous advances have been made in improving drug delivery from this much discussed yet so poorly understood delivery route. The sustained-release dosage form has matured to a high level of sophistication in the search for optimum drug release profiles.

While research on conventional dosage forms continues, attention is now focusing on new pathways and new routes of drug administration. Some routes are patently obvious and have been used for drug delivery, for therapeutic and other purposes, for some time. The mouth and lungs provide excellent absorption surfaces because of their rich blood supply, close proximity of the thin capillary networks adjacent to the external surface, and direct entry of substances into the general circulation by these routes. Other routes, such as the intranasal and transdermal, are less obvious for drug delivery, although the nasal route has been used, or abused, for some time. The possibility of administering small quantities of drugs via these dosage routes has provided the impetus for innovation and ingenuity in drug delivery systems. Despite the obstacles of local irritation and the relative impermeability of skin tissues, a number of successes have been achieved in transdermal drug delivery. If the present impetus continues, other successes are likely in the near future.

The physical and chemical forms in which a drug is produced, the type of formulation, and the route of administration may be decided at an early stage in drug development. In many cases the decision must be made at the discovery point as a result of the characteristics of the compound. Whenever the decision is made and for whatever reason, scientific or economic, a large and ever-increasing range of alternative dosage forms and delivery routes is becoming available. The intent of this chapter is to highlight some of the characteristics of the various dosage routes and some recent developments in their testing and clinical application.

I. CONVENTIONAL DOSAGE ROUTES IN DRUG DISCOVERY, DEVELOPMENT, AND CLINICAL PRACTICE

A. Oral Route

Despite the intense interest in alternative dosage routes, the oral route is still by far the most preferable from practically every viewpoint and is likely to continue to be so. The gastrointestinal tract is designed to selectively absorb substances. It has taken a while to develop to its present level of efficacy, and it is unwise not to make use of it. This is recognized throughout the drug discovery process, and "oral activity" is often a prerequisite when considering

a drug candidate for further development. The interest of those
concerned with marketing the final product often declines precipitously
if oral activity cannot be demonstrated at an early stage. Even then,
the possibility of animal models poorly predicting oral absorption in
humans is often of concern until the results of the first Phase I
clinical study are available.

1. Characteristics of the Gastrointestinal Tract

The anatomic and physiological characteristics of the gastrointestinal
tract, particularly as they pertain to drug absorption, have been
described elsewhere and are not discussed here (1-3). We know how
the gastrointestinal tract is constructed, but optimizing dosage forms
to take full advantage of the enormous absorption capability of the
gastrointestinal tract is not among our greatest achievements. Problems
associated with presystemic hepatic clearance of orally administered
drugs is now appreciated, but attempts to bypass hepatic clearance
by targeting drug absorption via the lymphatic system have been
disappointing. Similarly, the use of liposomes to promote gastrointestinal drug absorption via the splanchnic circulation or the lymphatic system has been unsuccessful.

2. Relationships Between Gastrointestinal Tract
and Novel Oral Dosage Forms

Although the major focus of product development and formulation is
to increase the rate and efficiency with which a drug is absorbed,
much attention is now paid to slowing the absorption process to
achieve less frequent dosing, flatter drug profiles, more consistent
therapeutic effects, and all the other advantages associated with
controlled drug release. Ideally, the rate of drug release must be
reduced without reducing absorption efficiency. This is difficult and
has often proven impossible to achieve.

Although a true anatomic absorption window has not been un-
equivocally demonstrated for any drug, it is clear that the absorption
efficiency of most substances, including drugs, declines as they pass
from proximal to distal regions of the gastrointestinal tract. Some
drugs exhibit this to a greater extent than others. Add to this the
thriving bacterial population in the large intestine and one has a
system that clearly favors proximal rather than distal drug absorption.
This may be why so few sustained-release formulations exhibit true
zero-order absorption in vivo, despite zero-order dissolution characteristics in vitro.

Reduced absorption is an intrinsic hazard with all oral controlled-release formulations. Apart from poor absorption and bacterial degradation in the distal intestine, the duration of drug absorption is limited by gastrointestinal residence time. Transit times within the gastrointestinal tract depend on both the dosage form and physiological factors (4, 5). Estimates of total gastrointestinal residence times vary from 12 to 24 hr. Residence time can be influenced by a variety of factors, including the pharmacological effect of the drug, food, disease, and stress. Changes in residence time invariably influence drug absorption.

Although possibly providing therapeutic advantages to the patient, and these advantages must justify the inevitable increase in cost, controlled-release dosage forms have presented problems for regulatory agencies and official compendia in terms of providing standards for their testing and assessment. The feasibility of establishing in vitro dissolution criteria to predict in vivo drug absorption characteristics has been debated for some time. For conventional products, dissolution criteria are based on the fatest dissolution rate. For controlled-release products, the optimum dissolution rate is some intermediate value. This gives rise to a dissolution window, and a controlled-release product may fail to meet a dissolution criterion by dissolving too slowly or too quickly. As a result of this, and also of the wide variety of controlled-release dosage forms that are currently available, it is not surprising that there are limited compendial guidelines for in vitro dissolution tests for controlled-release products (6).

A panel of experts appointed by the Academy of Pharmaceutical Scientists, the American Society of Clinical Pharmacology and Therapeutics, Drug Information Association, and the U.S. Food and Drug Administration, recently proposed guidelines for in vitro and in vivo testing of controlled-release products (7). The guidelines address several key issues, including in vitro-in vivo drug release relationships, design of pharmacokinetic studies, and the need for clinical studies. These guidelines do not resolve the issues but they provide a basis from which realistic general guidelines may evolve.

The major problem associated with developing general guidelines for testing is the wide variety of dosage forms. These include matrix tablets, encapsulated coated granules, resins, osmotic pumps, flotation devices, and adhesives. Although the in vivo release of drug from many of these devices can probably be described by conventional first-order or zero-order kinetics (8), there are sufficient exceptions to require that bioavailability and bioequivalence parameters most often need to be assessed on a case-by-case basis. More will be said on this subject from regulatory, industrial, and academic perspectives in the future.

3. Conditions of the Gastrointestinal Tract and Oral Drug Absorption

Conditions of the gastrointestinal tract that may influence drug absorption include disease, drug interactions, and the effect of food. With the increasing emphasis on global development of new chemical entities and rapid evolution of generic programs in many countries, more questions are being asked regarding the effect of these conditions on drug absorption. It may no longer be sufficient to prove bio-availability or bioequivalence in healthy young volunteers, although this will continue to be the standard test population.

The presence of food in the stomach can have a marked, and often unpredictable, effect on drug absorption (9-11). The intensity and variability of this interaction is recognized, and most New Drug Application (NDA) and Market Authorization Application (MAA) sub-missions include this type of information. There is no predictable animal model. Preliminary information may be obtained in preclinical studies, but definitive studies must be conducted in clinical Phase II or Phase III.

The result of some representative drug-food interactions are given in Table 1 (12), which demonstrates the broad spectrum of interactions. Food can affect drug absorption in a positive or negative way. Some compounds appear in more than one column in the table, indicating the variable influence of dosage form, type of meal, or some other factor, or perhaps divergent results from different laboratories.

A number of diseases have been shown to influence drug absorption (13, 14). These include diseases affecting gastrointestinal motility, diseases of the intestines, intestinal infections, and surgery. Although diseases of the gastrointestinal tract are very common, responsible for 11% of chronic illnesses and one-third of major operations in the United States (15), reports of the influence of gastrointestinal disease on drug absorption are scarce.

The rate of drug absorption may be influenced by changes in stomach emptying rate, achlorhydria, diseases of the small and large bowel, including celiac and Crohn's disease, changes in intestinal microflora, and intestinal infestations, but published information is limited to only a handful of drugs. This is an area that is likely to receive considerable attention in the future.

Drug-drug interactions affecting oral drug absorption are a major problem, particularly in patients receiving several medications simultaneously. Interactions may be indirect, by virtue of the action of one drug on the gastrointestinal tract, thereby affecting the absorption of another drug, or perhaps of itself. Interactions may also be direct: two compounds may interact chemically or physically to cause altered

TABLE 1 Effect of Food on Absorption of Some Drugs

Reduced	Delayed	Unaffected	Increased
Ampicillin	Acetaminophen	Bendroflume-thiazide	Carbamazepine
Aspirin	Aspirin	Bevantolol	Chlorothiazide
Atenolol	Cephalosporins (most)	Chlorpropamide	Diazepam
Captopril	Sulfonamides	Enoxacin	Dicoumarol
Ethanol	Diclofenac	Ethambutol	Diftalone
Hydrochloro-thiazide	Digoxin	Hydralazine	Griseofulvin
Penicillins (most)	Furosemide	Oxazepam	Labetalol
Tetracyclines (most)	Indoprofen	Oxprenolol	Metoprolol
Iron	Tolmesoxide	Phenazone	Propranolol
Levodopa	Valproate	Pivampicillin	Nitrofurantoin
Penicillamine		Propoxyphene	
Sotalol		Tolbutamide	
Warfarin		Tranexamic acid	

absorption characteristics. This is a critical factor in fixed drug
combination formulations. Some indirect and direct interactions are
listed in Table 2 (16).

Major indirect interactions that have been reported in the literature
include altered gastrointestinal motility by such agents as metoclopramide (17), propantheline (18), diamorphine (19), and diphenhydramine (20), causing altered absorption of other compounds. The
major direct interactions occur with antacid preparations, which
affect the absorption of a variety of drugs (21), and also with kaolin-
pectin (22), cholestyramine (23), and charcoal (24, 25). Many direct
and indirect interactions are somewhat predictable, but much information still remains to be collected or reported. Most NDA submissions
contain a number of interaction studies, and the number of these is
likely to increase as more information becomes available, but it is
impossible to anticipate the enormous variety of interactions that may
occur in the clinic. Animal models, particularly the dog, may be used

TABLE 2 Agents That Affect Absorption of Other Drugs

Agent	Effect on drug absorption
Indirect action	
Propantheline	Delayed (generally)
Metoclopramide	Increased rate (generally)
Neomycin	Reduced
Direct action	
Antacids	Reduced
Kaolin-pectin	Reduced
Charcoal	Reduced
Cholestyramine	Reduced
Metal ions	Reduced

to predict direct drug-drug interactions, but probably less so for indirect interactions owing to species differences in gastrointestinal physiology and anatomy, and also drug sensitivity.

Drug-drug interactions, both direct and indirect, may influence drug absorption from different oral formulations containing the same drug. This concept has given rise to much discussion, but there are few examples of this occurring with currently approved equivalent products.

B. Parenteral Route

The major conventional parenteral dosage routes are identified here as intravenous, intramuscular, subcutaneous, intra-arterial, intra-thecal, and intraperitoneal. These routes are differentiated in this chapter from buccal, nasal, inhalation, and transdermal as these latter delivery routes have undergone considerable investigation and expansion recently for administering drugs in less conventional dosage forms.

1. Intravenous Administration

Intravenously administered drugs enter the systemic circulation directly. Intravenous injection is thus used as a reference standard when determining absolute drug absorption efficiency from any other dosage route. As there is no absorption component and hence no question of bioavailability, intravenous administration should be used in all preliminary pharmacological screens for systemically acting compounds. If a compound is not active after intravenous administration, it is unlikely to be active by any other route, except in cases of presystemic metabolism of an inactive or less active oral precursor to an active substance. In many cases, intravenous dosing is precluded by low aqueous solubility, and the pharmacological activity of drugs is then determined after oral or intraperitoneal doses. However, in these cases drug absorption is being measured along with its intrinsic pharmacological activity. A major advantage of the intravenous dosage route, in drug discovery, development, or clinical practice, is the high degree of control that can be exercised in dose size and rate of administration. By applying simple pharmacokinetic principles, an infinite variety of drug profiles in plasma can be obtained and replicated. This is particularly useful when examining drug concentration-response relationships.

2. Intramuscular Injection

Intramuscular injection generally, but not always, results in quantitative absorption of drug into the bloodstream. Slow or incomplete absorption from intramuscular injection has been reported for a number of compounds, including chlordiazepoxide, diazepam, digoxin, phenytoin, and phenobarbital. Although phenobarbital appears to be completely bioavailable following intramuscular injections in children, it is only 80% bioavailable compared with oral doses in adults (26).

Absorption of drug from intramuscular sites is affected by drug solubility, the type of solvent, injection volume, molecular size of injected drug, and vascular perfusion. Sparingly soluble compounds may precipitate at the injection site. For example, quinidine base precipitates after intramuscular injection of quinidine hydrochloride solution. Drugs with low aqueous solubility may be administered in oily vehicles. In this case drugs may precipitate from these vehicles when introduced into the aqueous intramuscular environment, giving rise to slow and possibly incomplete absorption. Drugs are generally absorbed more readily from small injection volumes than from large volumes, due perhaps to mechanical compression of adjacent capillary beds, increased volume-surface area ratio, larger diffusion path traveled by molecules from the center of the injection site, and also a smaller concentration gradient with large injection volumes. Schriftman and Kondritzer (27) showed that atropine was absorbed faster from small injection volumes than from large injection volumes in guinea pigs.

Consistent with membrane theory, lipid-soluble molecules are more rapidly absorbed from intramuscular sites than water-soluble compounds, and absorption of the latter is dependent on molecular size. Small water-soluble compounds may enter the circulation directly via the capillaries, whereas larger molecules enter the circulation indirectly via the lymphatics. Thus absorption of the latter compounds is limited by lymph flow, which is only 0.1% of plasma flow.

Vascular perfusion is a rate-limiting factor in intramuscular drug absorption. Blood flows through muscular tissue at rates ranging from 0.02 to 0.07 ml/min per g. The faster the rate, the faster is the absorption. Lidocaine is absorbed more rapidly from arm muscle than from the gluteus maximus, insulin is absorbed faster from arm muscle than from thigh muscle, and cefuroxime and cephradine are absorbed faster from intramuscular doses to men than to women. The latter is presumably due to the greater fraction of adipose tissue in females (28, 29).

These comments show that, although intramuscular drug administration may generally be more reliable than oral administration, it is not without its problems. Complete and prompt absorption cannot be assumed in every case. The intramuscular dosage route is often used for sustained-release medication, and considerable attention has focused on the use of aqueous suspensions, oily vehicles, and complexes. An area of considerable potential is the use of microencapsulation and liposomes to achieve delayed delivery, with obvious potential for organ targeting. Although oral administration of liposomes has been unsuccessful, intramuscular administration has greater potential. The use of liposomes to target antitumor agents to cardiac tissue, central nervous system, and other tissues is being actively investigated. Microcapsules consisting of small drug particles coated with a biodegradable polymer gives rise to prolonged release after parenteral doses (30). Twofold increases in duration of activity of fluphenazine embonate and gold sodium thiosulfate have been achieved by intramuscular injection of microencapsulated drug (31, 32).

3. Subcutaneous Administration

Subcutaneous absorption is generally lower than intramuscular absorption because of less efficient regional circulation. As with intramuscular doses, however, low molecular weight molecules are absorbed primarily via the capillaries and larger molecules are absorbed primarily via the lymphatics. The subcutaneous route is used frequently for drug administration during early discovery and development stages. The route is ideal for prolonged delivery of suspensions or solutins. Further prolongation of drug release is achieved by subcutaneous implants of such devices as pellets (33). Drugs delivered by subcutaneous implants in commercial products include testosterone, progesterone, penicillin, gold, and sulfonamides. Silastic rubber implants have been examined for the release of progestogens, and marked differences in release rates have been demonstrated for different silastic polymers (34). This is illustrated in Figure 1, in which

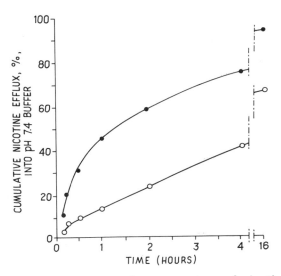

FIGURE 1 Cumulative percentage of nicotine base released from dimethylpolysiloxane (●) and dimethylpolysiloxane + fluorosilicone-laminated polysiloxane (○) tubing into pH 7.4 buffer at 37°C. (Reproduced by permission from *J. Pharm. Sci.* 63: 1849–1853, 1974.)

in vitro release of nicotine base into pH 7.4 buffer from a dimethyl-polysiloxane polymer was 95% in 6 hr, compared with only 65% from a fluorosilicone-laminate polymer. Different dosage forms of insulin are used to provide immediate and also sustained release from subcutaneous sites. Apart from the dosage form, the actual site of injection and the degree of exercise can also affect absorption rate. This is shown in Figures 2 and 3 (35, 36).

4. Intra-arterial Injection

Intra-arterial injection is used infrequently in drug discovery, development, and clinical practice. Its use is restricted largely to regional delivery of drugs to particular organs, particularly in cancer chemotherapy. Clinical reports have shown intra-arterial carmustine (BCNU) to be effective in treatment of metastatic brain tumors (37), and pelvic intra-arterial actinomycin D has been shown to be effective for malignant trophoblastic disease (38). Carotid artery infusion of vinblastine was more effective than intravenous vinblastine for the treatment of cerebral tumors in experimental animals (39). Despite its actual and potential advantages over the intravenous route for

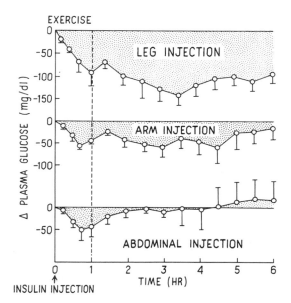

FIGURE 2 Influence of injection site on plasma glucose response to insulin during leg exercise. Shaded areas represent changes in plasma glucose levels (mean ± SD) following insulin injection during leg exercise compared with that with no exercise. The area for leg injection is significantly greater than those for both arm and abdominal injections. (Reproduced by permission from *N. Engl. J. Med.* 298: 79–83, 1978.)

organ targeting, intra-arterial administration is limited by its potential dangers. Such complications as embolization, arterial occlusion, bleeding, and local drug toxicity are common and require considerable care in drug administration.

5. Intrathecal Administration

Intrathecal administration is even more regionally specialized than intra-arterial and is used to deliver drug directly into cerebrospinal fluid (CSF). Intrathecally administered drugs are usually injected directly into the lumbar subarachnoid space, the subdural space, or the ventricals, the latter frequently via implanted reservoir. Lumbar puncture may cause leakage of drug into the epidural or subdural space. With this dosage route, drug must also ascend the spinal subarachnoid space against the descending flow of CSF, re-

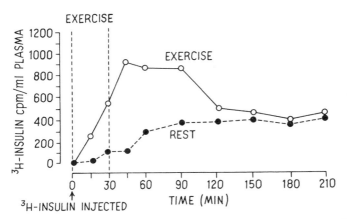

FIGURE 3 Effect of mild bicycle exercise on plasma [3H]insulin levels following subcutaneous injection of 4×10^5 cpm [3H]insulin per kg body weight into the leg of a juvenile patient. (Reproduced by permission from *Diabetes* (Suppl. I), 28: 53—57, 1979.)

sulting in low drug levels in the brain. Intraventricular administration is superior to intralumbar injection as the cerebral vesicles are the site of CSF production, allowing thorough mixing and distribution of drug throughout the CNS.

Whichever route is used, intrathecal injection ensures complete central nervous system (CNS) availability of drug that might have difficulty crossing the blood-brain barrier. This dosage route may be useful as a means of examining the intrinsic activity of CNS compounds in an in vivo setting. The technique is labor intensive however, and a variety of in vitro screens exist that are receptor site specific for CNS drugs. Many of these screens are high through-put and efficient and provide better dose-response relationships than intrathecal injection in vivo. Intrathecal injection can be used to produce regional spinal anesthesia and for treatment of meningial neoplasms and other forms of cancer affecting the CNS (40).

The volume of CSF in the human is about 140 ml. Transport of drug between CSF and plasma may be slow, governed by CSF turn-over rate and return of drug to the systemic circulation directly into adjoining capillaries or at the arachnoid villi. Intrathecal dosing thus gives rise to high CNS drug concentrations with reduced risk of systemic toxicity. Intrathecal injection of methotrexate yields CSF concentrations that are 100-fold higher than simultaneous plasma concentrations (41).

6. Intraperitoneal Injection

Intraperitoneal injection is used extensively in drug discovery and development, particularly in small animals. Despite the relative ease with which compounds are administered by this route, it can give rise to problems in data interpretation. Drugs administered into the intraperitoneal cavity are absorbed for the most part via the splanchnic circulation. This component of the circulation must pass through the liver before it joins the general circulation at the inferior vena cava. Intraperitoneally administered drugs are therefore subject to first-pass presystemic hepatic clearance to a similar extent to orally administered compounds. Thus for highly metabilized drugs intraperitoneal dosage may give rise to lower systemic drug concentrations than intravenous or intramuscular doses and may cause significant underestimation of intrinsic pharmacological activity. Clinically, the intraperitoneal route has been used to administer anticancer agents for tumors with extensive peritoneal involvement.

A novel aspect of intraperitoneal drug delivery has developed recently with the increased use of continuous ambulatory peritoneal dialysis (CAPD) for patients with renal impairment (42, 43). Peritoneal dialysis is intrinsically inefficient compared with hemodialysis, but owing to its continuous nature it works well on a self-administered basis. A major disadvantage of self-administered CAPD, one that may eventually be overcome with more refined techniques, is the frequent occurrence of peritonitis. CAPD-induced peritonitis is often accompanied by systemic infection so that eradication requires therapeutic antibiotic concentrations in both the bloodstream and the peritoneal cavity.

For treatment of CAPD-induced peritonitis, drug may be given orally or by a vascular route to achieve therapeutic plasma concentrations in the hope that sufficient drug will cross the peritoneum to achieve therapeutic levels in the peritoneal cavity. Alternatively, drug may be administered into the peritoneal cavity to obtain therapeutic levels locally, in the hope that sufficient drug will diffuse into the circulation to provide therapeutic systemic levels. Treatment by both these routes is complicated by the fact that drug is lost from the peritoneal cavity during each dialysis exchange. There have been a number of publications addressing the dynamics of peritoneal clearance and drug diffusion between blood and the fluids of the peritoneal cavity. One study has shown that vancomycin rapidly equilibrates across the peritoneum and that previous estimates of peritoneal vancomycin clearance underestimated the true value (44). The study showed that clinically effective concentrations of vancomycin can be achieved in the systemic circulation by administering a suitable loading dose, followed by lower maintenance doses, into the peritoneal cavity (Fig. 4). For example, a 2 g intraperitoneal loading dose of

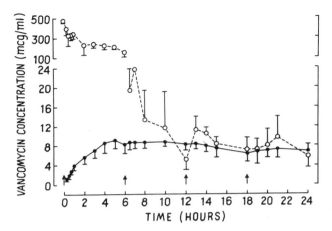

FIGURE 4 Mean (± 1 SD) plasma (●) and dialysate (○) vancomycin
concentrations in five subjects who received an initial intraperitoneal
1 g dose and three subsequent intraperitoneal 50 mg doses of vancomycin at 6 hr intervals. Vertical arrows indicate dialysate exchanges.
(Reproduced by permission from *Antimicrob. Agents Chemother.*,
27: 578–582, 1985.)

vancomycin would achieve plasma drug concentrations of about 16
μg/ml within 3 hr, and this level can be maintained with 50 mg doses
with each 6 hr fresh dialysate exchange. More information is likely
to be generated during the next year or so on drug dosage for CAPD-
associated peritonitis and on drug transport across the peritoneum
under normal and febrile conditions (45).

II. NOVEL DOSAGE ROUTES IN DRUG DISCOVERY,
DEVELOPMENT, AND CLINICAL PRACTICE

Novel dosage routes are defined here on the basis of the activity
associated with novel drug delivery systems and novel uses, rather
than the routes themselves. Current interest in delivery of drugs
by the buccal route, via nasal absorption, inhalation, and by the
transdermal route, has presented many new challenges to the pharmaceutical industry. The following sections do not attempt to provide
an exhaustive review of these subjects but rather to present information and achievements describing some of the more recent approaches
in these areas.

A. Buccal Route

Although the buccal and sublingual region has a surface area of only approximately 200 cm^2, it has high potential for drug absorption in that it provides a moist surface that is richly supplied with blood capillaries and lymphatics (46). A major advantage of buccal or sublingual routes is that absorbed drug passes directly into the circulation. Thus compounds that are subject to first-pass hepatic clearance may exhibit higher systemic bioavailability from buccal or sublingual doses compared with oral doses. This major advantage is offset by several disadvantages, including the problem of taste, inconvenience, and the need to retain the drug formulation in the mouth for prolonged periods. Regardless of these disadvantages, there is currently intense activity in the development of dosage forms for buccal drug delivery, particularly for controlled-release medication.

There is no really suitable animal model for buccal drug release, and it is unlikely that animals can be trained to retain drug delivery devices in the mouth for more than a few minutes. Even if they could, the presence of any device would provoke excessive buccal activity and salivation. Several animal models are used for buccal delivery of new chemical entities, but most of the testing of both conventional and controlled-release buccal formulations of marketed drugs is done in humans.

Apart from the organic nitrates, which are frequently administered by the buccal route and continue to provide a focus of activity for buccal controlled-release delivery, few other compounds have been administered by these routes. Despite this, one can confidently predict that there will be increasing activity in this area in the future. Developers of buccal dosage forms must recognize that drugs absorbed by this route must cross the membranes of the buccal cavity in order to enter systemic circulation. Buccally absorbed drugs are therefore subject to the same, or at least similar, lipophilicity requirements as those of any other route of administration. Some other compounds that have been considered or are being developed for buccal administration include buprenorphine, nifedipine, isoprenaline, isoproterenol, oxytocin, and steroids.

1. Organic Nitrates

Sublingual organic nitrates as capsules, tablets, or sprays are standard therapy for acute treatment of angina pectoris and other cardiac conditions. The small size and rapid membrane penetration of organic nitrates make them ideal for this dosage route. Peak plasma nitrate levels are achieved within minutes of administration,

and first-pass metabolism to less active compounds is avoided.
Organic nitrates currently available for sublingual doses include eryth-
rityl tetranitrate, isosorbide dinitrate, and nitroglycerine. Because
of the difficulty in measuring circulating nitrates, the systemic bioavailability of sublingual or buccal nitrates was until recently unknown
(47). Recent studies in healthy volunteers have shown that bioavailability may be extremely variable. Values in one study ranged
from 2.6 to 113% relative to intravenous infusion, with a mean of 36%
(48). Mean plasma concentrations of glyceryl trinitrate after sublingual
administration of 0.4 mg glyceryl trinitrate are shown in Figure 5 (49).

Development of buccal nitroglycerin for sustained action has com-
peted with transdermal release devices. Currently the transdermal
route appears to have been more successful, but the buccal route
has the advantage that the dosage form does not have to contain the
substantial excess of drug necessary to obtain efficient delivery
from transdermal dosage.

Several examples of controlled-release buccal nitroglycerin have
been described recently. They include Susadrin and Nitrogard (50).
These products incorporate the Synchron controlled-release technology.
Although oral controlled-release nitroglycerin has received both
positive (51) and negative (52) comments regarding its efficacy and
also susceptibility to hepatic clearance, buccal controlled-release
organic nitrates appear to be well accepted from a clinical viewpoint
(53—55).

2. Buprenorphine

Buprenorphine is a highly lipophilic compound, effective as an opiate
analgesic at submilligram doses, and is therefore an ideal candidate
for sublingual (and also topical) administration. Sublingual administration of buprenorphine is effective clinically. Even so it is absorbed
quite slowly, achieving peak levels in plasma at about 3 hr, and is
only 55% bioavailable following 0.4 and 0.8 mg doses (56). Plasma
levels of buprenorphine vary more widely between patients after
sublingual doses than after intramuscular injection (57). Good correlations have been reported between buprenorphine plasma concentrations and sublingual doses ranging from 0.4 to 3.2 mg, but no
correlation was obtained between plasma concentration and relief
of chronic pain (58).

3. Nifedipine

The calcium antagonist nifedipine has been shown to reduce blood
pressure associated with reduced peripheral resistance after sublingual
administration. Repeated 10 mg sublingual doses, four times a day
for 2 days, reduced systolic and diastolic blood pressure by 14% (59).

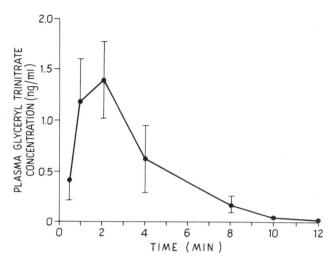

FIGURE 5 Mean (± 1 SD) plasma concentrations of glyceryl tinitrate after sublingual administration of 0.4 mg glyceryl tinitrate in five volunteers. (Reproduced by permission from *J. Cardiovasc. Pharmacol.* 4: 521–525, 1982.)

The antihypertensive action lasted for about 3 hr and was cumulative (Fig. 6). The peripheral dilatation effect of sublingual nifedipine was demonstrated by a 70% increase in forearm blood flow at 60 min after a single 10 mg sublingual dose (60).

4. Isoproterenol

Parenteral or sublingual isoproterenol is indicated for the treatment of bronchospasm. However, recent reports have claimed a dramatic benefit of sublingual isproterenol for long-term treatment of pulmonary artery hypertension. In one case, two patients with a favorable cardiac pulmonary response were maintained on 15 mg isoproterenol every 3-4 hr with marked improvement in pulmonary arteriolar resistance and cardiac index (61). In another case a patient was maintained with dramatic relief of symptoms and improved exercise capacity over a 6-year period (62). In a recent commentary on the remarkable efficacy of sublingual isoproterenol in the treatment of primary pulmonary hypertension. Ackroyd (63) points out that very little isoproterenol is absorbed through the buccal mucosa. Most of the drug is absorbed after being swallowed and is extensively metabolized presystemically. A sublingual dose of 20 mg isoproterenol

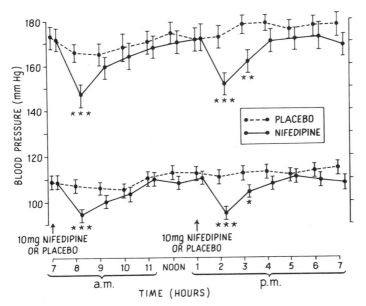

FIGURE 6 Systolic (upper graph) and diastolic (lower graph) pressure in the supine position from 7 am to 7 pm during sublingual placebo and nifedipine treatment (10 mg every 6 hr); *p < 0.05, **p < 0.01, ***p < 0.001. (Reproduced by permission from *Eur. J. Clin. Pharmacol.* 17: 161–164, 1980.)

caused a reduction in pulmonary artery pressure similar to that achieved by infusion of 3 μg/min into the pulmonary artery (64). The mechanism underlying the remarkable efficacy of sublingual isoproterenol in certain patients is not known. To the writer's knowledge, controlled sublingual dosage forms of isoproterenol for this type of condition have not been described.

5. Lormetrazepam

A sublingual dosage form of "sleeping wafer" has been described to deliver 1 mg doses of lormetrazepam (65). Drug is formulated as a solid solution in cellulose and a soluble cellulose derivative, packaged in a cellulose carrier. When placed under the tongue the formulation dissolved readily and completely. Lormetrazepam absorption rates after sublingual and oral administration are shown in Figure 7. It is claimed that faster release from the sublingual form should reduce the sleep latency observed with oral lormetrazepam. Clinical trials are ongoing.

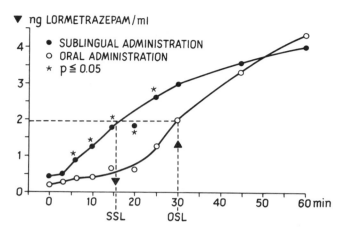

FIGURE 7 Mean lormetrazepam plasma levels after sublingual (●) and oral (○) administration of 1 mg lormetrazepam to 16 subjects. SSL = sublingual sleep latency; OSL = oral sleep latency. *p < 0.05. (Reproduced by permission from *Drug Dev. Ind. Pharm.* 10: 1587–1596, 1984.)

6. Peptides and Steroids

Oxytocin is the only peptide currently marketed in a sublingual form. It is used for induction or stimulation of labor, tablets being placed in alternte cheek pouches every 30 min until a dosage is found that produces the desired response. Absorption from the buccal cavity is probably inefficient as the buccal dose, 200–400 units, is about 100 times greater than intravenous or intramuscular doses. Swallowing the buccal tablets does not harm the patient because oxytocin is digested in the gastrointestinal tract. In a review of 50 cases in which buccal oxytocin was used, Miller (66) reported that the method was successful in 42 patients and the time required for effect was less than 7 hr.

Sublingual administration of steroids has not been examined extensively. 17β-Estradiol (E_2) for treatment of postmenopausal symptoms is readily absorbed sublingually. A 0.5 mg sublingual tablet gave rise to serum levels equivalent to those following a 2 mg oral dose of micronized E_2 (67, 68). However, serum levels of E_2 are transient and are followed by more prolonged levels of estrone (E_1). Serum levels of E_1 and E_2 and changes in serum follicle stimulating hormone (FSH) and lutenizing hormone (LH) following a single 0.5 mg sublingual dose of E_2 are shown in Figure 8 (68). Sublingual E_2 thus

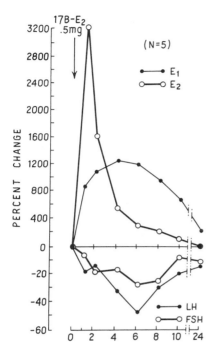

FIGURE 8 Relative changes in serum estrogen and gonadotropin
concentrations after sublingual administration of a single half-tablet
containing 0.5 mg of micronized 17β-estradiol. (Reproduced by permission from *Am. J. Obstet. Gynecol.* 140: 146–149, 1981.)

differs from vaginal administration which, for reasons yet to be explained, appears not to give rise to such extensive E_2-E_1 conversion.
Sublingual norethisterone has been shown to be significantly more
bioavailable compared with orally administered drug in monkeys (69).

B. Intranasal Route

Intranasal administration may be used for local or systemic effects.
Local effects are achieved with corticosteroids, antihistamines, and
other agents for such conditions as nasal allergy, rhinitis, and nasal
polyposis (70–73) and nasal decongestion (74). The mode of action
of corticosteroids in nasal allergy appears to be associated with
inhibition of basophilic cell accumulation in the mucosal surface (75).

The use of intranasal delivery for systemic effects is less well established but is currently the focus of considerable activity. This has been prompted by scattered reports of efficient drug absorption by this route, predominantly in animal models. These have been regarded as particularly promising for small peptide molecules that are inefficiently absorbed orally.

Despite the high interest in this area, no novel intranasal compounds have been successfully developed for systemic activity during the last several years, and existing marketed forms are restricted to vasopressin analogs and oxytocin. Cocaine is taken illicitly by the nasal route for its euphoric effect. The systemic availability of intranasal cocaine may be no greater and may also be no faster than after oral administration (76). Perhaps the rapid "high" after nasal dosing is related to particular circulatory pathways connecting the nasopharynx, sinus, and brain (77).

In considering why development of the nasal route for systemic drug effects has been relatively unsuccessful compared with buccal and transdermal routes, it is useful to consider the anatomy and physiology of the absorbing surfaces that are being exploited. The lateral wall of the nasal cavity, shown in Figure 9 (78), consists of several discreet anatomic and functional regions. Region A in the figure is the skin of the nasal vestibule, B is the region of squamous epithelium without microvilli, C is the transitional epithelium with short variable microvilli, D is stratified epithelium with some ciliated cells, and E is pseudostratified epithelium with many ciliated cells. The olfactory region is shaded in the figure.

The major function of these upper airways is to protect the delicate tissues of the lung from toxic and infectious agents in the inspired air. In addition to filtration, the nose also acts as a humidifier and heat exchanger (79). Air is moistened, filtered, and warmed during inspiration, and moisture and heat are conserved. The innervation of the nose is concerned primarily with regulation of nasal blood flow and secretions to enable it to perform its protective function. The mechanisms of the nose are exquisitely developed so that inspired or expired air can be handled, and the lungs protected in arctic or desert environments.

The sophisticated structure and finely balanced and specialized function of the airways and membranes associated with the nasal cavity and the limited surface area of this region raise questions, at least in the writer's mind, as to the capacity of this region for drug delivery and also the ability of these structures to withstand the insult of chronic drug exposure. Although research in this area continues, evidence is gathering that local toxicity may be the major limiting factor in intranasal drug delivery, particularly in view of the apparent need for addition of surfactants to assist drug absorption

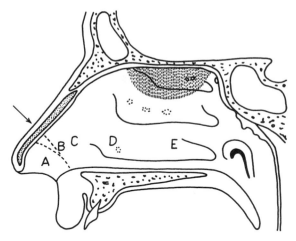

FIGURE 9 Lateral wall of the nasal cavity with the olfactory region
(hatched area). The arrow indicates the internal ostium. The different
types of epithelial cells are A, skin in nostril; B, squamous epithelium
without microvilli; C, transitional epithelium with short microvilli of
varying length; D, pseudostratified columnar epithelium with few
ciliated cells; and E, pseudostratifed columnar epithelium with many
ciliated cells. (Adapted by permission from *The Nose, Upper Airway
Physiology and the Atmospheric Environment,* Elsevier Biomedical
Press, New York, 1982, p. 72.)

by this route for systemic activity. Any advantage obtained by
systemic absorption and avoidance of presystemic clearance may be
offset by local toxicity.

1. Intranasal Dosage Forms

Given these qualifications, the physicochemical characteristics for
optimal intranasal drug absorption appear to be similar to those for
any other absorption route. The drug must be sufficiently water
soluble to be administered as a solution or to dissolve rapidly in the
fluids of the nasal mucosa and also must be sufficiently fat soluble
to penetrate the lipid membranes of the nasal epithelial cells. Nasal
absorption is facilitated by the high permeability of the small venules
and capillaries associated with the nasal mucosa (80).

A drug may be delivered to the nasal mucosa in the form of a
solution, formulated as drops or in a nebulized spray, or as an
aerosol. With nebulized sprays or particulate aerosols, the optimal
particle size for nasal deposition is 5–10 μm. Smaller particles do

not deposit as readily in the nasal mucosa but are deposited farther down the bronchial tree. A number of methods are available to determine particle size distribution in aerosol systems (81). A variety of devices continue to be described for accurate delivery of metered drug doses from aerosols and nebulizers (81–83).

2. Animal Models

The principal animal models used for intranasal drug delivery, apart from the human, are the rat and the monkey. In situ and in vivo rat models have been described (81, 84). These models appear to be useful to study nasal absorption from solutions, but not from aerosols. The latter have proven more difficult for two major reasons. The first is that it is not possible to train an experimental animal to sniff from a dispenser; the second is the natural reluctance of product development personnel to develop sophisticated aerosol delivery devices for animal testing at an early stage in drug development. A number of experiments in monkeys have utilized sprays (85, 86).

3. Compounds Administrated Intranasally

Nasal absorption has been examined for a wide variety of compounds, usually with limited success. Compounds examined include cardiovascular drugs, antimicrobials, anterior and posterior pituitary hormones, gonadotropin releasing hormones, adrenal and sex hormones, insulin, autonomic agents, CNS agents, prostaglandins, antihistamines, diagnostic agents, and inorganic salts. All these studies have recently been reviewed (87).

4. Peptides

There has been considerable interest in intranasal peptides and steroid hormones, as nasal absorption could present a substantial breakthrough in their systemic availability. These warrant further comment.

The peptides represent a major area of success in intranasal drug delivery. Vasopressin, desmopressin, and oxytocin are commercially available as nasal sprays. Other compounds being actively investigated include thyrotropin-releasing hormone (TRH), other vasopressin analogs, luteinizing hormone releasing hormone (LHRH) agonists and antagonists, adrenocorticotropic hormone (ACTH), and growth hormone releasing factor (GRF) (88). Intranasal administration of the immunomodulators *nor*-muramyl dipetide and muramyl tripeptide phosphatidylethanolamine has been examined in mice (77). Intranasal doses resulted in accumulation of both compounds in the brain compared with intravenous administration.

Intranasal interferon has been examined principally for local treatment of rhinovirus. Although efficacy is reported (89, 90), such side effects as bleeding, nasal discharge, and superficial lesions were observed after long-term treatment (91, 92). Prolonged intranasal treatment appears not to be feasible for prophylaxis of respiratory viral infection, at least not at the doses used in these studies. The new LHRH agonist buserelin is effective for treatment of endometriosis after prolonged intranasal administration of 100-400 μg/day (93) and may be an effective contraceptive at intranasal doses of 400-600 μg/day (94). Intranasal doses were apparently well tolerated.

5. *Insulin*

The intriguing possibility of administering insulin intranasally, rather than by injection, has prompted considerable activity in this area, with variable results. A number of studies have demonstrated hypoglycemic activity with intranasal insulin, but with relatively low efficacy. By addition of surfactants a hypoglycemic effect can be achieved that is approximately 1/10 that from an intravenous dose (95—97). Among the surfactants, bile salts, such as sodium deoxycholate (98), Carbopol 934 (99), and polyoxyethylene-9-laurylether (Laureth 9) (100), appear to be promising. Even so, this route of administration is considered only as an adjunct to injectable insulin, and there is little information on long-term toxicity.

6. *Steroids*

Intranasal studies with sex hormones in experimental animals have produced some interesting results. The bioavailability of intranasal testosterone in a rat model was 99 and 90% from 25 and 50 μg doses, respectively, compared with intravenous doses. Intraduodenal bio-availability was only 1% (101). Mean blood testosterone concentrations from the three dosage routes examined in this study are shown in Figure 10. In the same rat model, progesterone was also shown to be quantitatively absorbed compared with intravenous drug, with intraduodenal administration again yielding very poor absorption (102). However, in a monkey model, the bioavailability of intranasal progesterone when given as a spray or drops was significantly higher compared with intravenous or intramuscular doses (103, 104). Possible mechanisms are proposed, but it is unclear why intranasal progesterone would yield superior bioavailability to parenterally administered compound, particularly in view of the extensive metabolism of proges-terone in the nasal mucosa (105).

A number of studies have attested to the potency of intranasal estrogens to inhibit spermatogenesis, and this may be related to higher brain concentrations intranasally compared with other routes

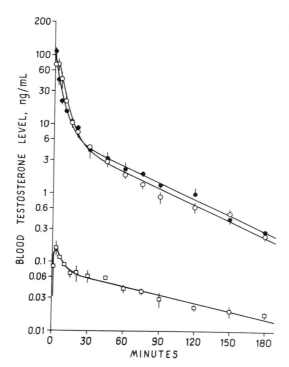

FIGURE 10 Mean (± SE) blood concentrations of testosterone in rats
following nasal (○), intravenous (●), and intraduodenal (□) administration of 25 μg testosterone per rat. (Reproduced by permission
from *J. Pharm. Sci.* 73: 1300–1301, 1984.)

(106). Other studies suggest, however, that high CSF concentrations
may be a function of the animal model. High brain levels of estradiol
relative to plasma levels were obtained after intranasal administration
in one monkey model (107) but not in another (108).

C. Inhalation

Inhalation, as with intranasal administration, is used predominantly
for local effect. Compounds administered by inhalation are intended
to treat asthma and other types of airway obstruction. During the
last 10 years, understanding of the difficulties associated with
aerosol drug delivery has increased and devices have been described
to improve drug delivery by this route. It is interesting that the
lung offers a potential absorption service of 72 m^2, a much larger

surface than the small intestine, and yet the lungs and associated airways are designed to deny access of administered compounds to this highly efficient absorption region. The respiratory system is designed to keep out particulate matter, and it does this very well. When compounds reach the central or peripheral regions of the lungs, absorption can be very efficient. This has been demonstrated repeatedly by toxic systemic effects from inhaled substances, such as β_2-adrenergic agents and corticosteroids.

1. Respiratory Tract

The human respiratory tract is shown diagrammatically in Figure 11. The objective of inhalation therapy is to reach that region of the respiratory tract where the drug may exert its maximum effect. The main problem lies in the uncertainty as to where that site is. Most proponents of inhalation drug delivery aim to achieve maximum drug penetration into peripheral lung airspaces, but the site for bronchodilatation is probably much higher in the airways of the tracheobronchial tree.

2. Anatomy and Physiology

The respiratory system consists of the upper respiratory tract (nose, nasal passages, sinuses, mouth, and larynx) and lower respiratory tract (tracheobronchial tree down to the pulmonary alveoli) (109, 110). Although the diameter of the airways decreases from about 2—3 cm in the pharynx to only 0.015 cm in the alveoli, airflow also decreases from 50—100 cm/sec in the pharynx to only 0.003 cm/sec in the alveoli. This is due to the huge increase in overall airway diameter in the alveolar region (109).

The degree to which inhaled substances penetrate into airway spaces is controlled by a number of factors, the major ones being particle size and velocity. It seems that the optimum particle size for airway penetration is 3—5 µm. Particles of larger size tend to be deposited in the upper respiratory tract by inertial impaction. Particles less than 2 µm tend not to deposit as effectively as larger particles, but there is some disagreement on this. The deposition of 3—5 µm particles in the lower respiratory tract is primarily by sedimentation (111—114). Drug deposition may also be influenced by individual variability in lung anatomy (115) and respiratory disease (116).

Three major mechanisms exist to remove particulate material, including undissolved drug, from the respiratory tract. A variety of ciliated cells line the trachea and bronchial tree. The motion of the cilia, together with the viscous mucous blanket lining the surface of the larger airways, constitutes an effective mechanism to remove

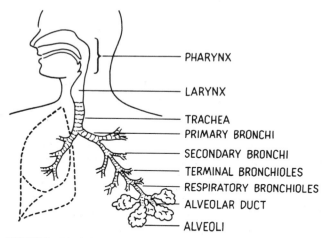

PHARYNX

LARYNX

TRACHEA
PRIMARY BRONCHI

SECONDARY BRONCHI

TERMINAL BRONCHIOLES

RESPIRATORY BRONCHIOLES

ALVEOLAR DUCT

ALVEOLI

FIGURE 11 The human respiratory tract. (Reproduced by permission from *Pharmacokinetics. Processes and Mathematics*. ACS Monograph 1986, pp. 7–19.)

particles from the airways toward the mouth or nose. The other major mechanisms are coughing and scavenging by alveolar macrophages (117, 118). Mucociliary clearance may be markedly affected by inhaled drugs, being increased by bromhexine, aminophylline, and predniso-lone and decreased by scopolamine. The commonly used β_2-adrenergic agents seem to have little effect (119).

Absorption from the lung appears to obey the same rules as that from the gastrointestinal tract. Absorption is related to lipophilicity, and there is little evidence of a specialized transport system (120). The lung permeability of hydrophilic substances in rabbits was shown to decrease as the animals matured (121).

Systemic absorption of inhaled compounds may be inhibited by first-pass pulmonary metabolism. The lungs contain a variety of drug-metabolizing enzymes of similar type, but in different proportions, to those present in liver (122, 123). These include microsomal mixed function and other oxidases, amine oxidase, monoamine oxidase, reductases, esterases, and a variety of conjugases. The activity of the primary defense mechanisms, the geometry of the bronchial tree, mucociliary activity, macrophage activity, and pulmonary metabolism combine to prevent access of drug to the peripheral pulmonary absorption sites, and systemic absorption. This has presented a sig-nificant obstacle to the development of effective inhalation dosages for both local and systemic activity.

3. Animal Models

A variety of animal models has been used to study drug inhalation.
These include the rat, rabbit (120) and dog (124, 125). In dog studies,
rapid systemic absorption of the lipophilic molecule fluorescein anion
was obtained after aerosol and intratracheal administration (125).
Inhaled drug as liquid aerosols was absorbed more rapidly than when
administered by intratracheal injection in rats (126).

4. Inhalation Delivery Systems

Several studies have confirmed that drug delivery devices for inhalation
deliver approximately 10% of the dose to the lower respiratory tract,
the balance being absorbed from the buccal cavity or swallowed
(127). For particles with mass median aerodynamic diameters of 2.7–
3.5 μm, less than 1% of the inhaled dose is lost in expired air (128).
Teflon particles labeled with $^{99}Tc^m$ have been used to demonstrate
changes in deposition with particle size (129) and also to show that,
of the 10% of an administered aerosol dose that penetrates the airways,
approximately two-thirds deposit in the conducting airways and only
one-third reaches the alveoli (130).

There have been several attempts to increase drug delivery to
peripheral pulmonary vessels. Newman et al. (131) achieved a maximum
effect with slow inhalation at 20% vital capacity and holding the breath
for 10 sec. The importance of monodisperse systems of optimal particle
size has long been recognized (132, 133), and delivery devices have
been devised to achieve optimal particle size distribution.

Pressurized metered-dose inhalers (MDI) have largely replaced
such early devices as the Spinhaler (134, 135). Even so, drug
delivery to the lung from MDI is inefficient, and a large number of
spacer devices have been proposed to improve delivery (136–140).
With one such device, which incorporated a spacer with a one-way
inhalation valve, 21% of the metered dose reached the lungs, and
only 16% was deposited in the oropharynx (141); 56% of the dose
was retained in the spacer. Lung deposition was thus increased while
oropharyngeal deposition was greatly reduced. The use of spacer
devices, together with patient education in the use of these and
other inhalation delivery systems, may improve the efficacy and
reliability of aerosol therapy (142–145). Arborelius (146) has described
a technique whereby the size of inhaled particles increases owing
to hygroscopic effects, promoting deposition in peripheral regions
of the lung.

Despite these advances, drug delivery to the lung is still very
inefficient. The following section briefly reviews the major compounds
administered by this route.

5. β₂-Adrenergic Agonists

β_2-Adrenergic agonists are playing an increasing role in the treatment of asthma and other obstructive airway diseases. They are administered by inhalation for local effect by modulating contraction and relaxation of bronchial smooth muscle. This is achieved through activation of adenyl cyclase to increase intracellular cyclic adenosine monophosphate (AMP). Increased concentrations of cyclic AMP inhibit smooth muscle contraction and facilitate relaxation by augmenting sequestration of calcium. The early β_2 agonists ephedrine and isoproterenol have a short duration of action. More recent compounds, albuterol, terbutaline, and fenoterol, have a longer duration of action and can be dosed less frequently (147—150).

6. Terbutaline

Terbutaline is used for the treatment of asthma, and its pharmacokinetics have been characterized, at least in part, in adults (151) and children (152). Some controversy exists as to the best dosage route for terbutaline. Earlier studies suggested that oral terbutaline had a greater effect on lung peripheral airways than inhaled terbutaline, and thus predosing with oral terbutaline may amplify the effect of inhalation treatment (153). More recent studies showed that inhaled terbutaline had a greater initial effect than oral drug, but there was no significant difference in the response to subsequently inhaled terbutaline (154). Pulmonary function tests, together with radioaerosol imaging, showed that terbutaline in particular, and perhaps bronchodilators in general, have a substantial relaxation effect on tracheobronchial smooth muscle in central airways and also that subcutaneous terbutaline is more effective than inhaled drug in dilating peripheral airways (155). Response to inhaled terbutaline sulfate was greatest from particle sizes less than 5 μm compared with larger sizes (156), but pulmonary absorption of terbutaline sulfate varied between 0.8 and 10.1% of the 1000 μg (4 × 250 μg) metered dose in healthy subjects (157). Studies using isocapnic hyperventilation suggest that inhalation doses greater than 1000 μg may be effective in exercise-induced asthma, but systemic side effects may be dose limiting (158).

A number of studies have recently examined ways to improve the delivery of terbutaline from nebulizers (159, 160) and metered dose aerosols (161—163), particularly the use of spacer devices. Marked improvements in forced expiratory volume (FEV_1) and forced vital capacity (FVC_1) by the use of tube extensions are shown in Figures 12 and 13.

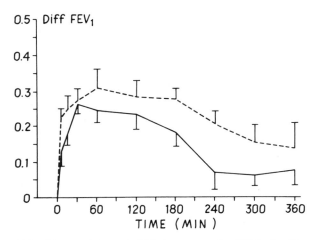

FIGURE 12 Mean (±SE) increase in FEV₁ in 12 patients who received 0.25 mg terbutaline sulfate aerosol inhaled via tube extension (---) and via ordinary actuator (—). (Reproduced by permission from *Eur. J. Clin. Pharmacol.* 20: 109—111, 1981.)

7. Metaproterenol

Metaproterenol is available as oral tablets, the usual adult dose being 20 mg three or four times daily, and as an inhalation, each puff delivering 0.65 mg. The dose response to inhaled metaproterenol is not well characterized, and a number of recent studies have addressed this issue. Problems associated with the use of sequential inhalation for dose-response determination were addressed by Heimer et al. (161), who showed that FEV₁ increased with subsequent doses of metaproterenol given at 10 min intervals. This is presumably the result of better penetration by aerosol into airways partially dilated by preceding treatments. Although this observation precludes dose-response determination by sequential dosing, it suggests improved therapeutic response by this dosage regimen. Other studies have described dose response to metaproterenol in asthma patients after bronchoprovocation with methacholine (162). The former study was used to explain why a treatment schedule may fail with increasing thermal burden or task severity. Task severity is claimed to have advantages over other bronchodilator response tests in that it measures nonspecific airway response and may thus relate more to clinical asthmatic situations.

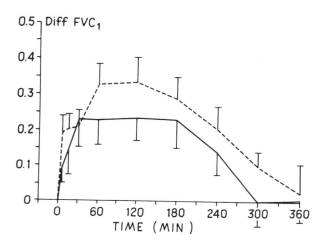

FIGURE 13 Mean (± SE) increase in FVC_1 in 12 patients who received 0.25 mg terbutaline sulfate aerosol inhaled via tube extension ($---$) and via ordinary actuator ($—$). (Reproduced by permission from *Eur. J. Clin. Pharmacol.* 20: 109–111, 1982.)

8. Albuterol

As with metaproterenol, there has been considerable interest in the dose-response characteristics of inhaled albuterol (salbutamol). In normal subjects, maximal bronchodilatation was achieved with a cumulative dose of 110 μg with a mean ED_{50} of 23 μg (163). In asthmatic patients, maximum effect was achieved with much higher doses ranging from 110 to 3210 μg, with a mean ED_{50} of 83 μg. Although these results were obtained with sequential doses at 15 min intervals, the carryover effect was apparently not sufficient to improve airway penetration in asthmatics. Alternatively, the disease process itself may have contributed. The need for high doses of albuterol, and doubtless other β_2 agonists, to treat severe asthma was confirmed in another study in which increasing responses were obtained from metered inhaled doses ranging from 86 to 688 μg and from nebulized doses ranging from 1.25 to 15 mg (164). Both data sets suggest that a greater response would have been obtained at even higher doses but systemic side effects may become dose limiting.

The possibility of selective sensitization of receptors in central airways to albuterol is suggested in a study showing reduced airway response in asthmatics following doses of 200 μg four times a day (165). This was more evident for specific airway conductance (SG_{aw})

than for maximum expiratory flow rate $MEF_{40\%(P)}$. Impaired SG_{aw} responses in this study contrast with previous results in which no subsensitization was obtained in asthmatics with an oral β_2 agonist (166). This discrepancy may be related to excessive deposition of inhaled drug in the central airways.

One study has claimed that between 61 and 89% of doses ranging from 119 to 359 μg [^{3}H]albuterol was inhaled (167). This value was obtained by subtracting mouth washings from the inhaled dose, and some of the dose may have been swallowed. Plasma levels and urinary excretion of radioactivity were dose related. Almost identical FEV_1 response values were obtained in asthmatics when albuterol was administered as a powder aerosol (0.2–4.8 mg) and a pressurized aerosol (0.1–2.4 mg) (168). It is suggested that the powder aerosol may be a useful alternative to the MDI for patients with poor inhalation techniques.

9. Fenoterol

A number of studies have attested to the efficacy of fenoterol for treatment of asthma (169–171), although the dose-response relationship is not well defined and the duration of bronchodilation effect is less than that of metaproterenol (169). Fenoterol is given orally as well as by inhalation, but systemic effects, as expected, are lower by inhalation. Dirksen (172) compared fenoterol activity when administered from a conventional MDI and an MDI with a spacer device (aerochamber) and found no significant difference between the two delivery systems.

Buccal (with no inhalation) administration of fenoterol effectively induced bronchodilatation in normal and asthmatic subjects, but to a lesser extent than inhalation (173). In a comparative study, fenoterol aerosol had a similar bronchodilator effect to albuterol, although fenoterol increased heart rate to a greater extent (174). Fenoterol had a greater inhibitory effect than albuterol on induced broncho-constriction from exercise-induced asthma (175). Fenoterol aerosol appeared to be at least as, if not more, effective than combined fenoterol and ipratropium, and also clenbuterol in exercise-induced bronchospasm in children (176).

10. Bitolterol

Bitolterol differs from the other β_2 agonists in that it is a prodrug. The compound is administered as the intact 3,4-diester that is then hydrolyzed by esterases to the active catecholamine N-t-butylarterenol (colterol), as shown in Figure 14 (177). This results in prolonged activity due to gradual hydrolysis of the administered substance to the active catecholamine. Comparative studies have shown bitolterol

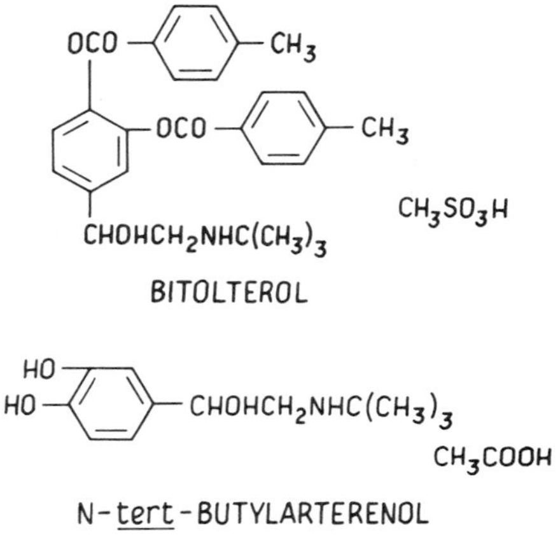

BITOLTEROL

N-<u>tert</u>-BUTYLARTERENOL

FIGURE 14 Chemical structures of bitolterol mesylate and *N-t*-butyl-arterenol. (Reproduced by permission from *Chest* 78: 283—287, 1980.)

to produce a greater and more prolonged response compared with isoproterenol in chronic obstructive pulmonary disease patients (178), and compared with albuterol in asthmatic patients (179).

11. Disodium Cromoglycate (DSG)

DSG has no intrinsic bronchodilator activity but exerts its effect by stabilizing the membrane of mast cells, preventing degranulation (180). The original dosage form for inhaled DSG was the Spinhaler (134, 135), but this is now replaced by the MDI. A number of studies have concluded in favor of one dosage form or the other (181—185). Some favor the MDI (182—184), others favor the powder (181), and other results are equivocal (185). Comparisons are difficult because of the wide disparity of dosage from the powder (20 mg) and the MDI (2 mg). Other studies have shown that oral DSG is ineffective against asthma (186), the inhaled substance presumably acting locally on mast cells in the bronchial lumen, and that the effect of aerosolized DSG on exercise-induced asthma is related to doses between 2 and 20 μg (187). This last result is in contrast to a previous study that failed to show dose-related protection with DSG aerosol against bronchoconstriction induced by airway cooling (188). The different results may be related to the methods of provoking bronchoconstriction (187).

12. Beclomethasone

After several years of use in other countries, beclomethasone dipropionate was approved for treatment of asthma in the United States in 1976. Beclomethasone administered as a topical aerosol causes symptomatic and functional benefit in asthma with reduced systemic effects compared with those of oral steroids (189). Despite some controversy, the efficacy of aerosol beclomethasone appears to be clearly dose related, particularly in severe asthmatics (190, 191). Currently, the largest daily recommended dose is 1 mg. It is used either alone or as a supplement to oral steroids (192—194).

The use of inhaled beclomethasone for the local treatment of severe asthma is not without its disadvantages. Oropharyngeal candidiasis and other fungal infections frequently accompany long-term therapy (195). Also, beclomethasone is well absorbed orally and much of the inhaled dose is doubtless swallowed. Side effects similar to those associated with oral corticosteroids, such as decreased eosinophil count and plasma cortisol levels, may be experienced. Adrenal function must be carefully monitored during transfer from oral corticosteroid therapy to aerosol beclomethasone (189). Frequent dosing of beclomethasone and other inhaled corticosteroids may increase their benefit-risk ratio (196). The C-21 ester corticoid fluocortin butyl is reported to have less systemic effect on adrenal function after inhalation than beclomethasone (197).

13. Atropine

Atropine is used in the clinical environment to increase airflow in chronic bronchitis, perennial childhood asthma, and cystic fibrosis (198, 199). A clear dose-response relationship for inhaled atropine sulfate has been established, but high doses are limited by systemic side effects (199). Inhaled atropine appears to be remarkably well absorbed into the bloodstream (200). Following 1 mg every 4 hr or every 6 hr dosing for a minimum of 48 hr, serum atropine levels were highly variable between subjects but exceeded 2 ng/ml in 2 of 11 subjects and reached 5.23 ng/ml in 1 subject.

In summary, despite considerable technical advances during the last decade, delivery of inhaled drugs to the lungs is still very inefficient. Most of the administered compound is deposited in the delivery vessel and wasted, deposited in the mouth and swallowed or perhaps absorbed buccally, or deposited in the upper respiratory tract and removed by mucociliary or other activity. More data are needed to characterize the deposition sites of inhaled drugs and their sites of action. Once compounds penetrate into central or peripheral air vessels they may be absorbed very efficiently, giving rise to systemic effects. With compounds currently administered by this

route, the systemic effects are for the most part undesirable and may
be dose limiting. Despite excellent absorption from the lungs, the
inability to deliver drugs to the optimal site and the intrinsic clearance
and metabolic defense mechanisms may preclude the use of this dosage
route for most systemically acting compounds.

D. Transdermal Drug Delivery

Since the introduction of transdermal scopolamine (201) there has
been intense interest in transdermal drug delivery for systemic effects.
The major advantages claimed for transdermal systems are based on
constant release of drug to the systemic circulation, reduced presystemic clearance, facile drug withdrawal by removing the delivery
device, and patient convenience and compliance. The major disadvantages
for transdermal systems—and these may effectively limit this delivery
route to a small drug population—are related to the barrier properties
of the skin and dose size. Skin has excellent barrier characteristics
and effectively inhibits the penetration of all but a small range of
lipophilic molecules. Even for molecules with the appropriate physicochemical characteristics, absorption through the skin is not very
efficient and there are frequent problems associated with local irritation
and toxicity. Transdermal delivery for systemic effects is a realistic
option only for drugs that are given in small doses ($\leqslant 10$ mg) and
that have optimum membrane penetration qualities. Four drugs are
currently approved in the United States for transdermal delivery:
clonidine, estradiol, nitroglycerin, and scopolamine. Many other
drugs are being examined. Many of these will probably fail, but
there are always the exceptions.

1. Skin

The anatomy, physiology, and biochemistry of the skin have been
extensively characterized (202, 203). The structure of skin is shown
schematically in Figure 15 (203). In order to reach the systemic
circulation, a drug must pass through the lipophilic stratum corneum
and also the more hydrophilic epidermis. Thus in order to be transdermally effective a drug must possess a balance of hydrophobic
and hydrophilic properties. For compounds with molecular weights
less than 600 daltons, absorption is controlled predominantly by
solubility. Absorption of larger molecules is limited primarily by their
bulk. Although transdermal delivery is often claimed to bypass presystemic metabolism, a large number of drug-metabolizing enzyme
systems are present in skin (203). These can carry out both Phase 1
and Phase 2 reactions. Although these enzymes systems may represent
a barrier to transdermal drug absorption, they may also be useful
in converting lipophilic prodrugs to active compounds during transdermal passage (204–206).

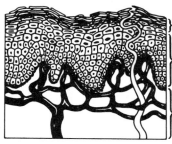

STRATEM CORNEUM

VIABLE EPIDERMIS

DERMIS (CONTAINS MICROVASCULATURE)

FIGURE 15 Skin structure (schematic). (Reproduced by permission from *J. Controlled Release* 4: 237–251, 1987.)

2. Absorption Models

In vitro systems are traditionally used as primary screens to test transdermal drug absorption (207, 208). These systems generally use human cadaver skin, hairless mouse or rat skin, or synthetic membranes. These systems may provide useful preliminary data, but they are notoriously unpredictable for in vivo absorption. In vivo animal models are more predictive of human absorption. Many species have been used, including the rabbit, monkey, dog, guinea pig, miniature pig, and rat. Of these the miniature pig is probably the most predictive.

3. Factors Affecting Transdermal Drug Delivery

Attempts to improve the bioavailability of transdermally administered compounds have generated a great number of delivery devices and delivery promoters. The main objective of the devices is to maintain intimate contact between the drug delivery surface and skin in an occluded environment and to deliver drug in a continuous fashion. The objective of the delivery promoters is to change the skin environment to facilitate drug passage, stopping short of solubilizing the skin. There is a tremendous literature on this subject, and much of the material has been described in recent reviews (202, 209–211). Azone (1-dodecylazacycloheptan-2-one) is a typical promoter that increases the absorption of both hydrophilic and, to a lesser extent, hydrophobic compounds (212, 213). Many other enhancers are being developed and tested. Liposomes have been examined to increase transdermal drug absorption (214, 215). Results of in vitro studies show that absorption of some lipophilic drugs is increased from liposome vehicles. The liposomes themselves do not diffuse across skin (214).

The two major types of transdermal drug delivery systems are shown in Figure 16 and 17 (203). The membrane-modulated system, as the name suggests, consists of a drug reservoir enclosed within an impermeable membrane, with a polymeric membrane on one side controlling drug transport from the reservoir to the skin via an adhesive layer. In the matrix device, drug is dispersed throughout a polymeric matrix, and transport through the matrix is intended to control release of drug to the skin. Despite the different mechanisms of drug release in these types of devices, and variations of these, the kinetics of drug release are similar. Penetration through the skin is often rate limiting (216). Much of the development of transdermal delivery systems is still empirical, and there is a need for a more systematic approach to their design and greater appreciation of the complexity of the systems (217). In this respect, a number of recent articles have addressed the evaluation of intrinsic diffusivity for membrane-controlled release (218), the pharmacokinetics of drug release from transdermal systems (219–222), kinetics associated with removal and reapplication of transdermal patches (223), and the pharmacokinetics of transdermal drug delivery to neonates (224). The last article focuses on the very high permeability of neonatal skin, facilitating transdermal drug absorption in this population. Some compounds currently administered transdermally, and others under investigation, are summarized in the next section.

4. Nitroglycerin

Nitroglycerin was early recognized as an ideal candidate for transdermal delivery owing to its physical properties, low dose, and poor oral systemic bioavailability. A number of transdermal systems are available (203, 225–227). Commercial formulations, which include both matrix and membrane-modulated systems, are Deponit-TTS, Nitrodisc, and Nitro-Dur (matrix systems) and Transderm-Nitro (membrane). All these devices give similar nitroglycerin plasma profiles (203). Most preparations claim a 24 hr duration of effect. Onset of action is generally 30 min after application, and effects continue for about 30 min after removal. Several studies have addressed the mechanisms of nitroglycerin relief from transdermal systems (228, 229) and the kinetics of transdermal nitroglycerin delivery (230–232).

Despite the popularity of transdermal nitroglycerin, questions regarding the possible development of tolerance to continuous drug exposure with these types of dosage forms for prophylaxis against angina are unresolved (233, 234). Similar concerns have been expressed for the closely related compound isosorbide dinitrate (235). Topical nitroglycerin has been associated with contact dermatitis (236), as have the transdermal dosage forms of a number of other compounds (237).

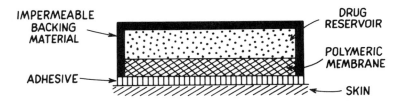

FIGURE 16 Diagram of a membrane-moderated transdermal drug delivery system. (Reproduced by permission from *J. Controlled Release* 4: 237–251, 1987.)

5. Scopolamine

Scopolamine was the first drug to be successfully administered transdermally, for the treatment of motion sickness. A membrane-controlled system is used to provide initial fast release of drug from the adhesive, followed by controlled zero-order release at a rate of 3.8 μg/cm^2 hr for 3 days (203). Scopolamine excretion patterns following transdermal

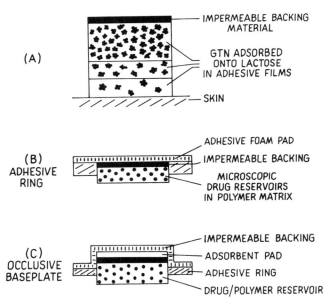

FIGURE 17 Diagrams of matrix-type transdermal nitroglycerin delivery systems: (A) Deponit-TTS, (B) Nitrodisc, (C) Nitro-Dur (Reproduced by permission from *J. Controlled Release* 4: 237–251, 1987.)

and intravenous infusion are shown in Figure 18 (201), which demonstrates rapid release of the scopolamine loading dose during the 12—14 hr after transdermal application. A number of studies have demonstrated the efficacy of transdermal scopolamine for motion sickness (238, 239).

6. Clonidine

The low oral therapeutic dose of this β-adrenergic antihypertensive agent, 0.1 mg twice a day, made it an excellent candidate for transdermal dosage. Devices with surface areas of 2.5—10.5 cm2 have achieved plasma concentrations of 0.6—1.2 ng/ml with release rates between 1.5 and 2.0 μg/cm2 per hr (240, 241). The efficacy of transdermal clonidine has been shown to be equivalent to conventional orla doses (242). Skin reactions, including irritation and sensitization, have been reported with transdermal clonidine (241).

7. Estradiol

Transdermal estradiol is intended for treatment of menopausal symptoms. Its efficacy at delivery rates of 0.025—0.1 mg/day (243) is equivalent to 20- 40-fold higher oral doses (244, 245). A membrane-controlled device, Estraderm, was recently shown to yield dose-related serum estradiol levels, as shown in Figure 19 (246). Another series of studies has examined simultaneous skin permeation and metabolism of lipophilic estradiol esters to estradiol (247, 248). This is an excellent example of the use of lipophilic prodrugs to enhance the transdermal delivery of active species. Other studies have examined the use of ester prodrugs to increase skin permeability of hydrocortisone (249) and complexation with γ-cyclodextrin to enhance percutaneous absorption of beclomethasone dipropionate (250).

8. β-Adrenergic Antagonists

The success achieved with transdermal delivery of the cardiovascular agents nitroglycerin and clonidine has prompted interest in other cardiovascular agents, particularly the β-adrenergic blocking agents. Initial results are promising. Timolol was shown to diffuse rapidly across rat skin in vitro and across dog skin in vivo (251). Preliminary human screenings support the results obtained in the animal studies (252). Other studies examined propranolol absorption from ethanol-propylene glycol gel ointments in rabbits (253) and the use of iontophoresis to induce transdermal delivery of metoprolol in human volunteers (254). In the latter study, delivery of drug from a 50 cm2 electrode pad on the forearm yielded therapeutic plasma concentrations that were maintained for a longer period compared with conventional oral administration.

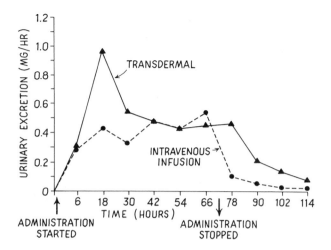

FIGURE 18 Mean scopolamine urinary excretion rates following trans-
dermal (n = 7) and intravenous (n = 6, 3.7—6.0 μg/hr) administration.
Drug input was stopped at 72 hr. (Adapted with permission from
Drug Dev. Ind. Pharm. 9: 627—646, 1983.)

9. *Theophylline*

The epidermis is poorly developed in preterm infants (224, 255).
The possibility of using this characteristic to advantage in terms of
transdermal drug delivery was examined by Evans et al. (256).
Theophylline gel equivalent to 17 mg anhydrous theophylline was
applied to 2 cm^2 of skin over the upper abdomen under an occlusive
dressing. Serum theophylline levels within the therapeutic range
of 4—12 μg/ml were obtained in 11 of 13 infants who had previously
received aminophylline infusion, therapeutic serum levels were
maintained by transdermal application. Transdermal theophylline
may thus be a useful alternative to oral theophylline in preterm infants with apnea in whom enteral feeding is not established and oral
absorption is erratic.

10. *Other Drugs*

Many other drugs are being investigated for transdermal delivery.
For some, preliminary data are appearing in the literature. Others
may remain unannounced for a while. Drugs mentioned in published
studies included ephedrine, indomethacin, and mitomycin C. Because
of its greater lipophilicity, ephedrine has a transdermal permeability

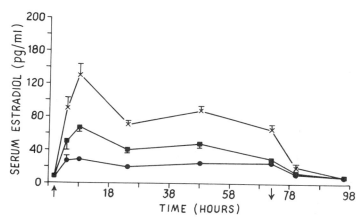

FIGURE 19 Mean (± 1 SE) serum concentrations of estradiol resulting from single 3-day topical applications of Estraderm 0.025 (●), Estraderm 0.05 (■), and Estraderm 0.1 (×). Corresponding surface areas are 5, 10, and 20 cm^3, respectively. (Reproduced by permission from *J. Controlled Release* 2: 89—97, 1985.)

120 times greater than that of scopolamine. Even in the protonated state ephedrine is 7-fold more permeable than scopolamine base and 110-fold more permeable than scolpolamine salt (202). A transdermal device has been described to deliver ephedrine at a rate of 370—380 μg/hr from a 10 cm^2 area, and urinary excretion profiles indicate that steady state is achieved by 9—10 hr in human subjects (257).

In vitro release of indomethacin has been shown to vary from different ointment bases, and in vitro release rates correlate with in vivo release through rabbit skin (258). In this study, indomethacin was absorbed rapidly from the ointment bases yielding peak plasma concentrations of 1.1—2.7 μg/ml at about 2 hr from 1—5% ointments. A 2 hr lag time reported earlier for percutaneous indomethacin (259) was not observed in this study.

Prodrug approaches have been used to improve transdermal delivery of a number of anticancer agents, including vidarabine (260), 5-fluorouracil (261), 6-thiopurines (262), and mitomycin C (263, 264). Most of these studies use lipophilic prodrugs that are converted to parent drug in the skin by either enzymatic or chemical lability. Some interesting results are being obtained. For example, lipophilic prodrugs of mitomycin C have enhanced transdermal delivery between three- and fivefold. The intense activity in this area is likely to result in some useful transdermal delivery forms for anticancer agents, for systemic and local effect.

In summary, there has been a tremendous increase in the investigation and development of transdermal drug delivery systems. This has resulted in marketed products for four drugs in the United States. This modest success reflects the problems inherent in this drug delivery approach. Transdermal delivery is limited to lipophilic molecules with excellent skin permeability that are not toxic to the skin. The prodrug approach is being used to increase the number of drugs that can be given by this route. A number of in vitro systems are available for preliminary testing, although these have variable predictability. A number of in vivo animal models are used.

Transdermal drug delivery is testing the ingenuity of pharmaceutical chemists and formulators and has generated a virtual industry focusing on membrane and matrix characteristics affecting transdermal absorption. Provided transdermal systems can do what they claim, to provide therapeutic effects with improved patient convenience, and are cost effective, they are likely to increase in number with a greater market share compared with that of conventional dosage forms.

REFERENCES

1. P. G. Welling. Pharmacokinetics, Processes and Mathematics. American Chemical Society, Washington D.C., 1986.
2. M. Rowland and T. N. Tozer. Clinical Pharmcokinetics: Concepts and Applications. Lea & Febiger, Philadelphia, 1980.
3. H. W. Davenport, Physiology of the Digestive Tract. Year Book Medical Publishers, Chicago, 1978.
4. A. F. Hoffmann, J. H. Dressman, C. F. Code, and K. F. Witztum. Controlled entry of oral administered drugs: Physiological Considerations. Drug Dev. Ind. Phar. 9: 1077—1109, 1983.
5. K. A. Kelly. Motility of the Stomach and Gastroduodenal junction. In Physiology of the Gastrointestinal Tract. Edited by L. R. Johnson. Raven Press, New York, 1981, pp. 393—410.
6. United States Pharmacopeia, Twenty-first revision. United States Pharmacopeial Convention, Inc., Rockville, Maryland, 1985.
7. J. P. Skelly, W. H. Barr, L. Z. Benet, J. T. Doluisio, et al. Report of the workshop on controlled release dosage forms. Sponsored by Academy of Pharmaceutical Sciences, American Society for Clinical Pharmacology and Therapeutics, Drug Information Association, and Food and Drug Administration, September-October, 1985.
8. P. G. Welling and M. R. Dobrinska. Dosing considerations and bioavailabilty assessment of controlled drug delivery systems. In Controlled Drug Delivery. Edited by J. R. Robinson and V. H. L. Lee. Marcel Dekker, New York, 1987, pp. 253—291.

9. P. G. Welling. Influence of food and diet on gastrointestinal drug absorption: A review. J. Pharmacokinet. Biopharm. 5: 291–334, 1977.

10. R. D. Toothaker and P. G. Welling, The effect of food on drug bioavailability. Annu. Rev. Pharmacol. Toxicol. 20: 173–199, 1980.

11. A. Melander. Influence of food on the bioavailability of drugs. Clin. Pharmacokinet. 3: 337–351, 1978.

12. P. G Welling and F. L. S. Tse. Factors contributing to variability in drug pharmacokinetics. I. Absorption. J. Clin. Hosp. Pharm. 9: 163–179, 1984.

13. P. G. Welling. Effects of gastrointestinal disease on drug absorption. In Pharmacokinetic Basis for Drug Treatment. Edited by L. Z. Benet, N. Massoud, and J. G. Gambertoglio. Raven Press, New York, 1984, pp. 29–47.

14. P. B. Andreasen, P. Dano, H. Kirk, and G. Greissen. Drug absorption and hepatic metabolism in patients with different types of intestinal shunt operations for obesity. A study with phenazone. Scand. J. Gastroenterol. 12: 531–535, 1977.

15. S. Bank, S. J. Saunders, I. N. Marks, B. H. Novis, and G. O. Barbezat. Gastrointestinal and hepatic diseases. In Drug Treatment, Principles and Practices of Clinial Pharmacology and Therapeutics. Edited by G. S. Avery. Adis Press, Sydney, 1980, pp. 683–759.

16. P. G. Welling. Absorption of drugs. In Encyclopedia of Pharmaceutical Technology, Marcel Dekker, in press.

17. J. Nimmo, R. C. Heading, P. Tothill, and L. F. Prescott. Pharmacological evaluation of gastric emptying: Effects of propantheline and metoclopramide on paracetamol absorption. Br. Med. J. 1: 587–589, 1973.

18. B. Beerman and M. Groschinsky-Grind. Enhancement of the gastrointestinal absorption of hydrochlorothiazide by propantheline. Eur. J. Clin. Pharmacol. 13: 385–387, 1978.

19. W. S. Nimmo, R. C. Heading, J. Wilson, P. Tothill, and L. F. Prescott. Inhibition of gastric emptying and drug absorption by narcotic analgesics. Br. J. Clin. Pharmacol. 2: 509–513, 1975.

20. J.-G. Lavigne and C. Marchand. Inhibition of gastrointestinal absorption of p-aminosalicylate (PAS) in rats and humans by diphenhydramine. Clin. Pharmacol. Ther. 14: 404–411, 1973.

21. M. A. Osman, R. B. Patel, A. Schuna, W. R. Sundstrom, and P. G. Welling. Reduction in oral penicillamine absorption by food, antacid, and ferrous sulfate. Clin. Pharmacol. Ther. 33: 465–470, 1983.

22. J. G. Wagner. Design and data analysis of biopharmaceutical studies in man. Can. J. Pharm. Sci. 1: 55–58, 1966.

23. R. L. Parsons and G. M. Paddock. Absorption of two antibacterial drugs, cephalexin and co-trimoxazole, in malabsorption syndromes. J. Antimicrob. Chemother. (Suppl.) 1: 59—67, 1975.

24. D. G. Corby and W. J. Decker. Management of acute poisoning with activated charcoal. Pediatrics 54: 324—328, 1974.

25. R. J. Neuvonen and E. Elonen. Effect of activated charcoal on absorption and elimination of phenobarbitone, carbamazepine and phenylbutazone in man. Eur. J. Clin. Pharmacol. 17: 51—57, 1980.

26. C. T. Vishwanathan, H. E. Booker, and P. G. Welling. Bio-availability of intramuscular and oral phenobarbital. J. Clin. Pharmacol. 18: 100—105, 1978.

27. H. Schriftman and A. Kondritzer. Absorption of atropine from muscle. Am. J. Physiol. 191: 591—594, 1957.

28. S. M. Harding, L. A. Eilon, and A. M. Harris. Factors affecting the intramuscular absorption of cefuroxime. J. Antimicrob. Chemother. 5: 87—93, 1979.

29. R. A. Vukovich, L. J. Brannick, A. A. Sugerman, and L. S. Neiss. Sex differences in the intramuscular absorption and bio-availability of cephradine. Clin. Pharmacol. Ther. 18: 215—220, 1975.

30. V. H. L. Lee and J. R. Robinson. Methods to achieve sustained drug delivery. The physical approach: Oral and parenteral dosage forms. In Sustained and Controlled Release Drug Delivery Systems. Edited by J. R. Robinson and V. H. L. Lee. Marcel Dekker, New York, 1978, pp. 123—209.

31. A. T. Florence, A. W. Jenkins, and A. H. Loveless. Approaches to the formulation of long-acting intramuscular infection. J. Pharm. Pharmacol. (Suppl.) 25: 120—121, 1973.

32. J. D. Scheu, G. J. Sperandio, S. M. Shaw, R. R. Landolt, and G. E. Peck. Use of microcapsules as timed-release parenteral dosage form: Application as radiopharmaceutical imaging agents. J. Pharm. Sci. 66: 172—177, 1977.

33. B. E. Ballard. Biopharmaceutical considerations in subcutaneous and intramuscular drug administration. J. Pharm. Sci. 57: 357—378, 1968.

34. T. S. Gaginella, P. G .Welling, and P. Bass. Nicotine base permeation through silicone elastomers: Comparison of dimethyl-polysiloxane and trifluoropropylmethylpoly-siloxane. J. Pharm. Sci. 63: 1849—1853, 1974.

35. M. Berger, P. A. Halban, J. P. Assal, R. E. Offord, M. Vranic, and A. E. Renold. Pharmacokinetics of subcutaneously injected tritiated insulin: Effects of exercise. Diabetes 28: 53—57, 1979.

36. V. A. Kovisto and P. Felig. Effects of leg exercise on insulin absorption in diabetic patients. N. Engl. J. Med. 298: 77—83, 1978.

37. K. Yamada, A. M. Bremer, C. R. West, J. Ghoorah, H. C. Park, and H. Takita. Intra-arterial BCNU therapy in the treatment of metastatic brain tumor from lung carcinoma. Cancer, 44: 2000—2007, 1979.

38. J. A. Goldman, D. Peleg, M. Agmon, and G. Shapiro. Arteriography and chemotherapy in localized trophoblastic disease, by means of local-(pelvic-) intraarterial infusion. Acta Obstet. Gynaecol. Scand. 58: 415—416 (1979).

39. H. A. Norell and C. B. Wilson. Chemotherapy of experimental brain tumors by arterial infusion. Surg. Forum 16: 429—431, 1965.

40. F. L. S. Tse and P. G. Welling. Bioavailability of parenteral drugs II. Parenteral doses other than intravenous and intramuscular routes. J. Parenter. Drug Assoc. 34: 484—495, 1980.

41. W. A. Bleyer and R. L. Dedrick. Clinical pharmacology of intrathecal methotrexate. I. Pharmacokinetics in nontoxic patients after lumbar injection. Cancer Treat. Rep. 61: 703—708, 1977.

42. C. A. Johnson, S. W. Zimmerman, and M. C. Rogge. The pharmacokinetics of antibiotics used to treat peritoneal dialysis-associated peritonitis. Am. J. Kidney Dis. 4: 3—17, 1984.

43. C. M. Bunke, G. R. Aronoff, M. E. Brier, R. S. Sloan, and F. C. Luft. Vancomycin kinetics during continuous ambulatory peritoneal dialysis. Clin. Pharmacol. Ther. 34: 631—637. 1983.

44. M. C. Rogge, C. A. Johnson, S. W. Zimmerman, and P. G. Welling. Vancomycin disposition during continuous ambulatory perotoneal dialysis. A pharmacokinetic analysis of peritoneal transport. Antimicrob. Agents Chemother. 27: 578—582, 1985.

45. R. Gokal, D. M. A. Francis, T. H. J. Goodship, A. J. Bint, J. M. Ramos, L. E. Ferner, et al. Peritonitis in CAPD. Lancet 2: 1388—1399, 1982.

46. A. G. De Boer, L. G. J. De Leede, and D. D. Breimer. Drug Absorption by sublingual and rectal routes. Br. J. Anaesth. 56: 69—82, 1984.

47. M. G. Bogaert. Clinical pharmacokinetics of organic nitrates. Clin. Pharmacokinet. 8: 410—421, 1983.

48. P. K. Noonan and L. Z. Benet. Incomplete and delayed bioavailability of sublingual nitroglycerin. Am. J. Cardiol. 55: 184—187, 1985.

49. H. Colfer, P. Stetson, B. R. Lucchesi, J. Wagner, and B. Pitt. The nitroglycerin polymer gel matrix system: A new method for administering nitroglycerin evaluated with plasma nitroglycerin levels. J. Cardiovasc. Pharmacol. 4: 521—525, 1982.

50. FDC Reports (Pink Sheet). October 13, 1986, T&G 4—5.

51. J. Abrams. New nitrate delivery systems: Buccal nitroglycerin. Am. Heart J. 105: 848—854, 1983.

52. P. Needleman and E. M. Johnson, Jr. Mechanisms of tolerance development to organic nitrates. J. Pharmacol. Exp. Ther. 184: 709–715, 1973.

53. J. Abrams. Nitroglycerin and long-acting nitrates. N. Engl. J. Med. 302: 1234–1237, 1980.

54. A. Lahiri, T. N. Sonecha, J. W. Crawley, and E. B. Raferty. Efficacy of sustained release buccal nitroglycerine in patients with ischaemic cardiomyopathy. Clin. Sci. 63: 38, 1982.

55. W. D. Bussman, R. R. Dries, and W. Wagner (Series Editors). Controlled release nitroglycerin in buccal and oral form. Advances in Pharmacotherapy; Vol. 1. Karger, Basel, 1982, pp. 35–43 and 64–183.

56. R. E. S. Bullingham, H. J. McQuay, E. J. B. Porter, M. C. Allen, and R. A. Moore. Sublingual buprenorphine used post-operatively: Ten hour plasma drug concentration analysis. Br. J. Clin. Pharmacol. 13: 665–673, 1982.

57. M. V. Shah, D. I. Jones, and M. Rosen. "Patient demand" postoperative analgesia with buprenorphine. Br. J. Anaesth. 58: 508–511, 1986.

58. H. Andriansen, B. Mattelaer, and H. Vanmeenen. A long-term open, clinical and pharmacokinetic assessment of sublingual buprenorphine in patients suffering from chronic pain. Acta Anaesthesiol. Belg. 1: 33–40, 1985.

59. M. Thibonnier, F. Bonnet, and P. Corvol. Antihypertensive effect of fractioned sublingual administration of nifedipine in moderate essential hypertension. Eur. J. Clin. Pharmacol. 17: 161–164, 1980.

60. B. F. Robinson, R. J. Dobbs, and C. R. Kelsey. Effects of nifedipine on resistance vessels, arteries and veins in man. Br. J. Clin. Pharmacol. 10: 433–438, 1980.

61. E. Lupi-Hereera, D. Bialostozky, and A. Sobrino. The role of isoproterenol in pulmonary artery hypertension of unknown etiology (primary). Chest 79: 292–296, 1981.

62. D. A. Pietro, K. A. LaBresh, R. M. Shulman, E. D. Folland, A. F. Parisi, and A. A. Sasahara. Sustained improvement in pulmonary hypertension during six years of treatment with sublingual isoproterenol. N. Engl. J. Med. 315: 1032–1034, 1984.

63. J. F. Ackroyd. Sublingual isoprenaline in treatment of primary pulmonary hypertension: Discussion paper. J. R. Soc. Med. 78: 474–477, 1985.

64. U. R. Shettigar, H. N. Hultgreen, M. Specter, R. Martin, and D. H. Davis. Primary pulmonary hypertension: Favorable effect of isoproterenol. N. Engl. J. Med. 295: 1414–1415, 1976.

65. U. Tauber, J. W. Tack, R. Dorow, and J. Hilman. Plasma levels of lormetazepam after sublingual and oral administration of 1 mg to humans. Drug Dev. Ind. Pharm. 10: 1587–1596, 1984.

66. G. W. Miller. Induction of labor by administration of oxytocin: Review of 50 cases. J. Am. Obstet. Assoc. 72: 1100−1103, 1973.

67. R. F. Casper and S. S. C. Yen. Rapid absorption of micronized estradiol-17β following sublingual administration. Obstet. Gynecol. 57: 62−64, 1981.

68. A. M. Burnier, P. L. Martin, S. S. C. Yen, and P. Brooks. Sublingual absorption of micronized 17 beta-estradiol. Am. J. Obstet. Gynecol. 140: 146−149, 1981.

69. C. P. Puri, S. J. Dharwadkar, S. Betrabet, Y. K. Hamied, and T. C. Anand Kumar. Sublingual spraying of norethisterone enhances its bioavailability in bonnet monkeys as compared with its administration by gavage. Adv. Contraceptive Delivery Systems 1: 133−137, 1985.

70. P. Larochelle, P. Du Souich, E. Bolte, J. Lelorier, and R. Goyer. Tixocortol pivalate, a corticosteroid with no systemic glucocorticoid effect after oral, intrarectal, and intranasal application. Clin. Pharmacol. Ther. 33: 343−350, 1983.

71. R. L. Mabry. Practical applications of intranasal corticosteroid injection. Ear Nose Throat J. 60: 23−27, 1981.

72. J. Hillas, R. J. Booth, S. Somerfield, R. Morton, J. Avery, and J. D. Wilson. A comparative trial of intra-nasal beclomethasone in patients with chronic perennial rhinitis. Clin. Allergy. 10: 253−258, 1980.

73. A. Toft, J. A. Wihl, J. Toxman, and N. Mygind. Double-blind comparison between beclomethasone dipropionate as aerosol and as powder in patients with nasal polyposis. Clin. Allergy 12: 391−401, 1982.

74. C. Secher, J. Kirkegaard, P. Borum. A. Maansson, P. Osterhammel, and N. Mygind. Significance of H_1 and H_2 receptors in the human nose: Rationale for topical use of combined antihistamine preparations. J. Allergy Clin. Immunol. 70: 211−218, 1982.

75. M. Okuda, K. Sakaguchi, and H. Ohtsuka. Intranasal beclomethasone: Mode of action in nasal allergy. Ann. Allergy 50: 116−120, 1983.

76. P. Wilkinson, C. Van Dyke, P. Jatlow, P. Barash, and R. Byck. Intranasal and oral cocaine kinetics. Clin. Pharmacol. Ther. 27: 386−394, 1980.

77. W. E. Fogler, R. Wade, D. E. Brundish, and I. J. Fidler. Distribution and fate of free and liposome-encapsulated [3H]-muramyl tripeptide phosphatidylethanolamine in mice. J. Immunol. 135: 1372−1377, 1985.

78. N. Mygind, M. Pedersen, and M. H. Nielsen. Morphology of the upper airway epithelium. In The Nose, Upper Airway Physiology and the Atmospheric Environment. Edited by D. F. Proctor and I. B. Anderson. Elsevier, New York, 1982, pp. 71−97.

79. R. Eccles. Neurological and pharmacological considerations. In The Nose, Upper Airway Physiology and the Atmospheric Environment. Edited by D. F. Proctor and I. B. Anderson. Elsevier, New York, 1982, pp. 191–214.

80. K. Watanabe, Y. Saito, I. Watanabe, and V. Mizuhira. Characteristics of capillary permeability in nasal mucosa. Ann. Otol. 89: 377–382, 1980.

81. K. S. E. Su and K. M. Campanali. Nasal drug delivery systems requirements, development and evaluation. In Transnasal Systemic Medications. Edited by Y. W. Chien. Elsevier Scientific Amsterdam, 1985, pp. 139–159.

82. W. Petri, R. Schmiedel, and J. Sandow. Development of a metered dose nebulizer for intranasal peptide administration. In Transnasal Systemic Medications. Edited by Y. W. Chien, Elsevier Scientific, Amsterdam, 1985, pp. 161–181.

83. Y. Sato, N. Hyo. M. Sato. H. Takano, and S. Okuda. Intranasal distribution of aerosols with or without vibration. Z. Erkr. Atmungsorgane 157: 276–280, 1981.

84. A. Hussain, S. Hirai, and R. Bamanshi. Nasal absorption of propranolol from different dosage forms by rats and dogs. J. Pharm. Sci. 69: 1411–1413, 1980.

85. G. F. X. David, C. P. Puri, and T. C. Anad Kumar. Bioavailability of progesterone enhanced by intranasal spraying. Experientia 37: 533–534, 1981.

86. T. C. Anand Kumar, G. R. X. David, and V. Puhi. Ovulation in rhesus monkeys suppressed by intranasal administration of progesterone and norethisterone. Nature 270: 532–533, 1977.

87. Y. W. Chien and S. F. Chang. Historical development of intranasal systemic medications. In Transnasal Systemic Medications. Edited by Y. W. Chien. Elsevier Sientific, Amsterdam, 1985, pp. 1–99.

88. J. Sandow and W. Petri. Intranasal administration of peptides. Biological activity and therapeutic efficacy. In Transnasal Systemic Medications. Edited by Y. W. Chien. Elsevier Scientific, Amsterdam, 1985, pp. 183–199.

89. G. M. Scott, R. J. Phillpotts, J. Wallace, D. S. Secher, K. Cantell, and D. A. J. Tyrrell. Purified interferon as protection against rhinovirus infection. Br. Med. J. 284: 1822–1825, 1982.

90. F. G. Hayden and J. M. Gwaltney, Jr. Intranasal interferon alpha-2 for prevention of rhinovirus infection and illness. J. Infect. Dis. 148: 543–550, 1983.

91. T. C. Samo, S. B. Greenberg, R. B. Couch, J. Quarles, P. E. Johnson, S. Hook, and M. W. Harmon. Efficacy and tolerance of intranasally applied recombinant leukocyte A interferon in normal volunteers. J. Infect. Dis. 148: 535–542, 1983.

92. F. G. Hayden, S. E. Mills, and M. E. Johns, Human tolerance and histopathologic effects of long-term administration of intranasal interferon-alpha 2. J. Infect. Dis. 148: 914—921, 1983.

93. R. W. Shaw, H. M. Fraser, and H. Boyle. Intranasal treatment with luteinizing hormone releasing hormone agonist in women with endometriosis. Br. Med. J. 287: 1067—1069, 1983.

94. H. Koch. Buserelin: Contraception through nasal spray. Pharm. Int. 2: 99—100, 1981.

95. S. Hirai. T. Yashiki, and H. Mima. Effect of surfactants on the nasal absorption of insulin in rats. Int. J. Pharm. 9: 165—172, 1981.

96. S. Hirai, T. Yashiki, and H. Mima. Mechanisms for the enhancement of the nasal absorption of insulin by surfactants. Int. J. Pharm. 9: 173—184, 1981.

97. A. C. Moses, G. S. Gordon, M. C. Carey, and J. S. Flier. Insulin administered intranasally as an insulin-bile salt aerosol. Effectiveness and reproducibility in normal and diabetic subjects. Diabetes 32: 1040—1047, 1983.

98. R. D. Silver, A. C. Moses, M. C. Carey, and J. S. Flier. Insulin-bile salt nasal aerosol markedly reduces postprandial glycemic excursion in diabetics. Diabetes 33: 75A, 1984.

99. T. Nagai, Y. Nishimoto, N. Nambu, Y. Suzuki, and K. Sekine. Powser dosage form of insulin for nasal administration. J. Controlled Release 1: 15—22, 1984.

100. R. Salzman, J. E. Manson, G. T. Griffing, R. Kimmerle, N. Ruderman, A. McCall, E. I. Stoltz, C. Mullin, D. Small, J. Armstrong, and J. C. Melby. Intranasal aerosolized insulin. Mixed-meal Studies and long-term use in type I diabetes. N. Engl. J. Med. 312: 1078—1084, 1985.

101. A. A. Hussain, R. Kimura, and C. H. Huang. Nasal absorption of testosterone in rats. J. Pharm. Sci. 73: 1300—1301, 1984.

102. A. A. Hussain, S. Hirai, and R. Bawarshi. Nasal absorption of natural contraceptive steroids in rats-progesterone absorption. J. Pharm. Sci. 70: 466—467, 1981.

103. G. F. X. David, C. P. Puri, and T. C. Anand Kumar. Bioavailability of progesterone enhanced by intranasal spraying. Experientia 37: 533—534, 1981.

104. T. C. Anand Kumar, G. F. X. David, A. Sakaranarayanan, V. Puri, and K. R. Sundram. Pharmacokinetics of progesterone after its administration to ovariectomized rhesus monkeys by injection, infusion, or nasal spraying. Proc. Natl. Acad. Sci. 79: 4185—4189, 1982.

105. E. B. Brittebo. Metabolism of progesterone by the nasal mucosa in mice and rats. Acta Pharmacol. Toxicol. 51: 441—445, 1982.

106. T. C. Anand Kumar, A. Sehgal, G. F. X. David, J. S. Bajaj, and M. R. N. Prasad. Effects of intranasal administration of hormonal steroids on serum testosterone and spermatogenesis in rhesus monkey (*Macaca mulatta*). Biol. Reprod. 22: 935–940, 1980.

107. T. C. Anand Kumar, G. F. X. David, B. Umberkoman, and K. D. Saini. Uptake of radioactivity by body fluids and tissues in rhesus monkeys after intravenous injection or intranasal spray of tritium-labelled oestradiol and progesterone. Curr. Sci. 43: 435–439, 1974.

108. L. Ohman, R. Hahnenberger, and E. D. B. Johansson. 17β-Estradiol levels in blood and cerebrospinal fluid after ocular and nasal administration in women and female rhesus monkeys (*Macaca mulatta*). Contraception 22: 349–358, 1980.

109. R. F. Hounam and A. Morgan. Particle deposition. In Respiratory Defense Mechanisms, Part I. Edited by J. D. Brain et al. Marcel Dekker, New York, 1977, pp. 125–156.

110. B. G. Simonsson. Anatomical and pathophysiological considerations in aerosol therapy. Eur. J. Respir. Dis. 63(Suppl. 119): 7–14, 1982.

111. J. E. Agnew, D. Pavia, and S. W. Clarke. Airways penetration of inhaled radioaerosol: An index to small airways function? Eur. J. Respir. Dis. 62: 239–255, 1981.

112. M. B. Dolovich, J. Sanchis, C. Rossman, and M. T. Newhouse. Aerosol penetrance: A sensitive index of peripheral airways obstruction. J. Appl. Physiol. 40: 468–471, 1976.

113. J. D. Brain and P. A. Valberg. Deposition of aerosol in the respiratory tract. Am. Rev. Respir. Dis. 120: 1325–1373, 1979.

114. J. Heyder. Particle transport onto human airway surfaces. Eur. J. Respir. Dis. 63(Suppl. 119): 29–50, 1982.

115. E. D. Palmes and M. Lippmann. Influence of respiratory air space dimensions on aerosol deposition. In Inhaled Particles and Vapours, IV. Edited by W. H. Walton. Pergamon Press, Oxford, 1977, pp. 127–136.

116. G. V. Taplin, N. D. Poe, E. K. Dore, A. Greenberg, and T. Isawa. Radioaerosol inhalation scanning. In Pulmonary Investigations with Radionuclides. Edited by A. J. Gibson and W. M. Smoals. Charles C. Thomas, Springfield, Illinois, 1970, pp. 296–317.

117. M. Lippmann, D. B. Yeates, and R. E. Albert. Deposition, retention, and clearance of inhaled particles. Br. J. Ind. Med. 37: 337–362, 1980.

118. D. Pavia, J. R. M. Bateman, and S. W. Clarke. Deposition and clearance on inhaled particles. Bull. Eur. Physiopathol. Respir. 16: 335–366, 1980.

119. D. Pavia, P. P. Sutton, M. T. Lopez-Vidriero, J. E. Agnew, and S. W. Clarke. Drug effects on mucociliary function. Eur. J. Respir. Dis. 64(Suppl. 128): 304–317, 1983.

120. J. A. Burton and L. S. Schanker. Absorption of antibiotics from the rat lung (37889). Proc. Soc. Exp. Biol. Med. 145: 752–756, 1974.

121. B. E. Goodman and D. Wangensteen. Alveolar epithelium permeability to small solutes: Developmental changes. J. Appl. Physiol. Respir. Environ. Exercise Physiol. 52: 3–8, 1982.

122. D. J. Benford and J. W. Bridges. Xenobiotic metabolism in lung. In Progress in Drug Metabolism, Vol. 9. Edited by J. W. Bridges and L. F. Chasseaud. Taylor and Francis, 1986, pp. 53–94.

123. D. S. Davies. Pharmacokinetic studies with inhaled drugs. Eur. J. Respir. Dis. 63(Suppl. 119): 67–72, 1982.

124. P. R. Byron and A. R. Clark. Drug absorption from inhalation aerosols administered by positive-pressure ventilation. I. Administration of a characterized, solid disodium fluorescein aerosol under a controlled respiratory regime to the beagle dog. J. Pharm. Sci. 74: 934–938, 1985.

125. A. R. Clark and P. R. Byron. Drug absorption from inhalation aerosols adminsitered by positive-pressure ventilation II. Effect of disodium fluorescein aerosol particle size on fluorescein absorption kinetics in the beagle dog respiratory tract. J. Pharm. Sci. 74: 939–942, 1985.

126. R. A. Brown, Jr., and L. S. Schanker. Absorption of aerosolized drugs from the rat lung. Drug Metab. Dispos. 11; 355–360, 1983.

127. D. S. Davies. Pharmacokinetics of inhaled substances. Postgrad. Med. J. 51(Suppl 7): 69–75, 1975.

128. F. Moren and J. Andersson. Fraction of dose exhaled after administration of pressurized inhalation aerosols. Int. J. Pharm. 6: 295–300, 1980.

129. S. P. Newman, M. Killip, D. Pavia, F. Moren, and S. W. Clarke. The effect of changes in particle size on the deposition of pressurized inhalation aerosols. Int. J. Pharm. 19: 333–337, 1984.

130. S. P. Newman, D. Pavia, F. Moren, N. F. Sheahan, and S. W. Clarke. Deposition of pressurized aerosols in the human respiratory tract. Thorax 36: 52–55, 1981.

131. S. P. Newman, D. Pavia, and S. W. Clarke. How should a pressurized beta-adrenergic bronchodilator be inhaled? Eur. J. Respir. Dis. 62: 3–21, 1981.

132. I. Gonda. Study of the effects of polydispersity of aerosols on regional deposition in the respiratory tract. J. Pharm. Pharmacol. 33: 52P, 1981.

133. F. C. Hiller, M. K. Mazumder, D. Wilson, R. G. Renninger, and R. C. Bone. Physical properties of therapeutic aerosols. Chest (Suppl.)80: 901–903, 1981.

134. Fisons Corporation. Intal Cromolyn Sodium: A monograph. Bedford, Massachusetts, 1973.

135. G. K. Crompton. Clinical use of dry powder systems. Eur. J. Respir. Dis. (Suppl.)122: 96–99, 1982.

136. S. P. Newman, F. Moren, D. Pavia, F. Little, and S. W. Clarke. Deposition of pressurized suspension aerosols inhaled through extension devices. Am Rev. Respir. Dis. 124: 317–320, 1981.

137. M. Dolovich, R. E. Ruffin, R. Roberts, and M. T. Newhouse. Optimal delivery of aerosols from metered dose inhalers. Chest (Suppl.)80: 911–915, 1981.

138. J. H. Toogood, J. Baskerville, B. Jennings, N. M. Lefcoe, and S. Johansson. Use of spacers to facilitate inhaled corticosteroid treatment of asthma. Am. Rev. Respir. Dis. 129: 723–729, 1984.

139. S. Pedersen. Aerosol treatment of bronchoconstriction in children, with or without a tube spacer. N. Engl. J. Med. 308: 1328–1330, 1983.

140. J. Morris, J. S. Milledge, H. Moszoro, and A. Higgins. The efficacy of drug delivery by a pear-shaped spacer and metered dose inhaler. Br. J. Dis. Chest 78: 383–387, 1984.

141. S. P. Newman, A. B. Millar, T. R. Lennard-Jones, F. Moren, and S. W. Clarke. Improvement of pressurized aerosol deposition with nebuhaler spacer device. Thorax 39: 935–941, 1984.

142. G. K. Crompton. Problem patients have using pressurised aerosol inhalers. Eur. J. Respir. Dis. 63(Suppl. 119): 101–104, 1982.

143. M. Dolovich, R. Ruffin, D. Corr, and M. T. Newhouse. Clinical evaluation of a simple demand inhalation MDI aerosol delivery device. Chest 84: 36–41, 1983.

144. C. Shim and M. H. Willimas, Jr. The adequacy of inhalation of aerosol from canister nebulizers. JAMA 69: 891–894, 1980.

145. J. S. Kelling, K. P. Strohl, R. L. Smith, and M. D. Altose. Physicians knowledge in the use of canister nebulizers. Chest 83: 612–614, 1983.

146. M. Arborelius, Jr. Generation of a microaerosol suitable for deposition in the peripheral airways. Eur. J. Respir. Dis. 63(Suppl. 119): 19–27, 1982.

147. H. W. Keely. Drug reviews. New beta 2-adrenergic agonist aerosols. Clin. Pharm. 4: 393–403, 1985.

148. S. P. Galant. Current Status of beta-adrenergic agonists in bronchial asthma. Pediatr. Clin. North Am. 30: 931–942, 1983.

149. C. Shim. Adrenergic agonists and bronchodilator aerosol therapy in asthma. Clin. Chest Med. 5: 659–668, 1984.

150. R. M. Sly. Beta-adrenergic drugs in the management of asthma in athletes. J. Allergy Clin. Immunol. 73: 680—685, 1984.
151. W. van der Berg, J. G. Leferink, R. A. A. Maes, J. Krenkniet, and P. L. B. Bruynzeel. Correlation between terbutaline serum levels, c-AMP plasma levels and FEV_1 in normals and asthmatics after subcutaneous administration. Ann. Allergy 44: 2335—239, 1980.
152. G. Lonnerholm. T. Foucard, and B. Lindstrom. Oral terbutaline in chronic childhood asthma; effects related to plasma concentrations. Eur. J. Respir. Dis. 65(Suppl. 134): 205—210, 1984.
153. K. Svedmyr and N. Svedmyr. Combined therapy with theophylline and beta-2-adrenostimulants in asthmatics. Br. J. Dis. Chest 73: 424—428, 1979.
154. R. J. S. Shaw, J. F. Waller, M. R. Hetzel, and T. J. H. Clark. Do oral and inhaled terbutaline have different effects on the lung? Br. J. Dis. Chest 76: 171—176, 1982.
155. D. P. Tashkin, E. Trevor, S. K. Chopra, and G. V. Taplin. Sites of airway dilatation in asthma following inhaled versus subcutaneous terbutaline. JAMA 68: 14—26, 1980.
156. P. J. Rees and T. J. H. Clark. The importance of particle size in response to inhaled bronchodilators. Eur. J. Respir. Dis. 63(Suppl. 119): 73—78, 1982.
157. D. S. Davies. The fate of inhaled terbutaline. Eur. J. Respir. Dis. 65(Suppl. 119): 141—147, 1984.
158. P. M. O'Byrne, M. Morris, R. Roberts, and F. E. Hargreave. Inhibition of the bronchial response to respiratory heat exchange by increasing doses of terbutaline sulphate. Thorax 37: 913—917, 1982.
159. J. B. Andersen and N. O. Klausen. A new mode of administration of nebulized bronchodialtor in severe bronchospasm. Eur. J. Respir. Dis. 63(Suppl. 119): 97—100, 1982.
160. K. G. Hidinger and J. Perk. Clinical trial of a modified inhaler for pressurized aerosols. Eur. J. Clin. Pharmacol. 20: 109—111, 1981.
161. D. Heimer, C. Shim, and H. Williams, Jr. The effect of sequential inhalations of metaproterenol in asthma. J. Allergy Clin. Immunol. 66: 75—77, 1980.
162. R. C. Ahrens, A. C. Bonham, G. A. Maxwell, and M. M. Weinberger. A method for comparing the peak intensity and duration of action of aerosolized bronchodilators using bronchoprovocation with methacholine. Am. Rev. Respir. Dis. 129: 903—906, 1984.
163. P. J. Barnes and N. B. Pride. Dose-response curves to inhaled β-adrenoceptor agonists in normal and asthmatic subjects. Br. J. Clin. Pharmacol. 15: 677—682, 1983.

164. H. S. Nelson, S. L. Spector, T. L. Whitsett, R. B. George, and J. H. Dwek. The bronchodilator response to inhalation of increasing doses of aerosolized albuterol. J. Allergy Clin. Immunol. 72: 371–375, 1983.

165. M. E. Conolly, D. P. Tashkin, K. K. P. Hui, M. R. Littner, and R. N. Wolfe. Selective subsensitization of beta-adrenergic receptors in central airways of asthmatics and normal subjects during long-term therapy with inhaled salbutamol. J. Allergy Clin. Immunol. 70: 423–431, 1982.

166. D. P. Tashkin, M. E. Conolly, R. I. Deutsch, K. K. Hui, M. Littner, P. Scarpace, and I. Abrass. Subsensitization of beta-adrenoceptors in airways and lymphocytes of healthy and asthmatic subjects. Am. Rev. Respir. Dis. 125: 185–193, 1982.

167. C. Lin, J. Magat, B. Calesnick, and S. Symchowicz. Absorption, excretion and urinary metabolic pattern of ^{3}H-albuterol aerosol in man. Xenobiotica 2: 507–515, 1972.

168. N. Svedmyr, C. G. Lofdahl, and K. Svedmyr. The effect of powder aerosol compared to pressurized aerosol. Eur. J. Respir. Dis. 63(Suppl. 119): 81–88, 1982.

169. P. Konig, N. L. Hordvik, and C. W. Serby. Fenoterol in exercise-induced asthma. Effect of dose on efficacy and duration of action. Chest 85: 462–464, 1984.

170. J. Rivlin, C. Mindorff, H. Levison, F. Kazim, P. Reilly, and G. Worsley. Effect of administration technique on bronchodilator response to fenoterol in a metered-dose inhaler. J. Pediatr. 102: 470–472, 1983.

171. C. A. Mitchell, J. G. Armstrong, M. A. Bartholomew, and R. Scicchitano. Nebulized fenoterol in severe asthma: Determinants of the dose response. Eur. J. Respir. Dis. 64: 340–346, 1983.

172. H. Dirksen. Addition of a spacer device as an alternative in treatment with a metered dose inhaler. Eur. J. Respir. Dis. 64(Suppl. 130): 42–47, 1983.

173. D. Rodenstein and D. C. Stanescu. Mouth spraying versus inhalation of fenoterol aerosol in healthy subjects and asthmatic patients. Br. J. Dis. Chest 76: 365–373, 1982.

174. M. K. Tandon. Cardiopulmonary effects of fenoterol and salbutamol aerosols. Chest 77: 429–431, 1980.

175. A. Bundgaard and A. Schmidt. Pretreatment of exercise-induced asthma by disodium cromoglycate and fenoterol. Eur. J. Respir. Dis. 64(Suppl. 128): 521–525, 1983.

176. M. Agostini, G. Barlocco, and G. Mastella. Protective effect of fenoterol spray, ipratropium bromide plus fenoterol spray, and oral clenbuterol, on exercise-induced asthma in children. Double blind controlled and randomized clinical trial. Eur. J. Respir. Dis. 64(Suppl. 128): 529–532, 1983.

177. I. Kass and T. S. Mingo, Bitolterol mesylate (WIN 32784) aerosol. A new long-acting bronchodilator with reduced chrono-tropic effects. Chest 78: 283—287, 1980.

178. T. L. Petty, C. H. Scoggin, D. R. Rollins, and L. H. Repsher. Bitolterol compared to isoproterenol in advanced chronic obstructive pulmonary disease. Chest 86: 404—408, 1984.

179. H. A. Orgel, J. P. Kemp, D. G. Tinkelman, and D. R. Webb, Jr. Bitolterol and albuterol metered-dose aerosols: Comparison of two long-acting beta2-adrenergic bronchodilators for treatment of asthma. J. Allergy Clin. Immunol. 75: 55—62, 1985.

180. B. A. Berman. Cromolyn: Past, present, and future. Pediatr. Clin. North Am. 30: 915—930, 1983.

181. R. A. Robson, B. J. Taylor, and B. Taylor. Sodium cromoglycate: Spincaps or metered dose aerosol. Br. J. Clin. Pharmacol. 11: 383—384, 1981.

182. S. Y. So and D. Y. C. Yu. Sodium cromoglycate delivered by pressurized aerosol in the treatment of asthma. Clin. Allergy 11: 479—482, 1981.

183. E. Bar-Yishay, I. Gur, M. Levy, D. Volozni, and S. Godfrey. Duration of action of sodium cromoglycate on exercise induced asthma: Comparison of 2 formulations. Arch. Dis. Child. 58: 624—627, 1983.

184. R. E. Schoeffel, S. D. Anderson, and D. A. Lindsay. Sodium cromoglycate as a pressurised aerosol (Vicrom) in exercise-induced asthma. Aust. N.Z. J. Med. 13: 157—161, 1983.

185. A. Bundgaard, N. Bach-Mortensen, and A. Schmidt. The effect of sodium cromoglycate delivered by Spinhaler and by pressurized aerosol on exercise-induced asthma in children. Clin. Allergy, 12: 601—605, 1982.

186. R. Dahl and J. M. Henriksen. Effect of oral and inhaled sodium cromoglycate in exercise-induced asthma. Allergy 35: 363—365, 1980.

187. W. M. Tullett, K. M. Tan, R. T. Wall, and K. R. Patel. Dose-response effect of sodium cromoglycate pressurised aerosol in exercise induced asthma. Thorax 40: 41—44, 1985.

188. K. M. Latimer, R. Roberts, M. M. Morris, and F. E. Hargreave. Inhibition by sodium cromoglycate of bronchoconstriction stimulated by respiratory heat loss: Comparison of pressurized aerosol and powder. Thorax 39: 277—281, 1984.

189. M. H. Williams, Jr. Beclomethasone dipropionate. Ann. Intern. Med. 95: 464—467, 1981.

190. J. H. Toogood, N. M. Lefcoe, D. S. M. Haines, L. Chuang, B. Jennings, N. Errington, L. Baksh, and M. Cauchi. Minimum dose requirements of steroid-dependent asthmatic patients for aerosol beclomethasone and oral prednisone. J. Allergy Clin. Immunol. 61: 355—364, 1978.

191. M. J. Smith and M. E. Hodson. High-dose beclomethasone inhaler in the treatment of asthma. Lancet 1: 265—269, 1983.

192. M. Weinberger. Steroids in asthma. Lancet 1: 316—317, 1980.

193. E. Bacal and R. Patterson. Long-term effects of beclomethasone dipropionate on prednisone dosage in the cortico-steroid dependent asthmatic. J. Allergy Clin. Immunol. 62: 72—75, 1978.

194. G. Davies, P. Thomas, I. Broder, S. Mintz, F. Silverman, A. Leznoff, and C. Trotman. Steroid-dependent asthma treated with inhaled beclomethasone dipropionate. A long-term study. Ann. Intern. Med. 86: 549—553, 1977.

195. J. H. Toogood, N. M. Lefcoe,D. S. M. Haines, B. Jennings, N Errington, L. Baksh, and L. Chuang. A graded dose assessment of the efficacy of beclomethasone dipropionate aerosol for severe chronic asthma. J. Allergy Clin. Immunol. 59: 298—308, 1977.

196. J. H. Toogood, J. C. Baskerville, B. Jennings, N. M. Lefcoe, and S. A. Johansson. Influence of dosing frequency and schedule on the response of chronic asthmatics to the aerosol steroid, budesonide. J. Allergy Clin. Immunol. 70: 288—298, 1982.

197. P. H. Vlasses, R. K. Ferguson, J. R. Koplin, R. A. Clementi, and P. J. Green. Adrenocortical function after chronic inhalation of fluocortin butyl and beclomethasone dipropionate. Clin. Pharmacol. Ther. 29: 643—649, 1981.

198. W. A. Kradjan, S. Lakshminarayan, P. W. Hayden, S. W. Larson, and J. J. Marini. Serum atropine concentrations after inhalation of atropine sulfate. Am. Rev. Respir. Dis. 123: 471—472, 1981.

199. C. C. F. Pak, W. A. Kradjan, S. Lakshminarayan, and J. J. Marini. Inhaled atropine sulfate. Dose-response characteristics in adult patients with chronic airflow obstruction. Am. Rev. Respir. Dis. 125: 331—334, 1982.

200. W. A. Kradjan, R. C. Smallridge, R. Davis, and P. Verma. Atropine serum concentrations after multiple inhaled doses of atropine sulfate. Clin. Pharmacol. Ther. 38: 12—15, 1985.

201. S. K. Chandrasekaran. Controlled release of scopolamine for prophylaxis of motion sickness. Drug Dev. Ind. Pharm. 9: 627—646, 1983.

202. Y. W. Chien. Novel Drug Delivery Systems. Marcel Dekker, New York, 1982, pp. 149—217.

203. R. H. Guy and J. Hadgraft. Transdermal drug delivery: A perspective. J. Controlled Release 4: 237—251, 1987.

204. D. A. W. Bucks. Skin structure and metabolsim: Relevance to the design of cutaneous therapeutics. Pharm. Res. 1: 148—153, 1984.

205. C. D. Yu, J. L. Fox, N. F. H. Ho, and W. I. Higuchi. Physical model evaluation of topical prodrug delivery—simultaneous transport and bioconversion of vidarabine-5'-valerate. I. Physical model development. J. Pharm. Sci. 68: 1341—1346, 1979.

206. A. Hoelgaard and B. Møllgaard. Dermal drug delivery—improvement by choice of vehicle or drug derivative. J. Controlled Release 2: 111—120, 1985.

207. E. W. Merritt and E. R. Cooper. Diffusion apparatus for skin penetration. J. Controlled Release 1: 161—162, 1984.

208. K. Tojo, M. Ghannam, Y. Sun, and Y. W. Chien. In vitro apparatus for controlled release studies and intrinsic rate of permeation. J. Controlled Release 1: 197—203, 1985.

209. B. Idsen. Vehicle effects in percutaneous absorption. Drug Metab. Rev. 14: 207—222, 1983.

210. S. I. Yum and R. M. Wright. Drug delivery systems based on diffusion and osmosis. In Controlled Drug Delivery, Vol 2, Clinical Applications. Edited by S. D. Bruck. CRC Press, Boca Raton, Florida, 1983, pp. 63—87.

211. J. E. Shaw and C. Mitchell. Dermal drug delivery systems: A review. J. Toxicol. Cutan. Ocular Toxicol. 2: 249—266, 1983—1984.

212. K. Sugibayashi, K.-I. Hosoya, Y. Morimoto, and W. I. Higuchi. Effect of the absorption enhancer, Azone, on the transport of 5-fluorouracil across hairless rat skin. J. Pharm. Pharmacol. 37: 578—580, 1985.

213. R. B. Stoughton and W. O. McClure. Azone: A new non-toxic enhancer of cutaneous penetration. Drug Dev. Ind. Pharm. 9: 725—744, 1983.

214. M. G. Ganesan, N. D. Weiner, G. L. Flynn, and N. F. H. Ho. Influence of liposomal drug entrapment on percutaneous absorption. Int. J. Pharm. 20: 139—154, 1984.

215. N. F. H. Ho, N. G. Ganesan, N. D. Weiner, and G. L. Flynn. Mechanisms of topical delivery of liposomally entrapped drugs. J. Controlled Release 2: 61—65, 1985.

216. W. P. O'Neill. Membrane systems. In Controlled Release Technologies: Methods, Theory, and Applications, Vol. 1. Edited by A. F. Kydonieus. 1980. pp. 129—182.

217. H. P. Merkle, A. Knoch, and G. Gienger. Release kinetics of polymeric laminates for transdermal delivery: Experimental evaluation of physical modelling. J. Controlled Release 2: 99—110, 1985.

218. R. H. Guy and J. Hadgraft. The prediction of plasma levels of drugs following transdermal application. J. Controlled Release 1: 177—182, 1985.

219. R. H. Guy and J. Hadgraft. Transdermal drug delivery: A Simplified pharmacokinetic approach. Int. J. Pharmaceutics 24: 267—274, 1985.

220. B. Berner. Pharmacokinetics of transdermal drug delivery. J. Pharm.Sci. 74: 718—721, 1985.

221. Y. W. Chien. Controlled drug release from polymeric systems. In Drug Delivery Systems. Edited by R. L. Juliano. Oxford University Press, New York, 1980, pp. 62—70.

222. K. Tojo, Y. Sun, M. Ghannam, and Y. W. Chien. Simple evaluation method of intrinsic diffusivity for membrane-moderated controlled release. Drug Dev. Ind. Pharm. 11: 1363—1371, 1985.

223. B. Berner. The pharmacokinetics of the removal and re-application of transdermal patches. J. Controlled Release 1: 127—135, 1984.

224. N. Evans, R. H. Guy, J. Hadgraft, G. D. Parr, and N. Rutter, Transdermal drug delivery to neonates. Int. J. Pharm. 24: 259—265, 1985.

225. A. Karim. Transdermal absorption: A unique opportunity for constant delivery of nitroglycerin. Drug Dev. Ind. Pharm. 9: 671—689, 1983.

226. Y. W. Chien. Pharmaceutical considerations of transdermal nitroglycerin delivery: The various approaches. Am. Heart J. 108: 207—216, 1984.

227. D. D. Mar. New topical nitroglycerin preparations. Am. J. Nurs. 82: 462—463, 1982.

228. P. R. Keshary and Y. W. Chien. Mechanisms of transdermal controlled nitroglycerin administration. I. Development of a finite-dosing skin permeation system. Drug Dev. Ind. Pharm. 10: 883—913, 1984.

229. P. R. Keshary and Y. W. Chien. Mechanism of transdermal controlled nitroglycerin administration. II. Assessment of rate-controlling steps. Drug Dev. Ind. Pharm. 10: 1663—1699, 1984.

230. R. H. Guy and J. Hadgraft. Kinetic analysis of transdermal nitroglycerin delivery. Pharm. Res. 2: 206—211, 1985.

231. E. D. Bennett and A. L. Davis. A haemodynamic and pharmacokinetic study to assess a new transdermal nitroglycerin preparation in normal subjects. Eur. J. Clin. Pharmacol. 26: 293—296, 1984.

232. M. Wolff, G. Cordes, and V. Luckow. In vitro and in vivo release of nitroglycerin from a new transdermal therapeutic system. Pharm. Res. 2: 23—29, 1985.

233. S. Scheidt. Update of transdermal nitroglycerin: An overview. Am. J. Cardiol. 56: 31—71, 1985.

234. J. Abrams. New nitroglycerin formulations: Transdermal and transmucosal nitroglycerin. Z. Kardiol. 74(Suppl. 4): 10—15, 1985.

235. J. O. Parker, K. A. von Koughnett, and H.-L. Fung. Transdermal isosorbide dinitrate in angina pectoris: Effect of acute and sustained therapy. Am. J. Cardiol. 54: 8–13, 1984.
236. A. A. Hendricks and G. W. Dec, Jr. Contact dermatitis due to nitroglycerin ointment. Arch. Dermatol. 115: 853–855, 1979.
237. C. Benezra, C. C. Sigman, L. R. Perry, C. T. Helmes, and H. I. Maibach. A systemic search for structure-activity relationships of skin contact sensitizers: Methodology. J. Invest. Dermatol. 85: 351–356, 1985.
238. S. Noy, S. Sapira, A. Zilbiger, and J. Ribak. Transdermal therapeutic system scopolamine (TTSS), dimenhydrinate, and placebo—a comparative study at sea. Aviat. Space Environ. Med. 55: 1051–1054, 1984.
239. W. F. von Marion, M. C. M. Bongaerts, J. C. Christiaanse, H. G. Hofkamp, and W. van Ouwerkerk. Influence of transdermal scopolamine on motion sickness during 7 days' exposure to heavy seas. Clin. Pharmacol. Ther. 38: 301–305, 1985.
240. D. Arndts and K. Arndts. Pharmacokinetics and pharmacodynamics of transdermally delivered clonidine. Eur. J. Clin. Pharmacol. 26: 79–85, 1984.
241. T. R. MacGregor, K. M. Matzek, J. J. Keirns, R. G. A. van Wayjen, A. van den Ende, and R. G. L. van Tol. Pharmacokinetics of transdermally delivered clonidine. Clin. Pharmacol. Ther. 38: 278–284, 1985.
242. A. A. H. Lawson. Clinical and pharmacological studies with transdermal clonidine. In Rate Control in Drug Therapy. Edited by L. F. Prescott and W. S. Nimmo. Churchill Livingstone, Edinburgh, 1985, pp. 215–219.
243. M. L. Padwick, J. Endacott, and M. I. Whitehead. Efficacy acceptability, and metabolite effects of transdermal estradiol in the management of postmenopausal women. Am. J. Obstet. Gynecol. 152: 1085–1091, 1985.
244. J. Holst, S. Cajander, K. Carlström, M. G. Damber, and B. von Schoultz. A comparison of liver protein induction in postmenopausal women during oral and percutaneous estrogen replacement therapy. Am. J. Obstet. Gynocol. 90: 355–360, 1983.
245. M. S. Powers, L. Schenkel, P. E. Darley, W. R. Good, J. C. Balestra, and V. A. Place. Pharmacokinetics and pharmacodynamics of transdermal dosage forms of 17β-estradiol: Comparison with conventional oral estrogens used for hormone replacement. Am. J. Obstet. Gynecol. 152: 1099–1106, 1985.
246. W. R. Good, M. S. Powers, P. Campbell, and L. Schenkel. A new transdermal delivery system for estradiol. J. Controlled Release 2: 89–97, 1985.

247. K. Tojo, K. H. Valia, G. Chotani, and Y. W. Chien. Long-term permeation kinetics of estradiol. IV. A theoretical approach to the simulatenous skin permeation and bioconversion of estradiol esters. Drug Dev. Ind. Pharm. 11: 1175–1193, 1985.

248. Y. W. Chien, K. H. Valia, and U. B. Doshi. Long-term permeation kinetics of estradiol. V. Development and evaluation of transdermal bioactivated hormone delivery system. Drug Dev. Ind. Pharm. 11: 1195–1212, 1985.

249. N. Bodor and K. B. Sloan. Improved delivery through biological membranes. XII. The effect of incorporation of biphasic solubilizing groups into produgs of steroids. Int. J. Pharm. 15: 235–250, 1983.

250. K. Uekama, M. Otagiri, A. Sakai, T. Irie, N. Matsuo, and Y. Matsuoka. Inprovement in the percutaneous absorption of beclomethasone dipropionate by γ-cyclodextrin complexation. J. Pharm. Pharmacol. 37: 532–533, 1985.

251. R. Cargill, K. Engle, G. Rork, and L. J. Caldwell. Systemic delivery of timolol after dermal application: Transdermal flux and skin irritation potential in the rat and dog. Pharm Res. 3: 225–229, 1986.

252. P. H. Vlasses, L. G. T. Ribeiro, H. H. Rotmensch, J. V. Bondi, A. E. Loper, M. Hichens, M. C. Dunlay, and R. K. Ferguson. Initial evaluation of transdermal timolol: Serum concentrations and beta-blockade. J. Cardiovasc. Pharmacol. 7: 245–250, 1985.

253. T. Nagai, Y. Santoh, N. Nambu, and Y. Machida. Percutaneous absorption of propranolol from gel ointment in rabbits. J. Controlled Release 1: 239–246, 1985.

254. K. Okabe, H. Yamaguchi, and Y. Kawai. New iontophoretic transdermal administration of the beta-blocker metoprolol. J. Controlled Release 4: 79–85, 1986.

255. V. A. Harpin and N. Rutter. Barrier properties of newborn infant's skin. J. Pediatr. 102: 419425, 1983.

256. N. J. Evans, N. Rutter, J. Hadgraft, and G. Parr. Percutaneous administration of theophylline in the preterm infant. J. Pediatr. 107: 307–311, 1985.

257. J. E. Shaw, S. K. Chandrasekaran, A. S. Michaels, and L. Taskovich. Controlled transdermal delivery, in vitro and in vivo. In Animal Models in Dermatology. Edited by H. Maibach. Churchill Livingstone, Edinburgh, 1975, pp. 138–146.

258. S. Kazmi, L. Kennon, M. Sideman, and F. M. Plakogiannis. Medicament release from ointment basis. I. Indomethacin, in vitro and in vivo release studies. Drug Dev. Ind. Pharm. 10: 1071–1083, 1984.

259. S. Naito and Y. H. Tsai. Percutaneous absorption of indomethacin from ointment basis in rabbits. Int. J. Pharm. 8: 263–276, 1981.

260. J. L. Fox, W. I. Higuchi, and N. F. H. Ho. General physical model for simultaneous diffusion in biological membranes. The computational approach for the steady-state case. Int. J. Pharm. 2: 41—57, 1979.

261. B. Møllgaard, A. Huelgaard, and H. Bundaard. Pro-drugs as drug delivery systems. XXIII. Improved dermal delivery of 5-fluorouracil through human skin via N-acyloxymethyl pro-drug derivatives. Int. J. Pharm. 12: 153—162, 1982.

262. K. B. Sloan, M. Hashida, J. Alexander, N. Bodor, and T. Higuchi. Prodrugs of 6-thiophenes: Enhanced delivery through the skin. J. Pharm. Sci. 72: 372—378, 1983.

263. H. Sasaki, E. Mukai, M. Hashida, T. Kimura, and H. Sezaki. Development of lipophilic prodrugs of mitomicin C. I. Synthesis and antitumor activity of la-N-substituted derivatives with aromatic pro-moiety. Int. J. Pharm. 15: 49—59, 1983.

264. E. Mukai, K. Arase, M. Hishida, and H. Sezaki. Enhanced delivery of mitomycin C prodrugs through the skin. Int. J. Pharm. 25: 95—103, 1985.

4

Nonclinical Pharmacokinetics in Drug Discovery and Development

FRANCIS L. S. TSE *Sandoz Research Institute, East Hanover, New Jersey*

I. INTRODUCTION

In the early stage of the drug discovery process, one may have an interesting new chemical that is yet to be proven useful for any medical purpose. Nonetheless, available physicochemical data have suggested the compound to be sufficiently promising to warrant the great deal of work that will follow. From the moment of decision to pursue to the actual submission of a Notice of Claimed Investigational Exemption for a New Drug (IND), as much information as possible will be sought concerning the efficacy and safety of the compound. Relevant pharmacological and toxicological assessments will be conducted in laboratory animals, with the presupposition of a reasonable transposition to humans of results obtained in animals, which is generally but certainly not always the case. It is for the purpose of supporting these animal pharmacological and toxicological data, and also properly interpreting such data for projection to humans, that the discipline of pharmacokinetics has become an integral part of the modern preclinical drug development process. Preclinical pharmacokinetic studies, together with additional studies in animals that are performed concurrently with clinical trials in the post-IND phase, constitute the typical nonclinical program. Although the majority of nonclinical studies consist of in vivo tests in various animal species, in vitro experiments, such as the determination of plasma protein binding of drugs, also fall into this category.

Under current regulations of the U.S. Food and Drug Administration (FDA), no specific type of preclinical test data is required for IND submission. However, it is generally expected that the results of animal pharmacology, drug disposition, and toxicology studies are included in order to provide adequate background knowledge to guide decision-making during the proposed clinical investigations. To this end, ADME (absorption, distribution, metabolism, and excretion) studies in at least two species, commonly the rat and the dog, are often conducted in the pre-IND phase. The minimum expectation typically includes testing at one oral dose level plus an intravenous reference dose. Considerable variations exist at present within the pharmaceutical industry in the specific conduct of studies and therefore in the type and extent of data obtained. In order to facilitate the drug evaluation process, there is an increasing desire by both industry and regulatory agencies for more precise, consistent, and practical guidelines for preclinical drug metabolism and disposition studies. Guideline proposals containing rather specific recommendations have been published (1, 2), and many of the suggested procedures have already been implemented by pharmaceutical companies to varying degrees. To better understand the rationale of the numerous studies constituting the nonclinical ADME package, it would be appropriate first to outline the overall objectives of pharmacokinetic research as applied to nonclinical drug development.

II. OBJECTIVES OF NONCLINICAL PHARMACOKINETIC STUDIES

A. Support for Pharmacology

It has long been recognized that the intensity and duration of the pharmacological effect of a systemically acting drug are functions not only of the intrinsic activity of the drug but also of its absorption, distribution, and elimination characteristics. Pharmacokinetic data obtained from the pharmacological test species are often useful in the interpretation of drug effects. A typical example is a drug that is active following intravenous administration but is considerably less active after comparable oral doses. Having the appropriate pharmacokinetic results could reveal whether the drug is poorly absorbed to yield subtherapeutic circulating levels or experiences presystemic biotransformation to an inactive metabolite. This would provide guidance for subsequent decisions, for example to improve drug absorption by altering the salt form or formulation, to investigate the possibility of making prodrugs, or to abandon the oral route of administration.

Many drugs show a direct correlation between drug concentration at the target site and pharmacological effect. For example, present knowledge suggests that the bacteriocidal action of antibiotics is directly related to the drug levels at the site of infection, and the bacteriocidal effect is lost when antibiotic levels fall below the minimum inhibitory concentration of the invading organisms. The β blockade induced by sotalol in dogs correlates significantly with the log plasma sotalol concentration (3). Following an intravenous dose of ^{14}C-labeled bromocriptine, the time course of drug-induced hypothermia in cold-room acclimatized rats parallels plasma bromocriptine concentrations but not total radioactivity levels, thus confirming the parent drug as the pharmacologically active entity (4).

Any knowledge of the effective blood or plasma concentration in animals can be used to guide later studies in humans as the drug trial progresses into the clinical phase. Specifically, a drug should not be considered inefficacious in humans prior to achieving circulating levels that approach the effective concentrations in the pharmacological species. Thus, potentially valuable therapeutic agents will not fall into unwarranted disrepute because of underdosing.

For drugs with an extravascular site of dynamic action, there is sometimes a more complicated relationship in the time course of plasma levels and the pharmacological effect produced. Simultaneous modeling of the pharmacokinetics and pharmacodynamics of these drugs is relatively complex, and numerous integrated models have been introduced with varying degrees of success (5-8). This type of elaborate analysis is usually not attempted during the preclinical phase of drug development, although the greater accessibility of tissue drug concentration data in small animals should render them attractive models for testing the applicability of this modeling approach.

B. Support for Toxicology

Perhaps the most important function of animal ADME studies is in the support of preclinical drug safety evaluation. In most subchronic toxicology studies, the drug is administered orally to the test species, often in large doses with no assurance of absorption or dose proportionality. Because the question of absorption or exposure is a crucial parameter in the validation of toxicology studies from both a scientific and a regulatory perspective, it must be carefully addressed for each animal model and the specific mode of administration. The importance of this point is exemplified by the hypocholesterolemic agent probucol. In rhesus monkeys administration of probucol in diets containing large amounts of cholesterol and saturated fat resulted in the death of four of eight animals after several weeks, whereas monkeys maintained on low-fat chow and receiving comparable doses of probucol showed no adverse effects over an 8-year period of continuous drug administration (9). This difference was associated with a significant increase in absorption and resulting blood levels of probucol by lipids (10), a phenomenon that has also been observed in other species (11).

Determination of pharmacokinetic characteristics during the course of a toxicology study may help interpret certain toxicological findings. For example, tissue distribution data may be useful in explaining local toxic manifestations. The occurrence of enzyme inhibition or capacity-limited metabolism may lead to drug accumulation accompanied by toxicity.

Pharmacokinetic data obtained from acute or subchronic studies during the pre-IND phase are useful in the selection of a proper dose range for subsequent chronic toxicological trials. Again the objective is to assure dose-proportional exposure of drug to the test species.

Comparison of the ADME data obtained from animals with those from humans may enable the rational selection of an appropriate animal model for additional toxicity testing, such as carcinogenicity and teratogenicity studies, that will give a more reliable prediction of human safety. Emphasis is often placed on qualitative similarity in overall metabolic pathways between the human and the test species in order to ensure that both are exposed to the parent drug as well as the same metabolites, any of which may contribute to toxicity. Additionally, it is desirable that the selected laboratory species demonstrate absorption and excretion characteristics similar to those of humans.

C. Prediction of Human Pharmacokinetics

Preclinical data on drug absorption and disposition can support and guide informed decisions concerning initial clinical trials during a period when human response to the drug is rudimentary. The animal data may also be helpful in the design of human ADME studies. For a large variety of drugs, the extent of absorption is remarkably consistent between different animal species and the human (12). The actual form of the drug reaching the systemic circulation, however, may differ among species. The following example concerns the hypolipidemic and antiatherosclerotic agent 58-035, an inhibitor of acyl-coenzyme A-cholesterol acyltransferase (13). Compound 58-035 is strongly lipophilic and virtually insoluble in water. In the rat and the dog, gastrointestinal absorption of 58-035 is relatively low; the greatest extent, approximately 20%, is obtained when the dose is administered in corn oil (14). Since the oral absorption of this type of compound is known to be affected by administration in lipid vehicles (15), it is possible that a similar lipid effect may apply to the absorption of 58-035 in humans. With this information at hand, a group of subjects was included in the subsequent human ADME study to receive single oral doses of 58-035 immediately following a high-fat meal, in addition to others that were given the drug on an empty stomach (16). The results indicated that compound 58-035 was poorly absorbed in the fasting state, and administration with the high-fat meal significantly increased the extent of absorption (by nearly 10-fold) to 15% of the dose. Indeed, in those subjects who received [3H]58-035 in the fasting condition, no measurable radio-activity levels were observed in blood at any time. Thus, careful planning with the help of animal data in this case not only served as a pharmacokinetic bridge by confirming an important absorption characteristic in humans, but also aided in interpreting the results of a costly human study that otherwise would have been difficult.

In contrast, the distribution and elimination characteristics of a drug tend to be more variable between species. For example, although the corticosteroid prednisolone is efficiently absorbed in both the dog and humans, its elimination half-life in the human (approximately 3 hr) is nearly three times that observed in the dog (17—19). Marked differences between species were also found in the serum protein binding of prednisolone (20), as illustrated in Figure 1.

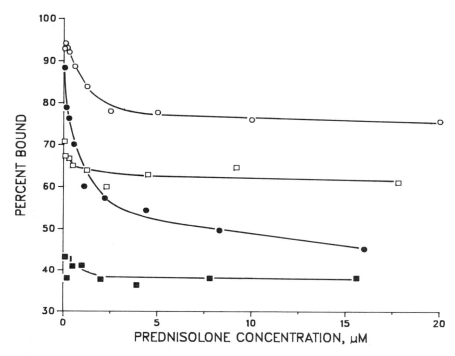

FIGURE 1 Percentage of serum protein binding of prednisolone as a function of concentration in the rabbit (○), dog (□), rat (■), and human (●). (Reproduced with permission from Ref. 20.)

A great deal of the interspecies variations in such important pharmacokinetic parameters as absolute bioavailability, clearance, and elimination half-life may be attributed to the vast qualitative and quantitative differences in the metabolism of a drug by the host organism (21). As a result, direct extrapolation of animal disposition data to humans may not be appropriate. This does not imply, however, that pharmacokinetic data obtained in animals cannot be mathematically manipulated to derive estimates of human pharmacokinetic parameters. As mammals, humans share with other mammalian species many similarities in anatomy, physiology, and biochemistry, which together form the basis of animal scale-up (22). Many anatomic and physiologic variables can be correlated among mammals as exponential functions of body weight, using the simple heterogonic equation (23)

$$Y = aW^b \tag{1}$$

or its logarithmic transformation

$$\log Y = \log a + b \log W \tag{2}$$

where Y is a physiological parameter, W is body weight, a is the allometric coefficient, and b is the allometric exponent. A few examples are shown in Table 1. It appears that the anatomic variables are nearly proportional to body weight but the physiologic processes tend to vary as the 0.7–0.8 power of body weight. Thus, physiologic function per unit of body weight or per unit of organ weight generally decreases as body size increases. In order to use a specific animal as a model for a physiologic or pharmacokinetic parameter, some sort of appropriate time scaling is required (24). Because the smaller species have greater clearance values (ml/min per kg body weight), chronological time in these species must be decelerated relative to the larger species. The concept of physiological or pharmacokinetic time, in which a physiological or pharmacokinetic event becomes the independent variable, has been discussed in detail (25). By using a biologic clock that measured physiological time (heartbeats) rather than chronological time (minutes), Mordenti (26) demonstrated that ceftizoxime half-life was identical in five mammals (Fig. 2). Thus, 50% of a dose of ceftizoxime was eliminated in approximately 7300 heartbeats regardless of the animal species. Similar interspecies correlations have been developed for a variety of drugs (27–29), and many of the current concepts on interspecies scaling were highlighted at a recent symposium organized by the American Pharmaceutical Association (30–34). A limiting factor in this type of pharmacokinetic scale-up appears to be the prerequisite of a relatively large data base. In order to project a pharmacokinetic parameter Y to humans, the values of Y in at least three or four animal species are needed to properly define the straight line described by Equation (2). Such information is often unavailable during the preclinical phase of drug development, which, ironically, is also the time when an accurate prediction of human response to the drug would be most helpful.

D. Screening New Dosage Forms and Formulations

During the process of developing a final drug product, the formulator develops one or more formulations that demonstrate desirable disintegration and dissolution characteristics in vitro. The dosage forms are then studied in humans to evaluate the in vivo release pattern based on the resulting blood level curves. If an adequate blood level profile is obtained, the dosage form is accepted. If no dosage form is acceptable, the entire process must be repeated. With

TABLE 1 Relationship Between Physiological Properties Y and Body
Weight W Among Mammals: $Y = aW^b$

Property Y	Exponent b
Creatinine clearance (ml/hr)	0.69
Inulin clearance (ml/hr)	0.77
PAH clearance (ml/hr)	0.80
Basal oxygen consumption (ml STP per hr)	0.73
Ventilation rate (ml/hr)	0.74
Weight (g)	
Kidneys	0.85
Heart	0.98
Lungs	0.99
Liver	0.87
Stomach and intestines	0.94
Blood	0.99

Source: Data from Reference 23.

sophisticated formulation designs, such as those used in some controlled-release drug delivery systems, repeated trial and error may
be needed before an acceptable product is identified. It should be
apparent that such a development process is not only costly but also
extremely time-consuming, since a typical human bioavailability study
requires the coordination of personnel from pharmacy, drug metabolism, and medical research departments, and often an off-site
study center as well. In order to eliminate unnecessary human studies
with formulations having potentially suboptimal in vivo performance,
a secondary screening procedure in addition to in vitro dissolution
tests can be included prior to clinical trials. One such screen, which
is based on simulated blood level-time curves using the product's in
vitro dissolution data and the drug's pharmacokinetic parameters
in conjunction with a classical pharmacokinetic model, has been described for the development of extended-release oral dosage forms
(35). A simpler and more direct approach is to perform in vivo
screening tests in animals. Thus, formulations with a desirable release

CHRONOLOGICAL CLOCK   BIOLOGICAL CLOCK

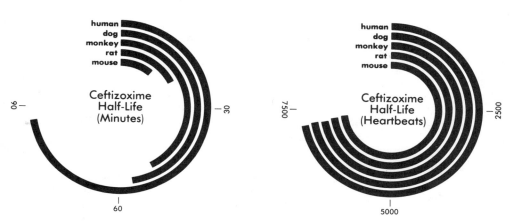

FIGURE 2 Ceftizoxime half-life in various mammals depends on the reference system used to denote time. Chronological clock for ceftizoxime half-life is based on chronological time. Biologic clock for ceftizoxime half-life is based on physiological time. (Reproduced with permission from Ref. 26.)

pattern in vitro are submitted for definitive bioavailability or bioequivalence testing in humans only if they also yield a favorable blood level profile in an animal model.

The key to the successful use of animal data in this manner is the selection of a proper model. Although there is limited information in the literature providing a direct comparison of drug absorption in humans and laboratory animals, the beagle dog has proven to be the most commonly used animal species in bioavailability studies for the following reasons:

1. Oral dosage forms intended for humans can generally be administered intact to dogs. However, it is important to first establish dose proportionality, since the resulting dose per unit body weight would be higher in the dog than in the human.
2. The beagle dog is relatively easy to maintain and handle. Its body weight is sufficiently stable over time to allow repeated studies in the same animal, that is, studies using a crossover design. Approximately 100 ml of blood can be withdrawn from a 10 kg beagle every week for 6 weeks without significantly affecting its normal physiology (36).

3. Dog and human share many similarities in gastrointestinal
    anatomy and physiology (37, 38). Although the dog may differ
    from the human in the absolute bioavailability of drugs owing
    to possible differences in first-pass metabolism, it appears
    to be a good indicator of the relative bioavailability of different
    dosage forms or formulations. Formulation-related absorption
    problems in the dog usually also exist in the human (39).

The suitability of the beagle dog or any other animal model, however, also depends on the specific drug product in question. For
example, owing to slightly higher gastric and intestinal pH values in
dogs than in humans, the absorption of a poorly soluble drug with
a pK_a in the 5—8 range may differ between the two species (40).
The bioavailability of a drug may show a distinct dependence on
gastric acidity in one species but not in the other (41). The extent
of absorption from certain slow-release products may be compromised
by the shorter small intestine of the dog (4 m) than that of humans
(6.5 m) (42). Discrepancies in certain bioavailability parameters
between dogs and humans have also been attributed to more rapid
gastric emptying and transition of drugs in the gastrointestinal
tract of the dog (43, 44). Beagles were found to be a useful model
for bioavailability studies of certain griseofulvin formulations, but
not ultramicrosized tablets (45). As shown in Figure 3, a good correlation of peak plasma concentrations C_{max} between humans and
beagles was obtained for three different microsized griseofulvin
tablets (B, C, and D) but not for the ultramicrosized tablet (A).
    Although bioavailability testing in the dog can provide useful
information on the best choice of formulation for early clinical studies,
the definitive bioavailability data should always be obtained in
humans. In rare occasions when such studies are not ethically permissible or desirable in humans, for example such cytotoxic agents
as methotrexate or cyclophosphamide, the FDA has accepted the use
of validated animal models for evaluating bioequivalence (46).

III. METHODOLOGY

A. Pre-IND Studies

The great majority of pre-IND pharmacokinetic studies are conducted
to support preclinical toxicological findings. Therefore, the discussions
in this section focus on this type of study. Periodically, pharmacokinetic studies are also performed to support other disciplines, that
is, pharmacology, although these normally do not constitute an
integral part of the drug development program.

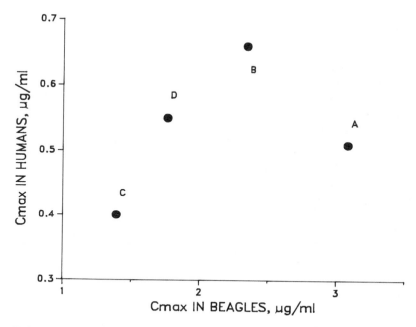

FIGURE 3 Correlation of C_{max} values after oral administration of four griseofulvin formulations between humans and beagles. (Reproduced with permission from Ref. 45.)

1. General Considerations for ADME Studies in Support of IND

a. Animals The species and strain should be the same as those employed in the subchronic toxicity study and should be matched as closely as possible with regard to age, weight, and sex. The rat and beagle dog are most commonly used, although under special circumstances disposition studies in additional species, such as the mouse and the monkey, may also be performed at this stage. The number of animals in each study should be adequate to indicate the variability to be expected within a given species.

b. Drug In order to support toxicological findings, at least two doses encompassing the dose range used in the subchronic toxicity study should be tested. These should be prepared in the same dosage form containing the same excipients in identical proportions as in the subchronic toxicity study and administered via the same

route. Additionally, an intravenous dose is usually included to serve
as a reference standard. Drug disposition should be studied after
a single dose and, preferably, also during multiple dosing.

ADME studies can be greatly facilitated by the use of drug substance appropriately labeled with radioactive isotopes, usually [14]C
or ^{3}H, since this method provides a simple means of obtaining material
balance and allows an estimation of the total exposure to drug-related
material. The decision to start radiosynthesis is usually made when
subchronic toxicity trials are scheduled as a result of promising
pharmacological activity and minimal toxicity in acute studies in
animals. During the synthesis of radiolabeled compounds, the label
should be introduced specifically into a metabolically stable and, in
the case of tritium, nonexchangeable position. Computer programs,
such as CAMP (computer-assisted metabolism prediction), with a
large data base of metabolic transforms have been found useful in
the prediction of biologically stable positions of the compound, thus
facilitating the selection of the most suitable precursor for the
introduction of the label (47). The in vivo stability of tritium labels
can be assessed by preliminary experiments measuring the extent
of tritiated water formation. The tritiated water concentration (dpm/ml)
in the distillate or lyophylisate of urine samples collected during a
designated time interval after dosing, presumably after equilibrium
is reached between urine and the body water pool, is determined.
The value is extrapolated from the midpoint of the collection interval
to zero time, based on the known half-life of tritiated water in the
given species. The percentage of the radioactive dose that is transformed to tritiated water ($\% \ ^{3}H_2O$) can be calculated using Equation
(3):

$$\% \ ^{3}H_2O = \frac{^{3}H_2O \text{ concentration at zero time} \times \text{exchangeable body water volume}}{\text{radioactivity dose}} \times 100\% \tag{3}$$

The exchangeable body water content as well as the half-life of
tritiated water in some mammalian species are shown in Table 2 (48,
49). The stability of ^{14}C labels, on the other hand, is usually determined by the extent of [^{14}C]carbon dioxide formation.

If the drug is likely to or is known to fragment into two major
portions, it may be advantageous to trace both fragments by providing
each with a different label.

The chemical and radiochemical purity of the labeled compound
must be assured prior to use. The desired specific activity of the
administered radioactive drug obviously depends on the dose to be
used as well as the species studied. Doses of ^{14}C of the order of 5

TABLE 2 Volume and Half-Life of Body Water in Some Mammalian Species

Species	Sex	Exchangeable body water (% body weight)	Half-life (days)
Mouse	F	58.5	1.13
Rat	M	59.6	3.53
Rabbit	F	58.4	3.87
Dog	M	66.0	5.14
Cynomolgus monkey	F	64.2	7.23
Rhesus monkey	M	61.6	7.80
Human	M, F	55.3	9.46

Source: Data from References 48 and 49.

μCi/kg for the dog and 20 μCi/kg for the rat yield measurable radio-activity levels in blood even when the oral absorption of the drug is relatively poor (14). Doses of ^{3}H are usually higher (approximately two to three times) than those of ^{14}C owing to lower counting efficiency of the former.

c. *Biologic Samples* Blood, urine, and feces should be collected from all species; bile and various tissues and organs should be collected at least from rats. Ideally, serial samples should be collected for an adequate duration to define the disposition kinetics of the compound and to achieve mass balance. Exhaled air should be collected for the determination of [^{14}C]carbon dioxide when difficulties in achieving mass balance are encountered.

d. *Analysis of Samples* Total radioactivity should be measured in all biologic samples. When methods are available, the parent drug in blood and other selected samples should also be determined. Metabolite patterns should be established in blood, urine, and feces (or bile), usually by liquid chromatography coupled with radioactivity monitoring (50). More definitive metabolism studies in animals, however, are usually not undertaken until phase I, that is, when the drug appears destined to undergo further development in humans. Concurrent human ADME studies at that stage provide the biologic

samples needed for the development of an optimal analytical method
that is suitable for the elucidation of metabolic pathways in animals
as well as humans.

2. Rat ADME Studies

a. *Study Design* If possible, the toxicological studies should be
designed so that extra animals are maintained in the control and the
various dose groups specifically for pharmacokinetic evaluation. After
allowing ample time to achieve steady-state conditions, the rats in
the control group are each given a single radioactive dose and biologic samples are collected to generate single-dose pharmacokinetic
data. The animals in the treatment groups are given four or five
successive doses of radiolabeled drug for the determination of multiple
dosing pharmacokinetic characteristics. Although the administration
of a single radioactive tracer dose to treatment animals at the end
of the toxicity study is sufficient to determine possible self-induced
changes in the pharmacokinetics of some compounds (51), it may not
be valid when applied to compounds that are slowly distributed,
redistributed, eliminated, or accumulated extensively in adipose
tissue (52). Furthermore, the superpositioning of a single radioactive
dose certainly does not reveal any potential accumulation of radioactivity in body tissues and fluids.

The number of rats per dose group and the samples to be collected
in a typical ADME study are shown in Table 3. In this example,
adequate information on the absorption, distribution, and elimination
of the drug would be obtained from 12 rats. Considering a protocol
calling for two dose levels, single and multiple dosing regimens, as
well as a single intravenous reference dose, it would require about
60 animals to study either the male or female alone. The total figure
is often larger since at least one or two of these studies should be
conducted in both genders in order to identify any sex-related differences in drug absorption and disposition (Table 4). The sequence
of the ADME studies outlined in Table 4 may vary, although it is
advisable to conduct the multiple high-dose studies as early as possible
in order to minimize the possibility of losing animals owing to drug-
related deaths. If the toxicologist should decide to increase the high
dose owing to lack of toxicity or decrease the low dose owing to
excessive adverse effects during the course of the toxicity trial,
the respective ADME studies, if already performed, should probably
be repeated at the adjusted dose level.

The applicability of such a program obviously depends on the
duration of the toxicological study. Although the full range of pharmacokinetic experiments can be conducted in parallel with a 26-week
toxicity study, it is virtually impossible to fit into the limited time

TABLE 3 Sample Collection from Each Dose Group in a Typical Rat ADME Study

Number of rats	Sample[a]
3	2 hr tissues[b]
3	24 hr tissues
3	48 hr tissues
3[c]	Serial blood; urine and feces in 12 or 24 hr intervals; tissues at end of study, e.g., 96 hr

[a]The samples are collected at designated times after a single radio-labeled dose or after the final dose during multiple dosing.
[b]Estimated peak time.
[c]During multiple dosing with tracer, predose blood specimens as well as complete urine and feces for each dose interval are also collected from these rats.

span of a 4-week toxicity trial. In the latter case, naive rats can be substituted in the single-dose experiments and can be tested independently of the toxicity study. Naive rats are also used in supplementary experiments, such as those for the determination of drug excretion in the bile or in exhaled air.

b. *Dosing* In most toxicological studies in the rat, the test drug is administered either by gavage or by incorporation in the diet. Dietary drug administration is usually the preferred mode during chronic toxicity studies because of the convenience of the method and the elimination of trauma and potential danger of pulmonary complications caused by intubation. On the other hand, administration by gavage provides a greater control over the amount of drug delivered and the time of dose and is the method of choice for obtaining pharmacokinetic data. There is now sufficient information in the literature to show that the absorption and/or metabolism of an orally dosed drug may be a function of the mode of administration. Boyd (53) suggested that the administration of the entire daily dose in a single gavage to animals is more likely to reveal the maximum toxic potential of chronic human dosing than administration of the compound in the diet. However, subsequent studies conducted by various investigators have produced conflicting results. Although the absorption and bio-availability of the anithypertensive agent captopril were greater after

TABLE 4 Rats Maintained in a Typical 26-Week Toxicity Study for
Pharmacokinetic Evaluation

Drug week to study pharmacokinetics	Sex and dose group	Number of rats	Pharmacokinetic study
10	Male, high	12	Multiple high oral dose
12	Male, low	12	Multiple low oral dose
14	Female, low	12	Multiple low oral dose
16	Male, control	12	Single high oral dose
17	Male, control	12	Single low oral dose
18	Female, control	12	Single low oral dose
19	Male, control	12	Single intravenous dose

gavage doses than after the same doses given in the diet (54), continuous dietary administration of cefatrizine, a cephalosporin antibiotic, yielded higher, albeit later, peak plasma concentrations and
greater overall bioavailability than administration of the same daily
dose once a day by gavage (55). In another study (56), the bioavailability of N-acetylprocainamide was unaffected when administered
in the diet compared with gavage. Therefore, it is apparent that
the effect of gavage or dietary administration on drug absorption
and bioavailability is dependent on the compound. Smyth et al. (57)
showed that the extent of absorption of water-soluble salts of acidic
and basic compounds was equivalent from diet and from oral solutions
but the availability of a water-insoluble, neutral compound incorporated
in the diet was 70% relative to an oral solution of the compound in
polyethylene glycol-400. Other factors, such as potential drug-diet
interactions or binding, must also be considered. Therefore, in order
for the pharmacokinetic data to determine accurately drug exposure
during the toxicity trial, it is important that the same mode of oral
administration be used in both studies.

     For administration by gavage, the correct amount of drug is
suspended or dissolved in an appropriate vehicle to allow a dose
volume of about 10 ml/kg body weight. In order to ensure consistency
throughout the entire dose range, a suspending agent, such as
sodium carboxymethylcellulose (CMC), is often used even if the drug
is readily soluble at the low dose level, since higher doses may exceed
the solubility limit of the drug. To prepare a drug-diet mixture, the

test compound should be incorporated into pulverized diet by geometric dilution (58) using a mortar and pestle. The drug-diet ratio is determined by the intended dose, the rat weight, and the average daily food consumption, whch is approximately 20 g for a 250 g rat. Because of the small amount of drug usually required for a comparatively large quantity of diet, thorough mixing is important and content uniformity must be confirmed by dose assays prior to starting the experiment. The design of the rat cage should be such that any spillage of the mixture is recovered and is not allowed to contaminate the excreta. The actual dose consumed is recorded at the end of each feeding cycle.

In addition to the oral doses, a single intravenous dose should also be administered as a reference standard for the calculation of oral bioavailability and absorption. The intravenous dose level is often selected to be near the lower end of the oral dose range, although its tolerability should first be established using nonradioactive drug. A simple way of intravenous dosing to the rat is by direct injection via the jugular vein exposed surgically under light ether anesthesia (59). Although this method requires surgical preparation of the rat, it appears to be one of the more reliable procedures for intravenous drug administration and, unlike most cannulation techniques, imposes no stress, which may affect at least some aspects of normal physiology resulting in altered drug kinetics (60—63). Intraperitoneal injection, commonly used for the administration of compounds to small animals, is different from intravenous dosing in that drug absorption from the peritoneal cavity is slower (64) and entails passage into the portal circulation, which can result in incomplete systemic bioavailability (65).

  c. *Data Collection* In rat studies, it is generally feasible to monitor concentrations of drug and related materials in blood as well as various tissues and organs. Furthermore, by confining the animals to properly designed cages, mass balance can be achieved as the potential loss of excreta is minimized.

With the development of sensitive analytical methods that require only microsamples of blood, pharmacokinetic data from individual rats can be obtained by serial sample collection. Several methods using a chronic indwelling catheter to facilitate repeated blood collection have been described (66—68), but the animal preparation procedures are elaborate and tedious and are incompatible with prolonged sampling periods in studies involving a large number of animals. A simple alternative to cannulation is the nonsurgical method of bleeding the rat from the cut end of its tail (69). The blood can be easily collected by capillary attraction into heparinized micropipettes of desired capacity (25—250 µl). Despite relatively low regional blood flow (61, 70), the tail vein has been shown to provide valid blood

concentration data for a variety of drugs (59, 71). The orbital sinus
is another commonly used vein for bleeding from the rat (69).

Designated tissues and organs are collected from sacrificed rats
by standard surgical procedures. Aliquots of homogenized tissues
can be combusted in a sample oxidizer, with capture of the radioactive
products in an appropriate absorption medium and incorporation into
a scintillation cocktail. Alternatively, the tissue sample may be dissolved
in a solubilizing agent before being added to the scintillant for radioactivity counting. It should be noted that certain biologic samples
yield colored solutions that may produce severe quenching and low
counting efficiencies. Such samples need to be decolorized prior to
counting. Bleaching agents that have been used for this purpose
include hydrogen peroxide, benzoyl peroxide, sodium borohydride,
sodium hypochlorite, and ammonium borohydride (72). If necessary,
tissue homogenates may be extracted for the isolation and quantitative
determination of parent drug and its metabolites.

The introduction of whole-body autoradiography (WBAR) (73)
provides an alternative method of examining tissue radioactivity.
Based on the photoradiographic localization of a radiolabeled compound
in sagittal sections of the whole animal prepared at appropriate times
postdose, a qualitative pattern of drug distribution and accumulation
in body tissues and fluids can be visualized (74). The technique
is useful in identifying organ or tissue structures with heretofore
unsuspected, high concentrations of drug or metabolite and thus
serves as a complement to pharmacokinetic studies. In recent years,
several methods have been described for the quantitative analysis
of isotope concentration using WBAR preparation and comparative
densitometry (75–77). Most of these methods are based on a comparison of the photographic impression produced by the unknown
sample with those produced by a radioactive chemical standard.
Since the extent of the photographic effect may vary between different
radioactive standards and also between different tissues, it is difficult to establish uniform standards. Thus, this approach requires
further refinement before it can be used in routine pharmacokinetic
studies. The relatively lengthy procedure involved in quantitative
whole-body autoradiography (QWBAR) may be another obstacle to
its wider acceptance. At present, approximately 2 months are required
from the time of sacrifice of the animal to the acquisition of concentration data, although this could be improved by the availability of
more sensitive x-ray films. Film development can also be accelerated
by increasing the dose of radioactivity. It should be noted, however,
that the usual dose required to conduct QWBAR, approximately 25–100
μCi per 200 g rat, is already substantially higher than that needed
for analysis by liquid scintillation counting.

Quantitative collection and analysis of urine and feces at designated intervals postdose provide useful information on the rate and extent of excretion of drug and/or metabolites via the renal and biliary pathways. Biliary excretion can also be studied directly by surgically exposing the common bile duct and inserting a cannula for bile collection (78). A recovery period of at least 24 hr should be allowed prior to administering the test drug in order to avoid possible delays in gastrointestinal transit associated with postoperative adynamic ileus (79). Since the loss of bile components may lead to impaired intestinal absorption, particularly for highly lipophilic drugs (80-86), a means of bile replenishment is usually needed in this type of experiment (87). Furthermore, prolonged depletion of bile can result in a 10- to 20-fold increase in bile salt synthesis and a decrease in biliary volume (88). These changes occur within 1-2 weeks of bile duct cannulation and could influence the biliary excretion and recycling of drugs. However, in experiments of relatively short duration (<1 day), the loss of bile appears to have little effect on the biliary excretion of xenobiotics (89).

A drug that is excreted in the bile enters the intestine, where some or all of the excreted dose may be reabsorbed to complete an enterohepatic cycle. Biliary secretion and intestinal reabsorption may continue until the drug is ultimately eliminated from the body via renal or fecal excretion or any other routes of disposition. Hence, enterohepatic circulation may result in unusually long persistence of drug in the body and may influence such pharmacokinetic parameters as the terminal half-life, the area under the blood level versus time curve (AUC), and possibly estimates of bioavailability (90-95). A direct approach to quantitatively examine the effect of enterohepatic circulation on drug pharmacokinetics is to monitor the biliary excretion and intestinal reabsorption in a "cascade" fashion (96-99). Thus, following drug administration, the bile obtained from a donor animal is administered intraduodenally to a recipient animal, also with a bile fistula, and the excreta from both animals are collected and assayed. Tse et al. (100) described an improved method using a pair of bile duct-duodenum cannula-linked rats. The method permits a realistic approximation of biliary excretion and reabsorption in intact animals and has been applied successfully to the evaluation of enterohepatic circulation of temazepam and metabolites in the rat (101).

For ^{14}C-labeled drugs, the tracer carbon may be incorporated in vivo into carbon dioxide, a potential metabolic product. In clinical investigation, the amount and rate of formation of labeled carbon dioxide as a metabolite have been used as an indicator of various physiologic functions, depending on the substrate used (102). The pharmacokinetic characteristics of a drug that affect the usefulness of carbon dioxide excretion specifically as a measure of liver function

have been examined (103). In nonclinical ADME studies, it is useful
to monitor the radioactivity in expired air if analyses of urine and
feces fail to yield complete recovery of the dose. Following drug
administration, the rat is placed in a special metabolism cage through
which room air is drawn by a vacuum pump. Exhaled breath exiting
the metabolism cage is passed through an appropriate trapping solution,
such as a mixture of 2-ethoxyethanol and 2-aminoethanol (2:1), which
captures the expired $^{14}CO_2$ (104). The trapping solution is replaced
and assayed at designated times postdose so that the total amount of
radioactivity expired as labeled carbon dioxide can be determined.

3. Dog ADME Studies

a. *Study Design* The rationale used for the design of rat ADME
studies as described previously is also generally applicable to studies
in the dog. However, both ethical and practical limitations often
preclude the allocation of a parallel group of dogs in the subchronic
toxicity study specifically for pharmacokinetic evaluation using radiolabeled drug. Instead, the same dogs undergoing toxicity trial can
be used for blood level monitoring if a "cold" assay is available.
Usually, concentrations of the parent drug alone are determined in
serial blood samples obtained after dosing on day 1 and toward the
end of the toxicity study when steady-state conditions can be assumed.
In a typical subchronic toxicity study that involves male and female
dogs and a wide range of oral dose levels (Table 5), this type of
effort provides information on the bioavailability and disposition of
the parent drug as a function of sex, dose, and repeated drug administration. The pharmacokinetic profile can be defined in each dog
and used to interpret toxic manifestations observed in the same animal.

In addition to the relative bioavailability study already described,
naive dogs unassociated with the toxicity trial are used for serial
blood and excreta collection after receiving single doses of radiolabeled drug orally or intravenously (Table 5). Data generated from
these experiments allow the estimation of absolute bioavailability
(of parent drug) and overall absorption (of radioactivity) as well as
describe the elimination pattern of the administered dose. Because
of the relatively long washout period often associated with residual
radioactivity, a crossover design is not usually employed in these
studies.

If necessary, supplementary experiments requiring specific
surgical procedures, for example bile-duct cannulation, may be conducted in the dog. These studies are usually designed to address
specific drug-related problems and are not within the normal routine
of the drug development program.

TABLE 5 Studies in a Typical Dog ADME Program

Study	Dose group	Sex	Number of dogs
Blood level monitoring after single and multiple doses in dogs undergoing subchronic toxicity trial	Control	Male	3
		Female	3
	Low, oral	Male	3
		Female	3
	Middle, oral	Male	3
		Female	3
	High, oral	Male	3
		Female	3
Blood, urine, and feces collection following a single radioactive dose in naive dogs unassociated with the toxicity study	Low, oral	Male	3
	High, oral	Male	3
	Intravenous	Male	3

b. *Dosing* The same high and low oral doses as well as the same dosage form used in the subchronic toxicity study should be chosen for the radioactive dose studies. If a solid dosage form is selected, it is important that the radiolabeled substance be identical to the nonradioactive drug used in the toxicity study with respect to crystal form and particle size. These factors may have a significant influence on the dissolution rate of the product, which in turn may govern the extent of absorption or bioavailability, especially for poorly soluble drugs (105–107). In general, drug absorption is inversely related to particle size when dissolution is rate limiting (108–112). As illustrated in Figure 4, the bioavailability of phenytoin from an encapsulated dose in the dog decreased by a factor of about 3 as the particle size increased from 0–32 to 100 μm (113).

The radiolabeled dose should be administered to dogs under the same condition, fasting or postprandial, as in the toxicity study. Depending on the drug, coadministration of food or fluids may profoundly influence the absorption of oral medications in the dog (114, 115) as it does in the human (116–120).

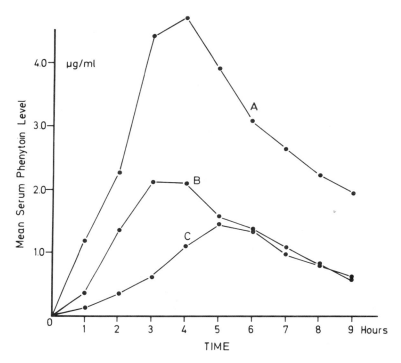

FIGURE 4 Mean serum phenytoin level as a function of time following oral administration of phenytoin (390 mg) of different particle size ranges to three dogs. (A) 0−32 μm, (B) 75 μm, (C) 100 μm. (Reproduced with permission from Ref. 113.)

A side effect frequently associated with the administration of large oral doses to dogs is the induction of emesis. Therefore, prior testing using nonradioactive drug in separate animals is advisable. In extreme cases, it may be necessary to reduce the high dose to a more tolerable level so that complete doses can be administered to, and data gathered from, a sufficient number of dogs. On the other hand, vomiting is not usually a problem in dogs in the toxicity study, as they tend to gain tolerance to the drug upon repeated dosing.

    c. *Data Collection* Serial blood samples can be obtained from the dog by direct venipuncture of the cephalic or femoral veins. Complete urine and feces are collected at designated intervals for a sufficiently long period to recover the administered radioactivity, usually 4−5 days. Fecal samples can be lyophilized and pulverized, or they can be homogenized while wet. Aliquots of homogenized feces are combusted in an oxidizer prior to liquid scintillation counting.

Bile is collected when necessary from dogs with cannulated bile ducts. Marshall et al. (121) described a chronic bile duct cannulation procedure that permits the bile to exteriorize for collection during an experiment but to drain into the intestine between experiments. The loss of bile over a short collection period (1 day) appears to have little or no effect on bile production in the dog (121), which is similar in this respect to the rat (89). As shown in Figure 5, the rate of bile flow in four dogs averaged 4.2 and 4.3 ml/hr, respectively, with and without replacement of bile into the duodenum (121).

Exhaled $^{14}CO_2$ can be collected by restraining the dog in a sling with an airtight plastic cover over its head. The plastic cover should have separate intake and exhaust ports, allowing the animal to breathe normally while simultaneously permitting the quantitative collection of expired air. Exhaled breath is passed through a series of traps in which radiolabeled carbon dioxide is captured.

B. Post-IND Studies

1. Additional ADME Studies

Two types of studies are included in this category: additional, definitive, metabolism studies in the subchronic toxicological species, that is, rat and dog, and ADME studies in additional species, such as mouse, rabbit, and monkey. The former usually entail blood and excreta collection following a single oral dose of radiolabeled drug; the latter are more complete pharmacokinetic studies conducted using single oral and intravenous doses. These studies should be scheduled in phase I, often concurrently with the single-dose human ADME study. At this stage, the optimal analytical methodology for unchanged drug and metabolites should become available for analyzing animal as well as human samples so that valid comparisons can be made between animal and human metabolic data. The primary goal of these studies is to identify one or more animal species in which the metabolic fate is similar to that in humans. If this is not attainable, it may suffice to have two species that between them display all the metabolic pathways present in the human. These species would then be good candidates for chronic toxicity studies to provide the best feasible prediction of human safety.

The additional ADME studies are usually conducted in either male or female animals. Rabbits and monkeys are studied in a manner similar to that used in studying dogs. The dosing and sampling procedures in the mouse are similar to those described for the rat, although

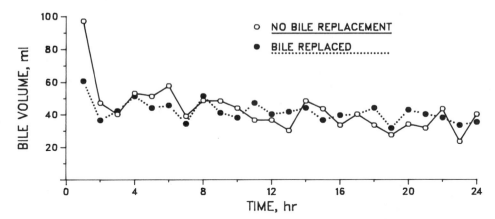

FIGURE 5 Average bile (hourly) collection from four dogs over a 24-hr period studied with and without bile replacements with 1 week between experiments. (Reproduced with permission from Ref. 121.)

serial blood collection is usually not attempted owing to the relatively small blood volume in this species [Table 6 (122–124)]. Instead, a given number of mice are sacrificed at each time point for blood and tissue collection and the mean results used to generate the concentration-time profiles.

In the absence of large interspecies differences in overall excretion pattern, specific excretion studies using bile duct-cannulated rabbits (125) or monkeys (126, 127) are normally not performed. Information on biliary excretion of the drug in these species is usually inferred from the data in rodents, that is, bile concentration from rats with bile fistulas and gallbladder content in the mouse.

2. Placental Transfer Studies

Among the various types of pharmacokinetic studies, those concerning the transfer of drugs from maternal blood to fetus have been most greatly facilitated by the use of laboratory animals. Owing to legal and ethical restrictions, placental transfer studies in humans have been largely confined to the comparison of drug concentrations in umbilical vein and maternal blood at birth. An often nondefinitive characterization of the time course of placental drug transfer can then be deduced by plotting fetal-maternal concentration ratios from different subjects as a function of the dose-delivery interval (128–130). In contrast, animal studies are not usually limited in this regard, and the increased flexibility of experimental design enables the

TABLE 6 Physiological Parameters in Several Species

Parameter	Mouse	Rat	Rabbit	Monkey	Dog	Human
Body weight (g)	22	500	2330	5000	12,000	70,000
Volume (ml)						
Blood	1.7	22.5[a]	—	367	670[b]	5400
Plasma	1.0	19.6	70	220	500	3000
Muscle	10.0	245	1350	2500	5530	35,000
Kidneys	0.34	3.7	15	30	60	280
Liver	1.3	19.6	100	135	480	1350
Gut	1.5	11.3	120	230	480	2100
Heart	0.095	1.2	6	17	120	300
Lungs	0.12	2.1	17	—	120	—
Spleen	0.1	1.3	1	—	36	160
Plasma flow rate (ml/min)						
Plasma	4.4	84.6	520	379	512	3670
Muscle	0.5	22.4	155	50	138	420
Kidneys	0.8	12.8	80	74	90	700
Liver	1.1	4.7	177	92	60	800
Gut	0.9	14.6	111	75	82	700
Heart	0.28	1.6	16	65	60	150
Lungs	4.4	2.3	520	—	512	—
Spleen	0.05	0.95	9	—	14	240

[a]Blood volume in 250 g rat.
[b]Blood volume in 10,000 g dog.
Source: Data from References 122 through 124.

collection of data that would permit the evaluation of a variety of
pharmacokinetic models (131, 132). Studies using ovine maternal-
fetal units have described the rate and extent of transplacental
passage of drugs from ewe to fetus and vice versa, thus providing
insight into important underlying mechanisms, such as the differential
binding of drug to maternal and fetal plasma proteins, placental drug

clearance, and fetal drug elimination (133–137). The major advantage of using sheep is the relatively large size of the fetus, which permits the implantation of catheters for fetal blood collection without sacrificing the animal. Similar studies in rats would necessitate sampling from sacrificed animals (138, 139).

To the scientist in the pharmaceutical industry, the primary purpose of placental transfer studies is to examine the overall extent of fetal exposure to drug that is administered to the pregnant mother, perhaps with less emphasis on the rate of the transfer process. It has been stated that, for both reversibly acting drugs and drugs that produce irreversible effects in the fetus, the ratio of the steady-state drug concentration in the fetus to that in the mother during chronic dosing throughout pregnancy may be used as the index of relative drug exposure (132). The studies are often conducted in rabbits, rats, or mice, the species commonly used for teratogenicity studies.

Female animals are mated with males of the same source and strain. A clear and concise description of the handling and mating of rats, mice, and rabbits can be found in a recent text by Taylor (140). Some breeding characteristics of these species are summarized in Table 7 (141). For rats and mice, mating is confirmed by the presence of vaginal plug, an approximately 3×5 mm coagulated mass of sperm, on the bottom of the cage or in the vagina. A vaginal smear is performed only if no plug is found. The day of mating is generally considered day 0 of gestation.

The test compound is usually administered once daily, beginning on day 6 postconception (PC) and continuing through days 15 or 18 PC depending on the species (Table 7). Dosing prior to day 6 PC may kill the embryo before it implants.

Groups of three or more animals are sacrificed during various stages of pregnancy, for example, at the same time after dosing on days 10 and 13 PC and after the final dose. Additional animals are sacrificed at designated times after the last dose in order to obtain an indication of the rate of drug removal from the body. From each sacrificed animal, maternal blood and major excretory organs, such as liver and kidneys, as well as amniotic fluid, placentas, ovaries, uterus, corpora lutea, and fetuses, are collected for analysis.

Extra animals should be mated and carried through the study to ensure the availability of a sufficient number of pregnant animals. This also allows for misdoses or spontaneous abortions.

3. Studies of Drug Passage into Milk

With the upsurge in breast-feeding in recent years, there has been an increasing concern for infant exposure to drugs via breast milk. The physiological principles of drug transfer to human breast milk

TABLE 7   Some Breeding Characteristics of the Mouse, Rat, and Rabbit

Species	Ovulation interval (days)	Detection of mating	Accepted period of dosing to cover organogenesis (days postconception)	Average duration of gestation (days)
Mouse	4—5	Vaginal plug, or sperm in smear	6—15	19
Rat	4—5	Vaginal plug, or sperm in smear	6—15	22
Rabbit	Induced by mating	Copulation	6—18	31

Source: Data from Reference 141.

have been reviewed (142), and compartmental models have been proposed to describe the kinetics of this process (142, 143). A primary determinant of relative drug concentrations in milk and plasma is the degree of drug ionization, although additional factors, such as lipid solubility and differential drug binding to maternal plasma and milk proteins, also need to be considered. Given that permeation of the mammary epithelium occurs primarily by passive diffusion, the ratio of unbound drug concentration in milk to that in plasma (M/P) for a lipid-soluble drug can be estimated by the following rearrangements of the Henderson-Hasselbach equation (144):

$$\frac{M}{P} = \frac{1 + 10^{(pH_m - pK_a)}}{1 + 10^{(pH_b - pK_a)}} \quad \text{acid} \tag{4}$$

$$\frac{M}{P} = \frac{1 + 10^{(pK_a - pH_m)}}{1 + 10^{(pK_a - pH_b)}} \quad \text{base} \tag{5}$$

where pH_m and pH_b represent the pH of milk (7.0) and blood (7.4), respectively.

For a variety of drugs that are commercially available, the human milk-plasma ratios have been reported based on clinical experience in nursing mothers even though the data are often scanty and somewhat qualitative in nature (145—147). In contrast, the applicability of Equations (4) and (5) to investigational new drugs can be evaluated only in laboratory animals because of obvious legal and ethical concerns.

Usually, drug excretion in milk is studied in a single animal species, such as rat, during phase III of drug development so that a projection of the potential risk to breast-fed infants can be made. In a typical study, approximately 30 rats in their first lactation are used. The litter size is adjusted to about 10 within 1—2 days following parturition. The test drug, usually radiolabeled to facilitate quantitative determination of the parent compound and metabolites, is administered to the mothers 8—10 days after parturition. The rats are then divided into groups for milk and blood collection at designated times postdose. All sucklings are removed from the mother rats several hours before milking. Oxytocin, 1 IU per rat, is given intravenously 5 min before each collection of milk to stimulate milk ejection. The usual yield of milk from each rat is about 1 ml. Immediately after milking, blood is obtained by exsanguination and plasma is separated by centrifugation.

The passage of drug into milk can be estimated as the milk-plasma ratio of drug concentrations at each sampling time or that of the AUC values. If total, that is, free plus protein-bound, drug concentrations are measured, the observed milk-plasma ratio must be adjusted for differential binding in milk and plasma before a valid comparison can be made with the predicted value based on Equation (4) or (5).

4. Blood-Plasma Ratio and Protein Binding Studies

Drugs are delivered to and from tissues in whole blood, yet the ability of a drug to enter extravascular spaces is largely determined by its distribution characteristics within the blood components. Drug in blood may be distributed into erythrocytes or plasma water or may be reversibly bound to plasma proteins. The extent to which a drug is protein bound depends upon the affinity of the protein for the drug, the number of binding sites on the protein molecule for that particular drug, and the concentrations of both drug and protein.

Protein-bound drugs are essentially confined to the plasma volume. In this state they may also be devoid of any pharmacological activity, as is the case for most antibiotics (148). Thus, both the pharmacokinetic and pharmacodynamic properties of a drug can be influenced by plasma protein binding. This subject has continued to generate a great deal of interest in recent years (149—156).

Blood-plasma distribution ratio and plasma protein binding are usually evaluated by in vitro studies. To avoid artifactual results, fresh blood prepared immediately after collection from animals (157) and humans (158) is preferred to preserved blood. The use of an indwelling venous catheter for blood collection (159) and the presence of heparin in the blood sample (160—163) are additional factors that can affect the results of protein binding studies. The importance of radiochemical purity of the radiolabeled drug used for determining plasma protein binding must also be stressed (164—166).

The fresh blood is spiked with radioactive drug and incubated at 37°C for about 30 min. Aliquots of blood are removed for liquid scintillation counting, and plasma is separated from the remaining blood by centrifugation. Aliquots of plasma are then pipetted for radioactivity determination. The fraction of drug in blood that is distributed to red blood cells f_{BC} is given by the equation (167)

$$f_{BC} = 1 - (1 - H) \frac{C_P}{C_B} \tag{6}$$

where H is the hematocrit and C_P and C_B are drug concentrations in plasma and whole blood, respectively. The binding of drug in plasma can be determined by a number of techniques, including equilibrium dialysis, ultrafiltration, ultracentrifugation, and gel filtration (168). Each of these methods has demonstrated certain advantages and disadvantages, but the first two appear to be most popular among routine users. After ultrafiltration or at dialysis equilibrium, the free fraction of drug in plasma is determined from the ratio of drug concentration in the ultrafiltrate or dialysate to that in the original plasma. With both methods, control experiments must be performed to correct for concentration-dependent adsorption of drug to the ultrafiltration filter or dialysis membrane (169). Other sources of error to which equilibrium dialysis may be especially prone include difficulties in attaining equilibrium (170—173) and volume shifts across the membrane due to osmotic differences between the buffer and plasma or serum (165, 174—176). The significance of these potential problems has been discussed, and some solutions offered, in Reference 170 through 176.

Drug-plasma protein binding is usually studied over a concentration range representative of the therapeutic drug levels in humans. This reveals any concentration dependency in the extent of binding. The protein responsible for the nonspecific binding of most drugs is albumin, which comprises about one-half of the total plasma proteins. Nonetheless, many basic drugs often bind to α_1-acid glycoprotein. For drugs that are extensively (>90%) bound, it is desirable to identify the principal drug-binding protein using specific protein solutions. The affinity of the protein for the drug as indicated by the association constant and the number of binding sites on each protein molecule can be deduced using mathematical models (177–179), although these specific parameters tend to have little practical value in drug development.

Protein binding studies are usually conducted in human plasma as well as plasma from various animal species since interspecies differences in drug binding are common (180). If the degree of binding in human plasma is high and if the therapeutic index of the drug is know to be low, competitive binding studies should be performed using plasma spiked with therapeutic agents that are likely to be administered concurrently with the test drug. Any effect of disease states on the protein binding of this type of drug could also be of particular clinical significance (181, 182) and therefore warrants further investigation.

5. Dosage Form Evaluation

The objective of screening new dosage forms and formulations in animal models is to weed out poorly performing candidates prior to bioavailability evaluation in humans. A rapid turnaround time is necessary for this testing procedure to be truly useful to the formulator. Therefore, the study should be designed to require the analysis of a minimum number of samples and sample types. Usually, three to six dogs are used and blood concentrations alone are measured for bioavailability determination (183). Otherwise the study would be similar to a typical human bioavailability study, which is described elsewhere in this book.

C. Miscellaneous Studies

In addition to the routine pharmacokinetic studies in the nonclinical program, animal models are also commonly used in experiments designed to address specific questions or problems that arise during the course of drug development. For example, isolated intestinal segments of the rat (184–186) or dog (187) have been used to study the mechanism and rate of drug absorption in situ when such information cannot be readily derived from blood concentration data following oral administration in conscious animals. Similar surgical preparations have enabled the determination of site-specific absorption from different segments of the gastrointestinal tract (188). This information can provide valuable guidance in the development of dosage forms, especially in the area of controlled-release drug delivery systems.

IV. DATA INTERPRETATION

The discussions in this section focus on the methods of pharmacokinetic analysis that are commonly used for interpreting the results
of nonclinical ADME studies. These studies ordinarily employ a limited
number of animals and therefore may be inadequate to characterize
the population as a whole, particularly in terms of variability. In
fact, individual data are not always available. For example, if the
parent drug is to be determined by reverse isotope dilution (189)
because of the lack of alternative methods, it is often necessary to
pool blood samples from individual animals to provide sufficient radioactivity for measurement. Thus, study conclusions should be formulated
within the context of these limitations, and often only qualitative
or semiquantitative statements can be made.

A. Absorption and Bioavailability

In the framework of the present discussion, absorption is defined
as the process by which a compound and its metabolites are transferred
from the gastrointestinal tract (or another site of application) to the
systemic circulation. Thus, the absorption of a dose in a given animal
reflects the total exposure of the animal to the parent drug as well
as all drug-related materials. In contrast, the bioavailability of a
drug concerns only the rate and extent to which the administered
drug reaches the systemic circulation intact or as the active ingredient.
For an orally dosed compound, the difference between absorption
and bioavailability could be due to chemical degradation in the gastrointestinal tract, microflora metabolism, gut wall metabolism, or presystemic metabolism in the liver. The extent of the first-pass effect
is variable between drugs and tends to be minimal for highly lipophilic
compounds that are preferentially absorbed via the intestinal lymphatic
system (190, 191).

The absolute bioavailability of a drug or drug product can be
estimated by comparison of the resulting plasma drug concentrations
or cumulative urinary excretion to those obtained from an intravenous
reference dose. The extent of bioavailability is often reflected by the
area under the plasma level versus time curve; the rate is indicated
by the peak concentration C_{max} and the time to peak t_{max} following
drug administration. Other methods of determining the rate of bioavailability, more sophisticated and less frequently applied to nonclinical data, were summarized in a recent review (192). Plasma
concentration data can also be evaluated by statistical moment analysis
in terms of mean residence time (MRT) and variance of residence
time (VRT) (193). These values, which are the first normal and
second central moments of the plasma drug profile, respectively, are
defined by Equations (7) and (8):

$$MRT = \frac{\int_0^\infty t \, C \, dt}{AUC} \tag{7}$$

$$VRT = \frac{\int_0^\infty (t - MRT)^2 C \, dt}{AUC} \tag{8}$$

where C is the drug concentration at time t. The MRT and VRT have advantages over other methods of calculating drug bioavailability in that they reflect not only the extent of availability but also the rate of transit of drug molecules through the body. They are also independent of the pharmacokinetic model (193).

On the other hand, the determination of total drug absorption in intact animals is a relatively complicated situation. Applicable information is usually gathered from the following sources.

1. Blood levels: A majority of the animal ADME studies are conducted during the preclinical phase of drug development when relevant metabolism data are either unavailable or fragmentary at best. Therefore, only the composite of all metabolites plus the parent drug can be monitored, that is, as total radioactivity. Although t_{max} and C_{max} of the radiotracer may be indicative of the rate of absorption, the complex nature of the AUC value for total radioactivity requires that this parameter be used only with caution. This point can be elucidated as follows. Assuming that a drug that is completely absorbed into the portal circulation is eliminated both via renal excretion and by hepatic metabolism to form a single metabolite, the AUC of the parent drug after oral administration will be smaller but that of the metabolite will be greater than the respective values after intravenous dosing because of first-pass metabolism. The magnitude of the difference is dependent on the ratio of renal versus hepatic clearances of the drug (194). The decrease in AUC of the parent drug may or may not be equal to the increase in AUC of the metabolite, depending on the relative distribution volumes of the two species. Consequently, the oral-intravenous AUC ratio of total radioactivity (drug + metabolite) can be smaller than, equal to, or even greater than unity, regardless of the extent of absorption. In fact, this ratio would be a true representation of the fraction of dose absorbed only if the drug demonstrates little or no first-pass effect and is studied in a dose range without saturating its usual elimination pathways.

2. Urinary excretion: The ratio of cumulative urinary recovery of radioactivity after oral and intravenous drug administration is a commonly accepted index of absorption (195–197), provided that the excretion pattern (urine-feces ratio) of absorbed radioactivity does not vary significantly with dose and route of administration. This condition can be verified to some extent by showing similar patterns of urinary metabolites following oral and intravenous doses. Under other circumstances, the urinary recovery of an orally administered radioactive dose can still provide useful information, as it represents the minimum amount of drug absorbed (198).

3. Parent drug in feces: Excluding biliary excretion of intact drug, any intact drug recovered in the feces can generally be assumed to represent the unabsorbed portion of dose. However, owing to the possibility of drug metabolism at the gut epithelium (199) or by intestinal microflora (200), the actual amount unabsorbed could be considerably greater. Therefore, unchanged drug in feces should not be used as the sole absorption index but may serve as a secondary, supportive indicator.

4. Excretion in bile duct-cannulated animals: If properly conducted to maintain physiologic conditions, experiments using bile duct-cannulated animals can yield definitive information concerning the extent of drug absorption (201). Following oral administration of a radiolabeled compound, the total recovery of radioactivity in urine and bile would indicate the minimum amount of drug absorbed; any radioactive material present in feces probably represents unabsorbed drug. In addition, the fraction of radioactivity excreted in the bile that undergoes enterohepatic circulation can be calculated after intravenous drug administration using the method of Tse et al. (202), as follows:

$$F_a = \frac{1 - AUC/AUC^*}{F_b} \tag{9}$$

where F_b is the fraction of drug in the body that is excreted in bile and F_a is the fraction of the excreted drug in bile subsequently reabsorbed from the gut. AUC* and AUC are the areas under blood level versus time curves after administering the same dose to control animals and to bile duct-cannulated animals in which biliary recycling is interrupted, respectively. Equation (9) has been used satisfactorily in determining the enterohepatic circulation of temazepam (202)

and diflunisal (203) in rats. F_a can also be estimated without
requiring blood concentration data, provided the cumulative
fecal and biliary excretion in control and bile duct-cannulated
animals, respectively, are measured (202):

$$F_a = \frac{F_b - F_f}{F_b(1 - F_f)} \tag{10}$$

In Equation (10), F_f is the fraction of the administered radioactivity that is recovered in the feces of control animals.
Even in the absence of bile samples, it may be possible to
evaluate biliary excretion indirectly using relative fecal
excretion data after oral and intravenous doses. For example,
if the amount of radioactivity recovered in feces after oral
administration is similar to that after intravenous dosing, it
is probably due to biliary excretion, not unabsorbed drug,
thus inferring complete absorption (204).

A combination of two or more of these indices is often necessary
to provide good insight into the absorption phenomenon. Although
blood concentration analysis can reveal the onset and rate of drug
absorption, the bile duct-cannulated animal model is usually more
reliable for the assessment of the extent of absorption. A potential
flaw associated with the latter, however, is the necessity of surgical
intervention, which could induce stress in the animal. The oral-
intravenous urine quotient in intact animals is a useful indicator of
absorption for drugs that are predominantly excreted in urine. This
method may not be appropriate if the renal route represents only a
minor pathway of drug excretion: any experimental error in urine
collection or analysis would tend to result in relatively large deviations
in absorption estimates.

As stated earlier in this chapter, animal data can usually provide
a good prediction of the extent of drug absorption, although not
necessarily of bioavailability, in humans. Therefore, the "no-effect"
dose found in preclinical toxicity trials should be qualified by the
fraction of dose absorbed in the same species before it is used in
selecting the initial human dose to be employed in clinical studies.

B. Distribution

The concentrations of drug-related material (total radioactivity) in
major tissues and organs reveal the degree of transient exposure
of specific organs to the drug. Comparison of tissue and circulating
concentrations can give a direct indication of the relative affinity

of the drug to tissue and blood components. With adequate sampling at appropriate intervals after a single dose, the half-life of radioactivity decline in each organ can be calculated. The results are useful in predicting the extent of drug accumulation in tissues and organs, which can be verified by multiple dosing experiments. Furthermore, selected tissue and biofluid concentrations obtained in placental transfer studies are used to determine the extent of fetal exposure to the drug taken during pregnancy.

Perhaps a more important use of tissue concentration and half-life data is for the projection of radioactivity exposure to human subjects during clinical ADME studies. The method of calculation is detailed in Chapter 5. This information is required by most institutional review boards before approving study protocols that involve the administration of radiolabeled drugs to humans.

C. Metabolism

The role of drug metabolism in the overall disposition of a foreign compound is discussed fully in Chapter 10, and a wealth of currently available methods for the isolation, identification, and quantitative determination of metabolites is presented in Chapter 11. The discussion here does not elaborate further on these topics but instead focuses on some of the characteristic features of metabolism work conducted in conjunction with animal ADME studies.

As indicated previously, the doses employed in nonclinical ADME studies usually encompass the relatively broad range used in the subchronic toxicity trial. This provides an excellent opportunity to examine the potential effect of dose size on drug metabolism (205–207). An increase in dose frequently leads to a change in the pattern of metabolites (208, 209). Furthermore, the influence of the route of administration on metabolite formation can also be investigated (210).

A variety of biologic samples, that is, blood, urine, feces, bile, liver, and so on, are usually collected in ADME studies and can be used for metabolism work. This not only facilitates the isolation of most of the metabolites formed but also provides information on the excretory pathways of these biotransformation products.

Typical ADME studies in the primary toxicological species, that is, rat and dog, often include a chronic dosing regimen. Comparison of the metabolite patterns following a single dose and at steady state indicates if the drug induces (211–213) or inhibits (214) its own metabolism.

The main objective of biotransformation studies in animals is to identify those species in which the metabolic fate of the drug is similar to that in humans. This is extremely important in the drug development process since the finding of similar metabolic pathways in animals and humans validates the use of certain animal species in lieu of humans in long-term tolerance studies. Additionally, similarities in biotransformation processes between animals and humans, coupled with similar absorption and excretion characteristics, justify the use of animal models in such areas as new dosage form development, evaluation of novel routes of administration, and drug-drug interaction studies.

D. Excretion

One of the primary objectives of ADME studies is to show that the administered dose is readily excreted from the body, presumably after exerting its intended therapeutic effect. In order to facilitate the achievement of mass balance, radiolabeled drug is almost always used in these studies. By quantitative collection of excreta at sufficient frequency, it is possible not only to provide information on the overall excretion pattern, that is, percentage of dose in urine, feces, and so on, but also to allow an assessment of the rate of elimination.

More often, however, the elimination rate of a drug is evaluated in terms of its terminal half-life in blood. The half-life is a useful kinetic parameter that indicates the time required to attain and decay from steady-state conditions after institution of a particular dosing regimen. Thus, blood concentration versus time data are plotted on semilogarithmic paper, and the terminal, log-linear phase of the curve is established. A linear regression analysis of the data points constituting this phase is performed, and the half-life can subsequently be calculated from the slope of the resulting line. The key to success with this method lies entirely in properly defining the terminal phase. As pointed out by Wagner (215), the true terminal phase is likely to be missed if blood samples are not collected for an adequate length of time or if a relatively insensitive assay method is used. These circumstances usually result in an underestimate of the elimination half-life. On the other hand, a problem almost unique to ADME studies using radiolabeled drugs has been attributed to the very high sensitivity of liquid scintillation counting. By adopting the proper counting strategy, that is, counting all samples to the same statistical error by accumulating the same number of total counts rather than the common, although incorrect, practice of counting all samples for a preset time period (216), reliable measurements can be obtained even at very low radioactivity levels. This has frequently led to a terminal phase of low but lasting blood concentrations, hence a relatively long half-life. The significance of this half-life on the accumulation of drug-related material upon chronic dosing is unfortunately difficult to determine. The simple method proposed by Benet (217), which judges the relevance of a half-life by its contribution to the total AUC, is not appropriate for evaluating total radioactivity data owing to the complex nature of the concentration value. Nonetheless, it is possible that the long half-life represents only a small fraction of the dose that is reversibly bound to and slowly released from a specific tissue depot, perhaps in the form of a metabolite. If such binding is saturable, the half-life will indeed not be predictive of accumulation. An interesting example of this phenomenon concerns the angiotensin-converting enzyme inhibitor enalaprilat. Enalaprilat is usually given as enalapril, the ethyl ester of enalaprilat that is well absorbed orally and rapidly and extensively hydrolyzed to the active diacid (218). In a recent study (219), repeated daily administration of enalapril to healthy volunteers resulted in little accumulation of enalaprilat inconsistent with the reported terminal half-life of approximately 35 hr following a single oral dose (220). The investigators postulated that the terminal phase of the enalaprilat serum profile represents binding of enalaprilat to angiotensin-converting enzyme and that this binding involves a finite amount of drug, regardless of the dose administered. Thus, the terminal phase would effectively have a fixed or "one-time" contribution to accumulation, contrary to the additive contribution by successive doses in a linear process. It was suggested that under such circumstances, steady-state blood level or urinary recovery data be used to estimate an effective half-life, that is, one that is consistent with the observed accumulation of drug during chronic dosing. In ADME studies that include a multiple dosing regimen, the effective half-life $t_{\frac{1}{2},\text{eff}}$ can be calculated as follows (221):

$$t_{\frac{1}{2},\text{eff}} = \frac{0.693}{\omega} \tag{11}$$

where

$$\omega = -\frac{\ln(1 - 1/R)}{\tau} \tag{12}$$

In Equation (12), τ is the dose interval and R is the accumulation ratio. The value of R is usually estimated by one of the following methods:

$$R = \frac{AUC_{0-\tau(ss)}}{AUC_{0-\tau(1)}} \tag{13}$$

$$R = \frac{C_{\min(ss)}}{C_{\min(1)}} \tag{14}$$

where $AUC_{0-\tau(1)}$ and $AUC_{0-\tau(ss)}$ are the AUC values during a dose interval following a single dose and at steady state, respectively, and $C_{min(1)}$ and $C_{min(ss)}$ are the blood concentrations immediately prior to the administration of the second dose and any dose at steady state, respectively (222). Equation (13) is the preferred method if sufficient serial blood samples are available after dosing on both day 1 and at steady state to determine the respective AUC values. Equation (14) is more susceptible to error in that excessive weight is placed on a single determinant $C_{min(1)}$, even though $C_{min(ss)}$ can usually be obtained as the mean of several predose concentrations at steady state.

Thus, the relevance of the half-life obtained from a single dose in predicting drug or radioactivity accumulation and the time required to reach steady state can be verified by multiple dosing experiments. It also should be noted that chronic administration of a drug can lead to altered elimination characteristics, such as induced metabolism, which may or may not be reflected in a change in its elimination half-life in blood. For example, increased first-pass metabolism without a significant effect on subsequent drug disappearance rate has been reported for drugs subject to a high hepatic (flow-limited) clearance (223).

The excretion data obtained from animals are useful in the design of human ADME studies. Despite the marked differences in the relative urine and bile flow rates among various species (Table 8), which could lead to differences in the relative importance of the renal and biliary excretory pathways, the total recovery of administered radio-activity is usually similar among species. Thus, if the combined recovery in animal urine and feces is considerably less than the amount administered, it would be advisable to collect additional sample types, such as exhaled air if the drug is ^{14}C-labeled, in the subsequent human ADME study. The half-lives in preclinical species can provide guidance in the selection of an adequate duration of sample collection.

Finally, it is appropriate to comment briefly on the projection of animal data to humans concerning the excretion of drugs via breast milk. First, the serial drug concentrations in milk and plasma of the animal model are used to calculate the respective AUC values, the ratio of which indicates the extent of drug passage into milk. This ratio is then applied to the average plasma concentration in humans to obtain the average milk level following a given dose. Based on an approximate milk consumption of 150 ml/kg per day by an average infant (224), the quantity of drug received in the milk can be readily calculated. For example, if data in the rat show a milk-plasma drug AUC ratio of 5, an average plasma concentration of 1 ng/ml observed after a 5 mg dose would correspond to an average milk level of 5 ng/ml. Therefore, the maximum amount of drug that an infant could be

TABLE 8 Average Bile and Urine Flow Rates in Different Species

Species	Bile flow (ml/kg per day)	Urine flow (ml/kg per day)
Mouse	100	50
Rat	90	200
Rabbit	120	60
Dog	12	30
Rhesus monkey	25	75
Human	5	20

Source: Data from Reference 12.

exposed to by ingesting 1 liter of milk per day would be 5 μg, that is, about 0.1% of the adult dose. Indeed, available data in humans have shown that the quantity of drug administered via nursing is considerably less than 1% of the adult dose in most cases (145).

V. SUMMARY

As stated in the introduction, there continues to be a lack of clearly defined regulatory guidelines in the area of nonclinical pharmaco-kinetic research. Attempts have been made here to describe a basic program of studies that appears to meet the usual requirements of nonclinical drug metabolism and pharmacokinetic input to IND and NDA applications. When appropriate, pharmacokinetic principles have been discussed with emphasis on the issues and problems that are more or less specific to these types of studies.

A current trend that will surely continue is the conduct of pharma-cokinetic studies in parallel with nonclinical safety assessment, if not in the same animals used in the toxicity trials. Thus, one can expect a growing need for good communication and close collaboration between the pharmacokineticist and the toxicologist. For example, a great deal of effort in planning and coordinating activities is required in order to assure the timely availability of the radiolabeled drug, a validated analytical method, and capacity in the pharma-cokinetics laboratory to handle the animals and biologic samples promptly upon their transfer from the toxicity study site. Furthermore, if pharmacokinetic data obtained using animals in the toxicity study are to be included in the toxicity study report as part of an IND or NDA application, the pharmacokinetic study then becomes an integral part of a toxicity trial and is no longer excluded from coverage under the Good Laboratory Practice (GLP) regulations (225). Special attention to assure compliance with the additional regulatory requirements in operating standards is warranted.

Since an overwhelming majority of nonclinical pharmacokinetic studies are conducted in living animals, it is appropriate to close this chapter with a few words on the sensitive and often controversial issue of laboratory animal welfare. Although normal experimental procedures used in drug metabolism and pharmacokinetic studies tend to cause minimum pain or distress, it is unlikely that this type of research in animals can completely escape the fire from animal welfare groups. Inasmuch as there is a growing public concern with the inhumane treatment of animals, scientists should begin planning how they might cope with an understandably increasing level of regulatory intervention in animal research. The latest amendments to the Animal Welfare Act, effective December 1986, strengthened standards for laboratory animal care and increased enforcement of the act (226). Every institution in the United States that utilizes animals for research is now required to appoint an institutional animal committee, whose primary responsibilities are to review all research protocols involving the use of animals, to assure the proper care and treatment of laboratory animals in accordance with federal, state, and local regulations, and to conduct frequent inspections of all animal facilities. Although the exact impact of these regulatory activities on the actual conduct of research is yet uncertain, one message comes across clearly: The use of animals in lieu of humans in preliminary and risky drug testing is a privilege, not a right. Only through a conscientious effort to avoid the misuse and unnecessary use of these animals can we continue to enjoy this privilege.

REFERENCES

1. V. C. Glocklin. General considerations for studies of the metabolism of drugs and other chemicals. Drug Metab. Rev. 13: 929–939, 1982.
2. V. C. Glocklin. Preclinical application of drug disposition data. PMA-Drug Metabolism Subsection Annual Meeting, Philadelphia, September 12, 1984.
3. T. Ishizaki and K. Tawara. Relationship between pharmacokinetics and pharmacodynamics of the beta adrenergic blocking drug sotalol in dogs. J. Pharmacol. Exp. Ther. 211: 331–337, 1979.
4. H. F. Schran, F. L. S. Tse, and S. I. Bhuta. Pharmacokinetics and pharmacodynamics of bromocriptine in the rat. Biopharm. Drug Dispos. 6: 301–311, 1985.

5. L. B. Sheiner, D. R. Stanski, S. Vozeh, R. D. Miller, and J. Ham. Simultaneous modeling of pharmacokinetics and pharmacodynamics: Application to d-tubocurarine. Clin. Pharmacol. Ther. 25: 358–371, 1979.

6. N. H. G. Holford and L. B. Sheiner. Pharmacokinetic and pharmacodynamic modeling in vivo. Crit. Rev. Bioeng. 5: 273–322, 1981.

7. W. A. Colburn. Simultaneous pharmacokinetic and pharmacodynamic modeling. J. Pharmacokinet. Biopharm. 9: 367–388, 1981.

8. B. E. Dahlström, L. K. Paalzow, G. Segre, and Å. J. Agren. Relationship between morphine pharmacokinetics and analgesia. J. Pharmacokinet. Biopharm. 6: 41–53, 1978.

9. Physicians' Desk Reference, 40th ed. Medical Economics Co., Oradell, New Jersey, 1986, p. 1230.

10. H. A. Eder. The effect of diet on the transport of probucol in monkeys. Artery 10: 105–107, 1982.

11. K. J. Palin and C. G. Wilson. The effect of different oils on the absorption of probucol in the rat. J. Pharm. Pharmacol. 36: 641–643, 1984.

12. B. Clark and D. A. Smith. Pharmacokinetics and toxicity testing. Crit. Rev. Toxicol. 12: 343–385, 1984.

13. J. D. Veldhuis, J. F. Strauss, S. L. Silavin, and L. A. Kolp. The role of cholesterol esterification in ovarian steroidogenesis: Studies in cultured swine granulosa cells using a novel inhibitor of acyl coenzyme A:cholesterol acyltransferase. Endocrinology 116: 25–30, 1985.

14. F. L. S. Tse and J. M. Jaffe. Disposition of a silicon-containing amide, an inhibitor of acyl-CoA:cholesterol acyltransferase, in dog and rat. Biopharm. Drug Dispos. 8: 437–448, 1987.

15. K. J. Palin. Lipids and oral drug delivery. Pharm. Int. 6: 272–275, 1985.

16. F. L. S. Tse and J. M. Jaffe. Influence of high-fat meal on the absorption of a silicon-containing amide, an inhibitor of acyl-CoA:cholesterol acyltransferase, in man. Biopharm. Drug Dispos., in press.

17. F. L. S. Tse and P. G. Welling. Prednisolone bioavailability in the dog. J. Pharm. Sci. 66: 1751–1754, 1977.

18. M. E. Pickup. Clinical pharmacokinetics of prednisone and prednisolone. Clin. Pharmacokinet. 4: 111–128, 1979.

19. J. G. Gambertoglio, W. J. C. Amend, Jr., and L. Z. Benet. Pharmacokinetics and bioavailability of prednisone and prednisolone in healthy volunteers and patients: A review. J. Pharmacokinet. Biopharm. 8: 1–52, 1980.

20. M. L. Rocci, Jr., N. F. Johnson, and W. J. Jusko. Serum protein binding of prednisolone in four species. J. Pharm. Sci. 69: 977–978, 1980.

21. B. B. Brodie. Of mice, microsomes and men. Pharmacologist 6: 12–26, 1964.

22. R. L. Dedrick. Animal scale-up. J. Pharmacokinet. Biopharm. 1: 435–461, 1973.

23. E. F. Adolph. Quantitative relations in the physiological constitutions of mammals. Science 109: 579–585, 1949.

24. R. L. Dedrick, K. B. Bischoff, and D. S. Zaharko. Interspecies correlation of plasma concentration history of methotrexate (NSC-740). Cancer Chemother. Rep. Part 1 54: 95–101, 1970.

25. H. Boxenbaum. Interspecies scaling, allometry, physiological time, and the ground plan of pharmacokinetics. J. Pharmacokinet. Biopharm. 10: 201–227, 1982.

26. J. Mordenti. Forecasting cephalosporin and monobactam antibiotic half-lives in humans from data collected in laboratory animals. Antimicrob. Agents Chemother. 27: 887–891, 1985.

27. H. Boxenbaum. Interspecies variation in liver weight, hepatic blood flow, and antipyrine intrinsic clearance: Extrapolation of data to benzodiazepines and phenytoin. J. Pharmacokinet. Biopharm. 8: 165–176, 1980.

28. E. A. Swabb and D. P. Bonner. Prediction of aztreonam pharmacokinetics in humans based on data from animals. J. Pharmacokinet. Biopharm. 11: 215–223, 1983.

29. Y. Sawada, M. Hanano, Y. Sugiyama, and T. Iga. Prediction of the disposition of β-lactam antibiotics in humans from pharmacokinetic parameters in animals. J. Pharmacokinet. Biopharm. 12: 241–261, 1984.

30. F. E. Yates and P. N. Kugler. Similarity principles and intrinsic geometries: Contrasting approaches to interspecies scaling. J. Pharm. Sci. 75: 1019–1027, 1986.

31. J. Mordenti. Man versus beast: Pharmacokinetic scaling in mammals. J. Pharm. Sci. 75: 1028–1040, 1986.

32. E. J. Calabrese. Animal extrapolation and the challenge of human heterogeneity. J. Pharm. Sci. 75: 1041–1046, 1986.

33. R. L. Dedrick. Interspecies scaling of regional drug delivery. J. Pharm. Sci. 75: 1047–1052, 1986.

34. H. Boxenbaum. Time concepts in physics, biology, and pharmacokinetics. J. Pharm. Sci. 75: 1053–1062, 1986.

35. L. J. Leeson, D. Adair, J. Clevenger, and N. Chiang. The in vitro development of extended-release solid oral dosage forms. J. Pharmacokinet. Biopharm. 13: 493–514, 1985.

36. R. D. Smyth, K. A. Dandekar, F. H. Lee, A. F. DeLong, and A. Polk. Use of the dog in bioavailability and bioequivalence testing. In Animal Models for Oral Drug Delivery in Man: In Situ and In Vivo Approaches. Edited by W. Crouthamel and A. C. Sarapu. American Pharmaceutical Association, Washington, D.C., 1983, pp. 125–148.

37. W. J. Hamilton. Textbook of Human Anatomy. Macmillan, London, 1957, p. 508.

38. A. C. Anderson. The Beagle as an Experimental Dog. Iowa State University Press, Ames, Iowa, 1970, p. 226.

39. W. Crouthamel and I. Bekersky. Preclinical evaluation of new drug candidates and drug delivery systems in the dog. In Animal Models for Oral Drug Delivery in Man: In Situ and In Vivo Approaches. Edited by W. Crouthamel and A. C. Sarapu. American Pharmaceutical Association, Washington, D.C., 1983, pp. 107–123.

40. C. Y. Lui, G. L. Amidon, R. R. Berardi, D. Fleisher, C. Youngberg, and J. B. Dressman. Comparison of gastrointestinal pH in dogs and humans: Implications on the use of the beagle dog as a model for oral absorption in humans. J. Pharm. Sci. 75: 271–274, 1986.

41. H. Ogata, N. Aoyagi, N. Kaniwa, A. Ejima, T. Kitaura, T. Ohki, and K. Kitamura. Evaluation of beagle dogs as an animal model for bioavailability testing of cinnarizine capsules. Int. J. Pharm. 29: 121–126, 1986.

42. M. J. Swenson. Dukes Physiology of Domestic Animals. Cornell University Press, Ithaca, New York, 1970, p. 220.

43. H. Ogata, N. Aoyagi, N. Kaniwa, M. Koibuchi, T. Shibazaki, A. Ejima, T. Shimamoto, T. Yashiki, Y. Ogawa, Y. Uda, and Y. Nishida. Correlation of the bioavailability of diazepam from uncoated tablets in beagle dogs with its dissolution rate and bioavailability in humans. Int. J. Clin. Pharmacol. Ther. Toxicol. 20: 576–581, 1982.

44. N. Aoyagi, H. Ogata, N. Kaniwa, A. Ejima, H. Nakata, J. Tsutsumi, T. Fujita, and I. Amada. Bioavailability of indomethacin capsules in humans (III): Correlation with bioavailability in beagle dogs. Int. J. Clin. Pharmacol. Ther. Toxicol. 23: 578–584, 1985.

45. N. Aoyagi, H. Ogata, N. Kaniwa, M. Koibuchi, T. Shibazaki, A. Ejima, N. Tamaki, H. Kamimura, Y. Katougi, and Y. Omi. Bioavailability of griseofulvin from tablets in beagle dogs and correlation with dissolution rate and bioavailability in humans. J. Pharm. Sci. 71: 1169–1172, 1982.

46. E. D. Purich and J. P. Hunt. The use of animal models in new drug evaluation. In Animal Models for Oral Drug Delivery in Man: In Situ and In Vivo Approaches. Edited by W. Crouthamel and A. C. Sarapu. American Pharmaceutical Association, Washington, D.C., 1983, pp. 163–177.

47. R. Voges, B. R. Von Wartburg, and H. R. Loosli. Tritiated compounds for in vivo investigations: CAMP and ^{3}H-NMR-spectroscopy for synthesis planning and process control. In Synthesis and Applications of Isotopically Labeled Compounds 1985. Edited by R. R. Muccino. Elsevier, Amsterdam, 1986, pp. 371–376.

48. C. R. Richmond, W. H. Langham, and T. T. Trujillo. Comparative
    metabolism of tritiated water by mammals. J. Cell. Comp. Physiol.
    59: 45—53, 1962.
49. E. Azar and S. T. Shaw, Jr. Effective body water half-life and
    total body water in rhesus and cynomolgus monkeys. Can. J.
    Physiol. Pharmacol. 53: 935—939, 1975.
50. F. L. S. Tse, D. A. Orwig, T. Chang, L. Guarducci, and
    J. M. Jaffe. Effect of age on the disposition of ∝-[(dimethyl-
    amino)methyl]-2-(3-ethyl-5-methyl-4-isoxazolyl)-1H-3-indole-
    methanol in the rat. Drugs Exp. Clin. Res. 10: 225—234, 1984.
51. R. Hammer and G. Bozler. Pharmacokinetics as an aid in the
    interpretation of toxicity tests. Arzneimittel Forsch. 27: 555—557,
    1977.
52. W. A. Colburn and H. B. Matthews. Pharmacokinetics in the
    interpretation of chronic toxicity tests: The last-in, first-out
    phenomenon. Toxicol. Appl. Pharmacol. 48: 387—395, 1979.
53. E. M. Boyd. Predictive drug toxicity: Assessment of drug safety
    before human use. Can. Med. Assoc. J. 98: 278—293, 1968.
54. S. M. Singhvi, K. J. Kripalani, A. V. Dean, G. R. Keim, J. S.
    Kulesza, F. S. Meeker, Jr., J. J. Ross, Jr., J. M. Shaw, and
    B. H. Migdalof. Absorption and bioavailability of captopril in
    mice and rats after administration by gavage and in the diet.
    J. Pharm. Sci. 70: 885—888, 1981.
55. D. R. Van Harken and G. H. Hottendorf. Comparative absorption
    following the administration of a drug to rats by oral gavage and
    incorporation in the diet. Toxicol. Appl. Pharmacol. 43: 407—410,
    1978.
56. B. L. Kamath, A. Yacobi, S. D. Gupta, H. Stampfli, M. Durrani,
    and C.-M. Lai. Bioavailability of N-acetylprocainamide from
    mixed diet in rats. Res. Commun. Chem. Pathol. Pharmacol. 32:
    299—308, 1981.
57. R. D. Smyth, R. C. Gaver, K. A. Dandekar, D. R. Van Harken,
    and G. H. Hottendorf. Evaluation of the availability of drugs
    incorporated in rat laboratory diet. Toxicol. Appl. Pharmacol.
    50: 493—499, 1979.
58. L. L. Augsburger. Powdered dosage forms. In Sprowls' American
    Pharmacy, 7th ed. Edited by L. W. Dittert. J. B. Lippincott,
    Philadelphia, 1974, p. 313.
59. F. L. S. Tse, T. Chang, B. Finkelstein, F. Ballard, and J. M.
    Jaffe. Influence of mode of intravenous administration and blood
    sample collection on rat pharmacokinetic data. J. Pharm. Sci.
    73: 1599—1602, 1984.
60. D. M. Cocchetto and T. D. Bjornsson. Methods for vascular
    access and collection of body fluids from the laboratory rat.
    J. Pharm. Sci. 72: 465—492, 1983.

61. W. M. Johannessen, I. M. Tyssebotn, and J. Aarbakke. Antipyrine and acetaminophen kinetics in the rat: Comparison of data based on blood samples from the cut tail and a cannulated femoral artery. J. Pharm. Sci. 71: 1352–1356, 1982.

62. W. F. Bousquet, B. D. Rupe, and T. S. Miya. Endocrine modification of drug responses in the rat. J. Pharmacol. Exp. Ther. 147: 376–379, 1965.

63. R. E. Stitzel and R. L. Furner. Stress-induced alterations in microsomal drug metabolism in the rat. Biochem. Pharmacol. 16: 1489–1494, 1967.

64. F. L. S. Tse and P. G. Welling. Bioavailability of parenteral drugs. II. Parenteral doses other than intravenous and intramuscular routes. J. Parenteral Drug Assoc. 34: 484–495, 1980.

65. G. Lukas, S. D. Brindle, and P. Greengard. The route of absorption of intraperitoneally administered compounds. J. Pharmacol. Exp. Ther. 178: 562–566, 1971.

66. R. S. Pope. Small vessel cannulator. J. Appl. Physiol. 24: 276, 1968.

67. B. Scharschmidt and P. D. Berk. A simple device to facilitate rapid blood sampling in small animals. Proc. Soc. Exp. Biol. Med. 143: 364–366, 1973.

68. R. A. Upton. Simple and reliable method for serial sampling of blood from rats. J. Pharm. Sci. 64: 112–114, 1975.

69. H. B. Waynforth. Experimental and Surgical Technique in the Rat. Academic Press, London, 1980, p. 68.

70. R. P. Rand, A. C. Burton, and T. Ing. The tail of the rat, in temperature regulation and acclimatization. Can. J. Physiol. Pharmacol. 43: 257–267, 1965.

71. F. L. S. Tse, T. Chang, and J. M. Jaffe. Effect of butalbital and phenobarbital pretreatment on antipyrine clearance in the rat. Arch. Int. Pharmacodyn. Ther. 279: 181–194, 1986.

72. W. R. Hendee. Radioactive Isotopes in Biological Research. Wiley-Interscience, New York, 1973, p. 189.

73. S. Ullberg. Studies on the distribution and fate of S^{35}-labelled benzylpenicillin in the body. Acta Radiol. (Suppl.) 118: 1–110, 1954.

74. J. I. Williams, S. I. Bhuta, J. M. Jaffe, B. H. Migdalof, H. J. Schwarz, K. C. Talbot, J. F. Brouillard, P. Donatsch, C. Hodel, M. Lemaire, J. Meier, and A. Schweitzer. Absorption, distribution, and excretion of fluproquazone in several animal species. Arzneimittel Forsch. 31(I): 897–904, 1981.

75. R. D. Irons and E. A. Gross. Standardization and calibration of whole-body autoradiography for routine semiquantitative analysis of the distribution of ^{14}C-labeled compounds in animal tissues. Toxicol. Appl. Pharmacol. 59: 250–256, 1981.

76. F. Keller and P. G. Waser. Quantification in macroscopic auto-
     radiography with carbon-14. An evaluation of the method. Int.
     J. Appl. Radiat. Isot. 33: 1427—1432, 1982.
77. J. R. Unnerstall, D. L. Niehoff, M. J. Kuhar, and J. M.
     Palacios. Quantitative receptor autoradiography using [^{3}H]ultro-
     film: Application to multiple benzodiazepine receptors. J. Neurosci.
     Methods 6: 59—73, 1982.
78. P. W. Tomlinson, D. J. Jeffery, and C. W. Filer. A novel
     technique for assessment of biliary secretion and enterohepatic
     circulation in the unrestrained conscious rat. Xenobiotica 11:
     863—870, 1981.
79. J. B. Furness and M. Costa. Adynamic ileus, its pathogenesis
     and treatment. Med. Biol. 52: 82—89, 1974.
80. T. R. Bates, M. Gibaldi, and J. L. Kanig. Solubilizing properties
     of bile salt solutions. I. Effect of temperature and bile salt
     concentration on solubilization of glutethimide, griseofulvin, and
     hexestrol. J. Pharm. Sci. 55: 191—199, 1966.
81. T. R. Bates, M. Gibaldi, and J. L. Kanig. Solubilizing properties
     of bile salt solutions. II. Effect of inorganic electrolyte, lipids,
     and a mixed bile salt system on solubilization of glutethimide,
     griseofulvin, and hexestrol. J. Pharm. Sci. 55: 901—906, 1966.
82. S. Feldman and M. Gibaldi. Physiologic surface-active agents
     and drug absorption. I. Effect of sodium taurodeoxycholate on
     salicylate transfer across the everted rat intestine. J. Pharm.
     Sci. 58: 425—428, 1969.
83. S. Feldman and M. Gibaldi. Physiologic surface-active agents
     and drug absorption. II. Comparison of the effect of sodium
     taurodeoxycholate and ethylenediaminetetraacetic acid on sali-
     cylamide and salicylate transfer across the everted rat small
     intestine. J. Pharm. Sci. 58: 967—970, 1969.
84. K. Kakemi, H. Sezaki, R. Konishi, T. Kimura, and M. Murakami.
     Effect of bile salts on the gastrointestinal absorption of drugs.
     I. Chem. Pharm. Bull. 18: 275—280, 1970.
85. K. Kakemi, H. Sezaki, R. Konishi, T. Kimura, and A. Okita.
     Effect of bile salts on the gastrointestinal absorption of drugs.
     II. Mechanism of the enhancement of the intestinal absorption
     of sulfaguanidine by bile salts. Chem. Pharm. Bull. 18: 1034—
     1039, 1970.
86. S. Miyazaki, H. Inoue, T. Yamahira, and T. Nadai. Interaction
     of drugs with bile components. I. Effect of bile salts on the
     dissolution behavior of indomethacin and phenylbutazone. Chem.
     Pharm. Bull. 27: 2468—2472, 1979.
87. A. Rahman, J. A. Barrowman, and A. Rahimtula. The influence
     of bile on the bioavailability of polynuclear aromatic hydrocarbons
     from the rat intestine. Can. J. Physiol. Pharmacol. 64: 1214—1218,
     1980.

88. S. Eriksson. Bile acids and steroids. Biliary excretion of bile acids and cholesterol in bile fistula rats. Proc. Soc. Exp. Biol. Med. 94: 578–582, 1957.

89. F. L. S. Tse, F. Ballard, and J. M. Jaffe. Biliary excretion of [^{14}C]temazepam and its metabolites in the rat. J. Pharm. Sci. 72: 311–312, 1983.

90. K. S. Pang and J. R. Gillette. A theoretical examination of the effects of gut wall metabolism, hepatic elimination, and enterohepatic recycling on estimates of bioavailability and of hepatic blood flow. J. Pharmacokinet. Biopharm. 6: 355–367, 1978.

91. H.-S. G. Chen and J. F. Gross. Pharmacokinetics of drugs subject to enterohepatic circulation. J. Pharm. Sci. 68: 792–794, 1979.

92. W. A. Colburn. Pharmacokinetic and biopharmaceutic parameters during enterohepatic circulation of drugs. J. Pharm. Sci. 71: 131–133, 1982.

93. P. Veng Pedersen and R. Miller. Pharmacokinetics and bioavailability of cimetidine in humans. J. Pharm. Sci. 69: 394–398, 1980.

94. T. A. Shepard, R. H. Reuning, and L. J. Aarons. Interpretation of area under the curve measurements for drugs subject to enterohepatic cycling. J. Pharm. Sci. 74: 227–228, 1985.

95. T. A. Shepard, R. H. Reuning, and L. J. Aarons. Estimation of area under the curve for drugs subject to enterohepatic cycling. J. Pharmacokinet. Biopharm. 13: 589–608, 1985.

96. P. Johnson and P. A. Rising. Techniques for assessment of biliary excretion and enterohepatic circulation in the rat. Xenobiotica 8: 27–36, 1978.

97. D. Greenslade, M. E. Havler, M. J. Humphrey, B. J. Jordan, and M. J. Rance. Species differences in the metabolism and excretion of fenclofenac. Xenobiotica 10: 753–760, 1980.

98. R. J. Parker, P. C. Hirom, and P. Millburn. Enterohepatic recycling of phenolphthalein, morphine, lysergic acid diethylamide (LSD) and diphenylacetic acid in the rat. Hydrolysis of glucuronic acid conjugates in the gut lumen. Xenobiotica 9: 689–703, 1980.

99. D. Brewster, M. J. Humphrey, and M. A. McLeavy. Biliary excretion, metabolism and enterohepatic circulation of buprenorphine. Xenobiotica 11: 189–196, 1981.

100. F. L. S. Tse, F. Ballard, and J. M. Jaffe. A practical method for monitoring drug excretion and enterohepatic circulation in the rat. J. Pharmacol. Methods 7: 139–144, 1982.

101. F. L. S. Tse, F. Ballard, J. M. Jaffe, and H. J. Schwarz. Enterohepatic circulation of radioactivity following an oral dose of [^{14}C]temazepam in the rat. J. Pharm. Pharmacol. 35: 225–228, 1983.

102. A. F. Hofmann and B. H. Lauterburg. Breath test with isotopes of carbon: Progress and potential. J. Lab. Clin. Med. 90: 405–411, 1977.

103. E. A. Lane and I. Parashos. Drug pharmacokinetics and the carbon dioxide breath test. J. Pharmacokinet. Biopharm. 14: 29–49, 1986.

104. D. J. Paustenbach, G. P. Carlson, J. E. Christian, and G. S. Born. A comparative study of the pharmacokinetics of carbon tetrachloride in the rat following repeated inhalation exposures of 8 and 11.5 hr/day. Fundam. Appl. Toxicol. 6: 484–497, 1986.

105. S. Chakrabarti, R. Van Severen, and P. Braeckman. Influence of particle size and crystal shape on the dissolution rate of phenytoin. Farmacol. Tijdschr. Belg. 54: 403–411, 1977.

106. S. Chakrabarti, R. Van Severen, and P. Braeckman. Studies on the crystalline form of phenytoin. Pharmazie 33: 338–339, 1978.

107. F. Nimmerfall and J. Rosenthaler. Dependence of area under the curve on proquazone particle size and in vitro dissolution rate. J. Pharm. Sci. 69: 605–607, 1980.

108. H. A. Koeleman and M. C. B. Van Oudtshoorn. An evaluation of the biological availability of chloramphenicol. S. Afr. Med. J. 47: 94–99, 1973.

109. M. C. Meyer, G. W. A. Slywka, R. E. Dann, and P. L. Whyatt. Bioavailability of 14 nitrofurantoin products. J. Pharm. Sci. 63: 1693–1698, 1974.

110. R. D. Schoenwald and P. Stewart. Effect of particle size on ophthalmic bioavailability of dexamethasone suspensions in rabbits. J. Pharm. Sci. 69: 391–394, 1980.

111. M. Dam, J. Christiansen, C. B. Kristensen, A. Helles, A. Jaegerskou, and M. Schmiegelow. Carbamazepine: A Clinical biopharmaceutical study. Eur. J. Clin. Pharmacol. 20: 59–64, 1981.

112. G. T. McInnes, M. J. Asbury, L. E. Ramsay, J. R. Shelton, and I. R. Harrison. Effect of micronization on the bioavailability and pharmacologic activity of spironolactone. J. Clin. Pharmacol. 22: 410–417, 1982.

113. S. Chakrabarti, E. Moerman, and F. Belpaire. Bioavailability of phenytoin in dogs: Effect of crystal form and particle size. Pharmazie 34: 242–243, 1979.

114. A. D. J. Watson. Chloramphenicol in the dog: Observations of plasma levels following oral administration. Res. Vet. Sci. 16: 147–151, 1974.

115. F. L. S. Tse, J. M. Jaffe. K. A. Marty, and H. J. Schwarz. Effect of food, fluid and dosage form on the absorption of 52–522, a potential antianxiety agent, in the dog. J. Pharm. Pharmacol. 36: 56–58, 1984.

116. P. G. Welling. Influence of food and diet on gastrointestinal drug absorption: A review. J. Pharmacokinet. Biopharm. 5: 291–334, 1977.
117. A. Melander. Influence of food on the bioavailability of drugs. Clin. Pharmacokinet. 3: 337–351, 1978.
118. R. D. Toothaker and P. G. Welling. The effect of food on drug bioavailability. Annu. Rev. Pharmacol. Toxicol. 20: 173–199, 1980.
119. P. G. Welling and F. L. S. Tse. The influence of food on the absorption of antimicrobial agents. J. Antimicrob. Chemother. 9: 7–27, 1982.
120. P. G. Welling and F. L. S. Tse. Food interactions affecting the absorption of analgesic and anti-inflammatory agents. Drug-Nutr. Interact. 2: 153–168, 1983.
121. R. W. Marshall, O. M. Moreno, and D. A. Brodie. Chronic bile duct cannulation in the dog. J. Appl. Physiol. 19: 1191–1192, 1964.
122. L. E. Gerlowski and R. K. Jain. Physiologically based pharmacokinetic modeling: Principles and applications. J. Pharm. Sci. 72: 1103–1127, 1983.
123. R. L. Dedrick, D. D. Forrester, J. N. Cannon, S. M. El Dareer, and L. B. Mellett. Pharmacokinetics of 1-β-d-arabinofuranosylcytosine (Ara-C) deamination in several species. Biochem. Pharmacol. 22: 2405–2417, 1973.
124. R. J. Lutz, R. L. Dedrick, H. B. Matthews, T. E. Eling, and M. W. Anderson. A preliminary pharmacokinetic model for several chlorinated biphenyls in the rat. Drug Metab. Dispos. 5: 386–396, 1977.
125. R. Jimenez, A. Esteller, and M. A. Lopez. Biliary secretion in conscious rabbits: Surgical technique. Lab. Animals 16: 182–185, 1982.
126. R. H. Dowling, E. Mack, J. Picott, J. Berger, and D. M. Small. Experimental model for the study of the enterohepatic circulation of bile in rhesus monkeys. J. Lab. Clin. Med. 72: 169–176, 1968.
127. J. Meszaros, F. Nimmerfall, J. Rosenthaler, and H. Weber. Permanent bile duct cannulation in the monkey. A model for studying intestinal absorption. Eur. J. Pharmacol. 32: 233–242, 1975.
128. G. Tomson, N.-O. Lunell, A. Sundwall, and A. Rane. Placental passage of oxazepam and its metabolism in mother and newborn. Clin. Pharmacol. Ther. 25: 74–81, 1979.
129. L. Padeletti, M. C. Porciani, and G. Scimone. Placental transfer of digoxin (beta-methyldigoxin) in man. Int. J. Clin. Pharmacol. Biopharm. 17: 82–83, 1979.

130. O. M. Bakke and K. Haram. Time-course of transplacental passage of diazepam: Influence of injection-delivery interval on neonatal drug concentrations. Clin. Pharmacokinet. 7: 353—362, 1982.

131. G. Levy and W. L. Hayton. Pharmacokinetic aspects of placental drug transfer. In Fetal Pharmacology. Edited by L. O. Boréus. Raven Press, New York, 1973, pp. 29—39.

132. H. H. Szeto. Pharmacokinetics in the ovine maternal-fetal unit. Annu. Rev. Pharmacol. Toxicol. 22: 221—243, 1982.

133. H. H. Szeto, L. I. Mann, A. Bhakthavathsalan, M. Liu, and C. E. Inturrisi. Meperidine pharmacokinetics in the maternal-fetal unit. J. Pharmacol. Exp. Ther. 206: 448—459, 1978.

134. H. H. Szeto, R. F. Kaiko, J. F. Clapp, R. W. Larrow, L.I. Mann, and C. E. Inturrisi. Urinary excretion of meperidine by the fetal lamb. J. Pharmacol. Exp. Ther. 209: 244—248, 1979.

135. H. H. Szeto, J. F. Clapp, III, R. W. Larrow, C. E. Inturrisi, and L. I. Mann. Renal tubular secretion of meperidine by the fetal lamb. J. Pharmacol. Exp. Ther. 213: 346—349, 1980.

136. H. H. Szeto, J. F. Clapp, III, R. W. Larrow, J. Hewitt, C. E. Inturrisi, and L. I. Mann. Disposition of methadone in the ovine maternal-fetal unit. Life Sci. 28: 2111—2117, 1981.

137. G. W. Mihaly, D. J. Morgan, A. W. Marshall, R. A. Smallwood, S. Cockbain, D. MacLellan, and K. J. Hardy. Placental transfer of ranitidine during steady-state infusions of maternal and fetal sheep. J. Pharm. Sci. 71: 1008—1010, 1982.

138. T. Nanbo. Pharmacokinetics in maternal-fetal unit after intra-venous administration of p-phenyl benzoic acid to rat. J. Pharm. Dyn. 5: 213—221, 1982.

139. T. Nanbo. Change in pharmacokinetic character of p-phenyl benzoic acid in developing fetus of rat. J. Pharm. Dyn. 5: 222—228, 1982.

140. P. Taylor. Practical Teratology. Academic Press, London, 1986. pp. 3—9.

141. A. K. Palmer. The design of subprimate animal studies. In Handbook of Teratology. Edited by J. G. Wilson and F. C. Fraser. Plenum Press, New York, 1978, p. 224.

142. J. T. Wilson, R. D. Brown, D. R. Cherek, J. W. Dailey, B. Hilman, P. C. Jobe, B. R. Manno, J. E. Manno, H. M. Redetzki, and J. J. Stewart. Drug excretion in human breast milk: Principles, pharmacokinetics and projected consequences. Clin. Pharmacokinet. 5: 1—66, 1980.

143. G. P. Stec, P. Greenberger, T. I. Ruo, T. Henthorn, Y. Morita, A. J. Atkinson, Jr., and R. Patterson. Kinetics of theophylline transfer to breast milk. Clin. Pharmacol. Ther. 28: 404—408, 1980.

144. A. Goldstein, L. Aronow, and S. M. Kalman. Principles of Drug Action: The Basis of Pharmacology, 2nd ed. John Wiley and Sons, New York, 1974, pp. 145—146.

145. H. Vorherr. Drug excretion in breast milk. Postgrad. Med. 56: 97—104, 1974.

146. A. C. D. Platzker, C. D. Lew, and D. Stewart. Drug "administration" via breast milk. Hosp. Pract., September: 111—122, 1980.

147. J. W. A. Findlay, R. L. DeAngelis, M. F. Kearney, R. M. Welch, and J. M. Findlay. Analgesic drugs in breast milk and plasma. Clin. Pharmacol. Ther. 29: 625—633, 1981.

148. G. N. Rolinson. The significance of protein binding of antibiotics in antibacterial chemotherapy. J. Antimicrob. Chemother. 6: 311—317, 1980.

149. J. J. Vallner. Binding of drugs by albumin and plasma protein. J. Pharm. Sci. 66: 447—465, 1977.

150. P. J. McNamara, J. T. Slattery, M. Gibaldi, and G. Levy. Accumulation kinetics of drugs with nonlinear plasma protein and tissue binding characteristics. J. Pharmacokinet. Biopharm. 7: 397—405, 1979.

151. S. Øie, T. W. Guentert, and T. N. Tozer. Effect of saturable binding on the pharmacokinetics of drugs: A simulation. J. Pharm. Pharmacol. 32: 471—477, 1980.

152. L. R. Peterson and D. N. Gerding. Influence of protein binding of antibiotics on serum pharmacokinetics and extravascular penetration: Clinically useful concepts. Rev. Infect. Dis. 2: 340—348, 1980.

153. E. M. Faed. Protein binding of drugs in plasma, interstitial fluid and tissues: Effect on pharmacokinetics. Eur. J. Clin. Pharmacol. 21: 77—81, 1981.

154. P. J. McNamara, M. Gibaldi, and K. Stoeckel. Volume of distribution terms for a drug (ceftriaxone) exhibiting concentration-dependent protein binding. I. Theoretical considerations. Eur. J. Clin. Pharmacol. 25: 399—405, 1983.

155. P. J. McNamara, M. Gibaldi, and K. Stoeckel. Volume of distribution terms for a drug (ceftriaxone) exhibiting concentration-dependent protein binding. II. Physiological significance. Eur. J. Clin. Pharmacol. 25: 407—412, 1983.

156. J. Huang and S. Øie. Hepatic elimination of drugs with concentration-dependent serum protein binding. J. Pharmacokinet. Biopharm. 12: 67—81, 1984.

157. R. C. Chou and G. Levy. Changes in plasma protein binding of drugs after blood collection from pregnant rats. J. Pharm. Sci. 71: 471—473, 1982.

158. A. J. Jackson, A. K. Miller, and P. K. Narang. Human blood preservation: Effect on in vitro protein binding. J. Pharm. Sci. 70: 1168—1169, 1981.

159. N. Terao and D. D. Shen. Alterations in serum protein binding and pharmacokinetics of *l*-propranolol in the rat elicited by the presence of an indwelling venous catheter. J. Pharmacol. Exp. Ther. 227: 369—375, 1983.

160. M. Wood, D. G. Shand, and A. J. J. Wood. Altered drug binding due to the use of indwelling heparinized cannulas (heparin lock) for sampling. Clin. Pharmacol. Ther. 25: 103—107, 1979.

161. B. Silber, M. Lo, and S. Riegelman. The influence of heparin administration on the plasma protein binding and disposition of propranolol. Res. Commun. Chem. Pathol. Pharmacol. 27: 419—429, 1980.

162. C. A. Naranjo, J. G. Abel, E. M. Sellers, and H. G. Giles. Unaltered diazepam plasma binding using indwelling heparinized cannulae for sampling. Br. J. Clin. Pharmacol. 9: 103—105, 1980.

163. C. A. Naranjo, E. M. Sellers, V. Khouw, P. Alexander, T. Fan, and J. Shaw. Variability in heparin effect on serum drug binding. Clin. Pharmacol. Ther. 28: 545—550, 1980.

164. T. D. Bjornsson, J. E. Brown, and C. Tschanz. Importance of radiochemical purity of radiolabeled drugs used for determining plasma protein binding of drugs. J. Pharm. Sci. 70: 1372—1373, 1981.

165. F. D. Boudinot and W. J. Jusko. Fluid shifts and other factors affecting plasma protein binding of prednisolone by equilibrium dialysis. J. Pharm. Sci. 73: 774—780, 1984.

166. D. Mungall, Y. Y. Wong, R. L. Talbert, M. H. Crawford, J. Marshall, D. W. Hawkins, and T. M. Ludden. Plasma protein binding of warfarin: Methodological considerations. J. Pharm. Sci. 73: 1000—1001, 1984.

167. M. Ehrnebo, S. Agurell, L. O. Boréus, E. Gordon, and U. Lönroth. Pentazocine binding to blood cells and plasma proteins. Clin. Pharmacol. Ther. 16: 424—429, 1974.

168. J. Steinhardt and J. A. Reynolds. Multiple Equilibria in Proteins. Academic Press, New York, 1969, pp. 45—53.

169. C. J. Briggs, J. W. Hubbard, C. Savage, and D. Smith. Improved procedure for the determination of protein binding by conventional equilibrium dialysis. J. Pharm. Sci. 72: 918—921, 1983.

170. S. Øie and T. W. Guentert. Comparison of equilibrium times in dialysis experiments using spiked plasma or spiked buffer. J. Pharm. Sci. 71: 127—128, 1982.

171. P. J. McNamara and J. E. Bogardus. Effect of initial conditions and drug-protein binding on the time to equilibrium in dialysis systems. J. Pharm. Sci. 71: 1066–1068, 1982.

172. S. S. Hwang and W. F. Bayne. Dynamic method for estimating the extent of plasma protein binding in a dialysis experiment. J. Pharm. Sci. 73: 708–710, 1984.

173. W. F. Bayne and S. S. Hwang. Effect of nonlinear protein binding on equilibration times for different initial conditions. J. Pharm. Sci. 74: 120–123, 1985.

174. T. N. Tozer, J. G. Gambertoglio, D. E. Furst, D. S. Avery, and N. H. G. Holford. Volume shifts and protein binding estimates using equilibrium dialysis: Application to prednisolone binding in humans. J. Pharm. Sci. 72: 1442–1446, 1983.

175. J. Huang. Errors in estimating the unbound fraction of drugs due to the volume shift in equilibrium dialysis. J. Pharm. Sci. 72: 1368–1369, 1983.

176. J. J. Lima, J. J. MacKichan, N. Libertin, and J. Sabino. Influence of volume shifts on drug binding during equilibrium dialysis: Correction and attenuation. J. Pharmacokinet. Biopharm. 11: 483–498, 1983.

177. G. Scatchard. The attractions of proteins for small molecules and ions. Ann. N.Y. Acad. Sci. 51: 660–672, 1949.

178. J. E. Fletcher and A. A. Spector. Alternative models for the analysis of drug-protein binding. Mol. Pharmacol. 13: 387–399, 1977.

179. J. Romer and M. H. Bickel. A method to estimate binding constants at variable protein concentrations. J. Pharm. Pharmacol. 31: 7–11, 1979.

180. H. Kurz and G. Friemel. Artspezifische Unterschiede der Bindung an Plasmaproteine. Naunyn-Schmiedebergs Arch. Pharmacol. 257: 35–36, 1967.

181. J. P. Tillement, F. Lhoste, and J. F. Giudicelli. Diseases and drug protein binding. Clin. Pharmacokinet. 3: 144–154, 1978.

182. K. M. Piafsky. Disease-induced changes in the plasma binding of basic drugs. Clin. Pharmacokinet. 5: 246–262, 1980.

183. H. Nosaka, K. Takagi, T. Hasegawa, Y. Ogura, Y. Mizukami, and T. Satake. Pharmacokinetics of theophylline in beagle dogs and asthmatic patients after multiple oral doses of sustained-release theophylline tablet formulation. Int. J. Clin. Pharmacol. Ther. Toxicol. 24: 528–535, 1986.

184. L. S. Schanker, D. J. Tocco, D. B. Brodie, and C. A. M. Hogben. Absorption of drugs from the rat small intestine. J. Pharmacol. Exp. Ther. 123: 81–88, 1958.

185. J. T. Doluisio, N. F. Billups, L. W. Dittert, E. T. Sugita, and J. V. Swintosky. Drug absorption. I. An in situ rat gut technique yielding realistic absorption rates. J. Pharm. Sci. 58: 1196–1200, 1969.

186. N. Schurgers, J. Bijdendijk, J. J. Tukker, and D. J. A. Crommelin. Comparison of four experimental techniques for studying drug absorption kinetics in the anesthetized rat in situ. J. Pharm. Sci. 75: 117—119, 1986.

187. D. C. Taylor, R. Grundy, and B. Loveday. Chronic dog intestinal loop model for studying drug absorption as exemplified by β-adrenoreceptor blocking agents, atenolol and propranolol. J. Pharm. Sci. 70: 516—521, 1981.

188. V. S. Patel and W. G. Kramer. Allopurinol absorption from different sites of the rat gastrointestinal tract. J. Pharm. Sci. 75: 275—277, 1986.

189. F. L. S. Tse, J. M. Jaffe, and J. G. Dain. Pharmacokinetics of compound 58—112, a potential skeletal muscle relaxant, in man. J. Clin. Pharmacol. 24: 47—57, 1984.

190. R. C. Grimus and I. Schuster. The role of the lymphatic transport in the enteral absorption of naftifine by the rat. Xenobiotica 14: 287—294, 1984.

191. V. J. Stella and W. N. A. Charman. Mechanism of intestinal lymphatic transport of lipophilic drugs. Abstracts, Academy of Pharmaceutical Sciences 39th National Meeting, Minneapolis, Minnesota, October 20—24, 1985, p. 16.

192. W. A. Ritschel. What is bioavailability? Philosophy of bioavailability testing. Methods Find. Exp. Clin. Pharmacol. 6: 777—786, 1984.

193. K. Yamaoka, T. Nakagawa, and T. Uno. Statistical moments in pharmacokinetics. J. Pharmacokinet. Biopharm. 6: 547—558, 1978.

194. K. S. Pang. A review of metabolite kinetics. J. Pharmacokinet. Biopharm. 13: 633—662, 1985.

195. H. B. Hucker, S. C. Stauffer, A. J. Balletto, S. D. White, A. G. Zacchei, and B. H. Arison. Physiological disposition and metabolism of cyclobenzaprine in the rat, dog, rhesus monkey, and man. Drug Metab. Dispos. 6: 659—672, 1978.

196. J. E. Swagzdis, R. W. Wittendorf, R. M. DeMarinis, and B. A. Mico. Pharmacokinetics of dopamine-2 agonists in rats and dogs. J. Pharm. Sci. 75: 925—928, 1986.

197. H. B. Matthews, H. M. Chopade, R. W. Smith, and L. T. Burka. Disposition of 2,4-dinitroaniline in the male F-344 rat. Xenobiotica. 16: 1—10, 1986.

198. G. C. Bolton, G. D. Allen, C. W. Filer, and D. J. Jeffery. Absorption, metabolism and excretion studies on clauvlanic acid in the rat and dog. Xenobiotica 14: 483—490, 1984.

199. W. A. Colburn, I. Bekersky, B. H. Min, B. J. Hodshon, and W. A. Garland. Contribution of gut contents, intestinal wall and liver to the first-pass metabolism of clonazepam in the rat. Res. Commun. Chem. Pathol. Pharmacol. 27: 73—90, 1980.

200. H. G. Boxenbaum, I. Bekersky, M. L. Jack, and S. A. Kaplan. Influence of gut microflora on bioavailability. Drug Metab. Rev. 9: 259–279, 1979.

201. H. P. A. Illing and J. M. Fromson. Species differences in the disposition and metabolism of 6,11-dihydro-11-oxodibenz[be]-oxepin-2-acetic acid (isoxepac) in rat, rabbit, dog, rhesus monkey, and man. Drug Metab. Dispos. 6: 510–517, 1978.

202. F. L. S. Tse, F. Ballard, and J. Skinn. Estimating the fraction reabsorbed in drugs undergoing enterohepatic circulation. J. Pharmacokinet. Biopharm. 10: 455–461, 1982.

203. J. H. Lin, K. C. Yeh, and D. E. Duggan. Effect of entero-hepatic circulation on the pharmacokinetics of diflunisal in rats. Drug Metab. Dispos. 13: 321–326, 1985.

204. C. T. Gombar, K. Straub, P. Levandoski, L. Gutzait, J. Swagzdis, C. Garvie, G. Joseph, B. D. Potts, and B. A. Mico. Pharmacokinetics, metabolism, and disposition of 6-chloro-2, 3,4,5-tetrahydro-3-methyl-1H-3-benzazepine (SK&F 86466) in rats and dogs. Drug Metab. Dispos. 14: 540–548, 1986.

205. P. A. J. Reilly, T. Inaba, D. Kadar, and L. Endrenyi. Enzyme induction following a single dose of amobarbital in dogs. J. Pharmacokinet. Biopharm. 6: 305–313, 1978.

206. P. G. Dayton and J. E. Sanders. Dose-dependent pharmaco-kinetics: Emphasis on phase I metabolism. Drug Metab. Rev. 14: 347–405, 1983.

207. G. Powis. Dose-dependent metabolism, therapeutic effect, and toxicity of anticancer drugs in man. Drug Metab. Rev. 14: 1145–1163, 1983.

208. R. Mehta, P. C. Hirom, and P. Millburn. The influence of dose on the pattern of conjugation of phenol and 1-napthol in non-human primates. Xenobiotica 8: 445–452, 1978.

209. H. Koster, I. Halsema, E. Scholtens, M. Knippers, and G. J. Mulder. Dose-dependent shifts in the sulfation and glucuroni-dation of phenolic compounds in the rat in vivo and in isolated hepatocytes. The role of saturation of phenolsulfotransferases. Biochem. Pharmacol. 30: 2569–2575, 1981.

210. J. C. Kapeghian, G. A. Burdock, and L. W. Masten. Effect of the route of administration on microsomal enzyme induction following repeated administration of methadone in the mouse. Biochem. Pharmacol. 28: 3021–3025, 1979.

211. I. H. Patel, R. H. Levy, and W. F. Trager. Pharmacokinetics of carbamazepine-10,11-epoxide before and after autoinduction in rhesus monkeys. J. Pharmacol. Exp. Ther. 206: 607–613, 1978.

212. L. W. Masten, G. R. Peterson, A. Burkhalter, and E. L. Way. Tolerance to methadone lethality and microsomal enzyme induction in mice tolerant to and dependent on morphine. Drug Alcohol Depend. 5: 27–37, 1980.

213. L. W. Masten, S. R. Price, and C. J. Burnett. Microsomal enzyme induction following repeated oral administration of LAAM. Res. Commun. Chem. Pathol. Pharmacol. 20: 1–19, 1978.

214. D. W. Schneck and J. F. Pritchard. The inhibitory effect of propranolol pretreatment on its own metabolism in the rat. J. Pharmacol. Exp. Ther. 218: 575–581, 1981.

215. J. G. Wagner. Pharmacokinetics and bioavailability. Triangle 14: 101–108, 1975.

216. E. C. Long. Liquid Scintillation Counting Theory and Techniques. Beckman Instruments, Fullerton, California, 1976, p. 36.

217. L. Z. Benet. Pharmacokinetic parameters: Which are necessary to define a drug substance? Eur. J. Respir. Dis. (Suppl.) 65: 45–61, 1984.

218. E. H. Ulm. Enalapril maleate (MK-421), a potent, nonsulfhydryl angiotensin-converting enzyme inhibitor: Absorption, disposition, and metabolism in man. Drug Metab. Rev. 14: 99–110, 1983.

219. A. E. Till, H. J. Gomez, M. Hichens, J. A. Bolognese, W. R. McNabb, B. A. Brooks, F. Noormohamed, and A. F. Lant. Pharmacokinetics of repeated single oral doses of enalapril maleate (MK-421) in normal volunteers. Biopharm. Drug Dispos. 5: 273–280, 1984.

220. E. H. Ulm, M. Hichens, H. J. Gomez, A. E. Till, E. Hand, T. C. Vassil, J. Biollaz, H. R. Brunner, and J. L. Schelling. Enalapril maleate and a lysine analogue (MK-521): Disposition in man. Br. J. Clin. Pharmacol. 14: 357–362, 1982.

221. F. L. S. Tse and J. M. Jaffe. Pharmacokinetics of PN 200–110 isradipine, a new calcium antagonist, after oral administration in man. Eur. J. Clin. Pharmacol. 32: 361–365, 1987.

222. W. A. Colburn. Estimating the accumulation of drugs. J. Pharm. Sci. 72: 833–834, 1983.

223. G. Alvan, K. Piafsky, M. Lind, and C. von Bahr. Effect of pentobarbital on the disposition of alprenolol. Clin. Pharmacol. Ther. 22: 316–321, 1977.

224. P. N. Bennett. Drugs in breast milk—an assessment of risk to the infant. III World Conference on Clinical Pharmacology and Therapeutics, Stockholm, Sweden, July 27 to August 1, 1986.

225. Fed. Reg., 43: 60013, 1978.

226. U.S. Congress, Office of Technology Assessment, Alternatives to Animal Use in Research, Testing, and Education, U.S. Government Printing Office, OTA-BA-273, Washington, D.C., 1986, p. 280.

5

Clinical Pharmacokinetics in Drug Discovery and Development

JAMES M. JAFFE and HORST F. SCHRAN *Sandoz Research Institute, East Hanover, New Jersey*

I. INTRODUCTION

Prior to its first administration in humans, the safety of a new drug
entity will have been extensively tested in studies using in vitro
and animal systems. These studies, consolidated in a Notice of Claimed
Investigational Exemption for a New Drug (IND) and presented to the
U.S. Food and Drug Administration (FDA), provide the basis of
approval for limited, well-controlled studies of a new drug in humans.
Nevertheless, extrapolation from the preclinical to the clinical stage
of new drug development involves considerable uncertainty and
possible risk. Therefore, the progression of events from the initial
exposure of a small number of patients or normal volunteers to a
new drug to more extended clinical trials is necessarily a methodical,
consecutive process. The Investigational New Drug Development
Process as outlined in FDA form 1571 divides this progression into
three distinct phases: phase I, consisting of safety studies, usually
performed in less than 100 patients or normal volunteers; phase II,
which evaluates the effectiveness and common short-term side effects
in usually not more than several hundred patients; phase III, which
includes expanded controlled and uncontrolled clinical trials in
several hundred to several thousand patients to gather additional
information on safety and effectiveness. Pharmacokinetic and bioavailability studies should be an integral part of this consecutive
process. In the early stages of clinical development, PK studies provide
an assessment of intrinsic drug properties, such as rates of absorption
and elimination or the degree of exposure to and accumulation of drug
and/or its biotransformation products, as well as an evaluation of the
performance of dosage forms used and dosing schedule. In the latter
stages of clinical development such studies could explain safety or
efficacy issues, provide labeling information, and assess the performance
of dosage forms other than those used in the clinical trials.

The 1977 FDA bioavailability and bioequivalence regulations and
the subsequent interpretations of these regulations have elaborated
the scope and formalized the conduct of several types of pharmacokinetic studies (1--4). Although no official published "checklist"
exists of the pharmacokinetic studies required as part of a complete
New Drug Application (NDA, i.e., the regulatory basis for marketing
a prescription drug substance), an approvable biopharmaceutics
submission in an NDA normally consists of a core group of studies
of the type applicable to most new drugs as well as supplemental
studies related to the particular drug class or use. Table 1 outlines
the format of a typical biopharmaceutics submission. This format
has recently been instituted by the FDA and may further evolve
with time (5) [see also Guidelines for the format and content of the

TABLE 1 Format for Human Pharmacokinetics and Bioavailability Section (Biopharmaceutics Submission) of an NDA Application

Table of contents and summary of studies

Summary of bioavailability and pharmacokinetic data and overall conclusions

Summary of all formulations used in pivotal clinical trials and pharmacokinetic studies

Summary of analytical methodology employed

Summary description, specifications, and results of in vitro dissolution testing

Individual study reports

    Pilot or background studies
    Bioavailability and bioequivalence studies
    Pharmacokinetic studies
    Other in vivo studies using pharmacological or clinical end points
    In vitro dissolution studies

human pharmacokinetics and bioavailability section of an application (Docket 85D-0275), and Guideline for the format and content of the summary for new drug and antibiotic applications (Docket No. 85D-0247), Food and Drug Administration, Center for Drug and Biologics, 5600 Fishers Lane, Rockville, MD 20857]. Table 2 summarizes typical core and supplemental pharmacokinetic studies contained in a biopharmaceutics submission. The type, protocol, and conduct of the core studies, particularly those related to drug bioavailability and bioequivalence, are now well established, although scientific debate continues on such specific issues as the statistical methodology necessary for their evaluation (6—8). The type, protocol, and conduct of the supplemental studies is under active debate at present.

    Table 2 serves to illustrate, not to prescribe, various studies to be included in a biopharmaceutics submission. Such a submission should be designed within the context of the overall clinical and biopharmaceutical development program for, and take into consideration the specific characteristics of, the new drug entity in question. This chapter is divided into three general areas, each containing the pharmacokinetic studies typically performed during the clinical development phases I, II, and III, respectively. Within each area, a discussion of general issues characteristically of concern at that

TABLE 2 Pharmacokinetic Studies: Phase I Through III

Study	Clinical phase	Objective	Design	Comments
Pilot pharmacokinetic (single and multiple dose)	I	Validation of analytical method; preliminary pharmacokinetics	Parallel groups (n = 3-6/group); suspension or solution dosage form if possible; minimal number (n 6/subject) of blood samples collected	May be performed as part of single- and/or multiple-dose safety and tolerance studies
Pilot bioavailability	I	Pilot study to determine if sold dosage form adequate for phase II and III studies	Single-dose crossover (n = 6-12); solution or suspension versus solid dosage form	
Single-dose ADME	I	Obtain definitive pharmacokinetic data, excretion pattern, dose proportionality, definitive metabolism; project pharmacokinetic parameters upon multiple dosing	Single-dose parallel groups (n = 6/group); radiolabeled drug in solution or suspension at two dose levels; urine and feces as well as serial blood samples collected	
Intra- and inter-subject variability	II	Determine variability expected during phase III pharmacokinetic studies and determine number of subjects required in future pharmacokinetic studies to adequately (statistically) assess differences	Three-way crossover (n = 12) using same dose solution or suspension (doses one-half highest tolerated dose)	

Dose proportionality	II	Determine if bioavailability parameters (C_{max}, AUC) are linear over proposed dose range	Three-way crossover (n = 12); solution or suspension covering the therapeutic range for a single dose	
Multiple-dose ADME	II	Validate single-dose pharmacokinetic projections; determine ADME profile upon multiple dosing; obtain large quantities of biologic fluids for biotransformation studies	Single dose of radio-labeled drug in solution or suspension (n = 6) for 4–5 days; C_{min} values obtained during dosing and complete blood profile after last dose; urine and feces collected during entire study	
Bioequivalence of service and proposed marketed dosage forms	III	Determine if dosage form(s) used during clinical trials is bioequivalent to dosage form proposed for marketing; determine relative bioavailabilities of service and proposed market forms	Single-dose crossover (n based on results of dose proportionality and/or variability study using a power calculation); highest strength dosage form proposed for market evaluated	Pivotal study for registration
Dosage form proportionality	III	Determine if equipotent drug treatments administered as different dose strengths of one dosage form produce equivalent drug bioavailability	Single-dose crossover (n based on dose proportionality, variability, or prior bioequivalence studies); multiple strengths evaluated by bracketing, i.e., using lowest and highest strengths in study	Pivotal study for registration

TABLE 2 (Continued)

Study	Clinical phase	Objective	Design	Comments
Food interaction	III	Influence of food on bioavailability	Single-dose crossover (n = 9-12); dosage form proposed for marketing should be used if available	
Effect of age	III	Influence of age on pharmacokinetic parameters	Single dose in elderly volunteers (n = 25)	Results compared to those obtained from other pharmacokinetic studies using younger volunteers under the same experimental conditions
Renal insufficiency	III	Influence of renal function on pharmacokinetic parameters	Single dose in patients (n = 12) with creatinine clearance < 25 ml/min	Results compared to those obtained from other pharmacokinetic

				studies using subjects with normal renal function under similar experimental conditions; study not essential if renal excretion of drug and/or metabolites minimal
Hepatic insufficiency	III	Influence of hepatic function on pharmacokinetic parameters	Single dose in patients (n = 12) with confirmed hepatic insufficiency	Results compared to other pharmacokinetic studies using subjects with normal hepatic function under the same experimental conditions
Drug-drug interactions	III	Influence of concomitant medication on bioavailability parameters	Single-dose three-way crossover (n = 12–18); comparison is drug and codrug, drug, codrug	

juncture of development is followed by one or more specific examples of studies and methodological details. In order to provide a unifying thread among the three areas as well as to outline the decision-making processes at various stages of clinical drug development, most of the specific examples described in this chapter are based on work performed at Sandoz Pharmaceuticals with the new drug entity PN 200—110 (isradipine), although studies with other experimental drugs are included when PN 200—110 data were unavailable or less suited to illustrate a particular point. Figure 1 contains background information of the new drug entities discussed in this chapter.

II. GENERAL CONSIDERATIONS

It is paradoxical that pharmacokinetic studies have become an integral part of the clinical development program for a new drug since the relationship between the time course of drug concentration in the compartments commonly measured and the therapeutic effect is usually complex and seldom amenable to rigorous quantification (13, 14). This leads to the speculation that the utility of pharmacokinetic studies is less related to their own merits and more to the short-comings inherent in the clinical evaluation process. Thus, "regardless of whether a new therapeutic agent has been tested in a number of clinical trials, and regardless of the number of patients who have participated, the results cannot always be applied to the wider array of patients, clinical conditions, dosages and durations of exposure that will be encountered when the agent is made available for general use" (15). Therefore, even though pharmacokinetic studies may only imperfectly explain the time course and dynamics of clinical effects caused by a new drug, they can contribute to the process of extrapolating clinical safety and efficacy data to the general population via bioavailability assessment and drug disposition studies in various groups and situations.

In the absence of safety concerns, the conduct of pharmacokinetic studies with normal, healthy volunteers is preferred. Using such individuals can provide a much larger data pool compared to patients, because greater flexibility is allowed with respect to study entry criteria, scheduling of drug administrations, sampling of blood or other fluids, drug washout periods, changeover from one dosage form to another, and other such variables. With a relatively homogeneous panel of normal volunteers, obtained by appropriate entry restrictions with respect to sex, age, and other demographic variables, "baseline" pharmacokinetic parameters can be obtained. Any changes in these variables or other factors, such as the effect of a disease

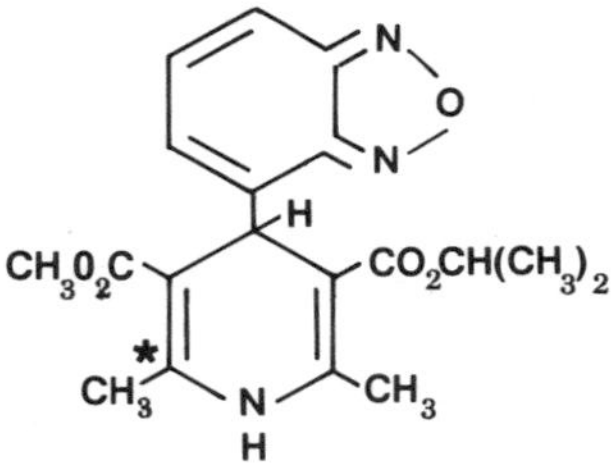

PN 200 - 110
(isradipine)
*position of carbon-14 label

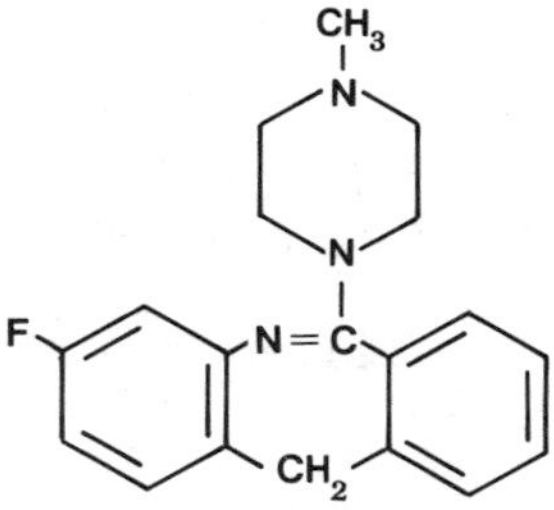

NB 106 - 689
(fluperlapine)

MeVal – C$_9$aa – Nva – Sar
  | |
MeLeu   MeLeu
  | |
MeLeu   Val
  | |
D-Ala – Ala – MeLeu

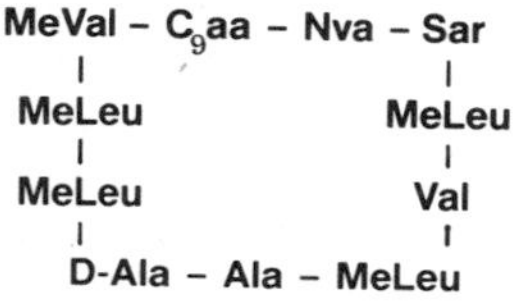

OG 37 - 325
(cyclosporine G)

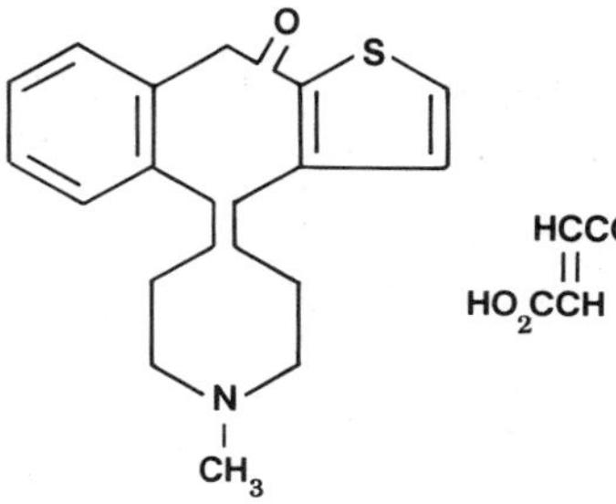

HCCO$_2$H
  ||
HO$_2$CCH

HC 20 - 511
(ketotifen fumarate)

FIGURE 1 Chemical structures of compounds discussed in this chapter. PN 200–110 (isradipine) is a dihydropyridine derivative with vaso- dilating activity caused by inhibition of calcium movement through calcium channels (9). NB 106–689 (fluperlapine) is an experimental tricyclic neuroleptic agent (10). OG 37–325 (cyclosporin G, CyG) is an analog of the cyclic undecapeptide cyclosporin A (CyA) used clinically as an immunosuppressant (11). HC 20–511 (ketotifen) is a potent orally active antianaphylactic agent (12).

state and specific organ function, can then be compared. Alternatively, comparisons of interest, such as the effect of a coadministered drug on the new drug's pharmacokinetics, can be performed under "baseline" conditions in a crossover design. Both approaches, in conjunction with a third, that of a general pharmacokinetic screen of the patient population used in the clinical trials, should contribute to the information needed for safe and effective general use of the new drug. Examples of the three approaches are cited in the latter parts of this chapter.

The success of pharmacokinetic studies in normal subjects or in patients depends upon prior careful weighing of the risks and benefits of the study, elaboration of clear objectives, and meticulous detailing in the study protocol of these objectives and all methodologies employed to achieve them. That portion of pharmacokinetic studies relating to safety should be evaluated by appropriate methods, which usually include physical examinations and determination of vital signs, electrocardiograms, and clinical laboratory parameters. Irrespective of the degree of "safety" of the drug to be administered, it is essential that the clinical portion of a pharmacokinetic study be supervised at several levels of hierarchy and accountability. Negligence in seemingly unimportant details, even those unrelated to safety, can have serious repercussions. For example, a pharmacokinetic study can be compromised by easily avoidable problems, such as illegible or missing specimen labels or thawed specimens due to improper shipment from the clinical site to the analytical laboratory. Additional factors for the successful completion of a pharmacokinetic study are the correct application of appropriately validated bioanalytical methodology in generating drug level data (see Chap. 2), and the proper choice of curve-fitting procedures and statistical techniques for the evaluation of these data. The stability of the analyte under various storage and handling conditions of the pharmacokinetic study must also be confirmed.

Curve-fitting and pharmacokinetic modeling are well accepted techniques for the evaluation of drug level data from pharmacokinetic studies. Particularly by simultaneous fitting of several compartments [e.g., blood, urine, and feces in ADME (absorption, distribution, metabolism, and excretion) studies as discussed below], meaningful model parameters can be calculated. However, the model chosen should be the simplest configuration that can explain the available data. A similar conservative approach applies to the use of statistical techniques. For example, the therapeutic equivalence of two dosage forms used by the patient population at large usually is inferred from the fact that these two forms produce similar rates and extents of bioavailability in a small group of normal subjects; that is, they are bioequivalent. Therefore, sound techniques to compare the individual and average rate and extent of bioavailability of the two forms in these normal subjects are mandatory (16).

III. CLINICAL PHASE I

The primary purpose of phase I clinical studies is to obtain short-term safety data for a new drug. Procurement of preliminary efficacy data is frequently a secondary objective. In an approach used widely by the pharmaceutical industry, the safety and tolerance of escalating single-dose treatments of the new drug are established, followed subsequently by escalating multiple-dose administrations generally not exceeding 1–2 weeks per dose level. These studies usually involve evaluation of parallel groups of healthy normal volunteers, frequently under placebo control and double-blind conditions. The initial dose administered to humans normally represents 1/10 or less of the maximum justifiable dose, which in turn is extrapolated from animal toxicity data. As outlined in the "grey book," a monograph issued in 1959 by the Division of Pharmacology of the FDA, "the rat should be able to tolerate without major toxicity ten or more times the maximum human dose and the dog a minimum of six times this dose on a milligram per kilogram basis." In the absence of more recent regulatory pronouncements, a safety factor of 10, 6, or 2 for rat, dog, and primate, respectively, based on the species that was found to be most sensitive to the toxicological effects of the new drug, is normally used to determine the maximum human dose. Such extrapolation from animals to humans is truly appropriate only if both show similar absorption, bioavailability, biotransformation, and sensitivity to toxic effects by the drug or its biotransformation products. This is frequently not the case. However, comparative pharmacokinetic and biotransformation (metabolite pattern) data from several animal species can provide a means to assess the reliability of the extrapolation to humans. Thus, for a new drug substance demonstrating in one or more animal species poor, erratic, and/or dosage form-dependent oral absorption, nonlinear accumulation of drug or biotransformation products, unusual retention of drug or biotransformation products, an abnormal dose-response profile, or a significantly dissimilar metabolite pattern compared with other species, the maximum human dose and, correspondingly, the initial dose should be lower than that extrapolated from the highest no-effect dose in the toxicity species. Particularly for this type of drug it is imperative that an evaluation of human pharmacokinetics during clinical phase I be performed. It has been suggested by the FDA (17) that the following information routinely be obtained in phase I:

1. Preliminary bioavailability and pharmacokinetic profile in humans. This provides information of potential bioavailability problems related to intrinsic drug properties or dosage form that may confound the evaluation of safety and subsequent efficacy studies.

2. Dose proportionality for single doses. Such data serve as a
   basis for designing multiple-dose regimens and may alert to
   potential safety or efficacy problems if nonlinearity is detected.
3. Preliminary drug metabolism in humans. Knowledge of the
   relative importance of various routes of drug elimination and
   the extent of biotransformation of the drug, as established by
   "metabolite patterns," enhances interspecies comparisons of
   pharmacological effect and drug toxicity.

Some of these evaluations may be done as a part of the usual
single- and multiple-dose safety and tolerance studies, although
logistical factors and concerns that additional blood sampling may
interfere with the clinical evaluations or compromise safety may either
preclude this altogether or severely limit the number of samples that
can be obtained. Alternatively, separate studies can be performed.
The potential benefit of more detailed pharmacokinetic data usually
provided by separate studies must be weighed against the greater
expenditure in time and resources with this approach. In any event,
studies utilizing radiolabeled drug, so called radioactive ADME studies
are conducted separately. As seen from the following examples, the
complexity of the pharmacokinetic program and choice of separate
or combined studies during clinical phase I should be a compromise
among considerations of safety, desired information, and available
resources.

A. Pharmacokinetic Monitoring as an Integral Part of the Safety and Tolerance Study

In animals, the experimental drug OG 37—325 (cyclosporin G) shows
immunosuppressive effects equal to the marketed immunosuppressant
cyclosporin A (CyA; see Fig. 1 for structures and abbreviations),
but renal and hepatotoxicity in the rat occur at doses two-to threefold higher than those at which such effects are seen with CyA.
However, the ratio of CyA dosage causing immunosuppression versus
renal toxicity is much lower in other animals than in humans (11).
Therefore, despite the two- to threefold higher safety factor for
CyG compared with CyA, concerns regarding the initial administration
of CyG to humans were warranted and are reflected by the conservative phase I study protocol detailed below. In a multiperiod, double-
blind, randomized, placebo-controlled escalating dose design, groups
of eight subjects each (five active and three placebo) received
single oral doses of CyG. The starting dose was 1.25 mg/kg. CyA
at this dose shows no adverse effects. The next scheduled dose
(2.5 mg/kg CyG) was to be administered only if the safety of the
previous dose level had been ascertained based on clinical laboratory

evaluations and CyG blood level profiles. Figure 2, containing the results of four dose levels of CyG, suggests that progression to the 5 and then 7.5 mg/kg dose levels was warranted by the proportional (or less than proportional) increase of AUC (area under the concentration-time curve) and C_{max} with dose. Increasing the dose from 1.25 to 2.5 mg/kg was justified by the absence of adverse findings in the follow-up evaluation of the one subject showing substantially higher CyG levels than the other four subjects (see Fig. 2). Escalating the dosages of CyG was also justified by the similar or lower blood levels compared with those of CyA. The results of this study demonstrate that both individual and mean pharmacokinetic parameters obtained in the course of a single-dose safety and tolerance study can be usefully applied to evaluate drug safety. Furthermore, the single-dose blood level profiles of CyG (data not shown) suggest possible advantages for administering CyG to humans in divided doses rather than the once daily regimen frequently used for CyA by providing higher trough levels and reducing the peak-trough ratio. A clinical phase I program should be sufficiently flexible to test such dosing issues, as exemplified by CyG, in the subsequent multiple-dose safety and tolerance study.

B. Incidental Monitoring of Safety and Tolerance Studies

The utility of incidental pharmacokinetic monitoring of a safety and tolerance study depends on the timing and frequency of sampling. The generation of complete drug level profiles at several dose levels as performed in the preceding example usually provides more detailed and reliable pharmacokinetic data than occasional sampling. However, with judicious selection of sampling times for the drug under investigation, even occasional blood sampling can yield useful information. The experimental drug NB 106—689 (fluperlapine; see Fig. 1) belongs to the class of tricyclic neuroleptic agents and therefore has the potential to adversely affect the hematopoietic system. Exposure to prolonged high levels of the drug represents a risk factor, and of particular concern would be a disproportionate increase of drug level with increasing doses. Early generation of drug level profiles and determination of pharmacokinetic parameters would be advantageous for this type of drug; however, frequent blood sampling is undesirable as part of a safety study in which the effects on the hematopoietic system are monitored. Although measuring urinary concentrations frequently represents an alternative approach, this was not considered appropriate for NB 106—689 since preclinical studies showed that the major route of elimination of the drug was in the bile. Consequently, in the multiple-dose safety and tolerance study of NB 106—689, a

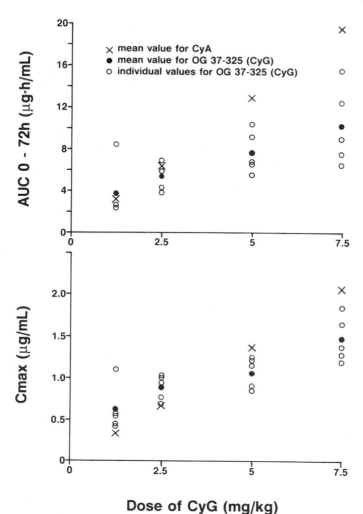

FIGURE 2 Derived pharmacokinetic parameters of CyG in sequential groups of healthy normal volunteers administered escalating single oral doses of CyG in a safety and tolerance study.

limited number of plasma samples for drug level analysis were obtained for each dose group. Five groups of 10 normal volunteers (8 active and 2 placebo) each received two or three daily doses of drug ranging from 30 to 200 mg/day for a period of 7 days. Progression to the next higher dose group occurred only upon evaluation of all safety data for the previous group. Blood for clinical laboratory evaluations was obtained during the baseline (predose) stage of the study, on the morning of dose day 3, on the morning of dose day 7, and during the washout phase of the study (day 10). Plasma levels of NB 106—689 were determined from aliquots of these blood specimens. The results are summarized in Figure 3. Irrespective of the dosing day, there was a linear relationship between the C_{min} values and the dose. Based on the increase in drug levels between days 3 and 7 and the decline in drug levels between days 7 and 10, a terminal elimination half-life of about 20 hr could be calculated for NB 106—689. This was confirmed in subsequent studies.

With a drug showing a substantially shorter half-life of elimination than NB 106—689, monitoring of the trough levels may be inappropriate. In such a case, monitoring on 3—4 dosing days at a fixed time point postdose (when adequate drug levels are expected to occur), should provide some information concerning possible nonlinear accumulation of drug.

C. Performance of Separate (Pilot) Bioavailability Studies and ADME Studies

As can be seen from the following examples for the drug PN 200—110 (isradipine, see Fig. 1), the performance of separate pharmacokinetic studies can substantially increase the quality of pharmacokinetic information. The safety and tolerance of PN 200—110 was demonstrated in a randomized, double-blind, parallel group, placebo-controlled study. The single oral doses administered ranged from 2.5 to 20 mg, 20 mg or about 0.4 mg/kg representing one-tenth of the highest no-effect dose of 4 mg/kg in the dog, the species most sensitive to the adverse effects of PN 200—110. Significant mean decreases in blood pressure were observed in the volunteers at the 10, 15, and 20 mg doses, the effect being greatest with the highest dose. Single oral doses of 15 mg or less were better tolerated than the 20 mg dose. Instead of directly monitoring this and subsequent phase I studies to evaluate the relationship among drug dose, plasma level, and effect, pharmacokinetic information on PN 200—110 was obtained from separate studies not hampered by the double-blind controls, presence of placebo-treated subjects, and limitations in blood sampling frequency posed by the safety and tolerance studies. These included one pilot pharmacokinetic bioavailability study and two studies with radiolabeled drug (see Table 1) described below.

1. Pilot Pharmacokinetic Study

In this study, six normal healthy male volunteers received single oral doses of PN 200—110 on six separate occasions as 5 and 20 mg capsules, 5 and 20 mg as an oral solution, and 5 and 20 mg in solution administered

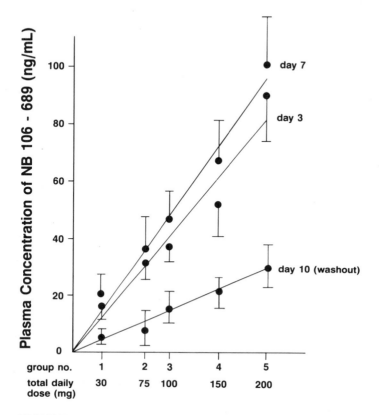

FIGURE 3 Mean plasma levels (±SD) of NB 106—689 in groups of
normal volunteers during the course of a 10-day regimen of the drug
involving various dose levels: group 1, 10 mg 3 times a day; group
2, 25 mg 3 times a day; group 3, 50 mg twice a day; group 4, 50 mg
three times a day; group 5, 100 mg twice a day. Solid lines represent
linear regression equation through the origin.

sublingually. Blood samples were obtained at fixed time points up
to 24 hr postdose. The following key information was obtained from
this pilot pharmacokinetic study: (1) there exists considerable intersubject variability for PN 200—110 bioavailability parameters (area
under the plasma level-time curve = AUC, peak plasma level = C_{max},
time to peak plasma level = t_{max}, and rate constants for absorption
and the biphasic elimination); (2) the oral and sublingual routes of
administration yield a similar rate and extent of bioavailability; (3)
the capsule formulation showed reduced AUC compared with the solution

and a C_{max} about one-half that of the solution; (4) PN 200—110 AUC and C_{max} show rough dose proportionality irrespective of formulation; and (5) very low plasma levels of PN 200—110 are achieved and the elimination of drug from plasma is rapid. The following conclusions and consequences for further development of PN 200—110 resulted from this pilot pharmacokinetic study. (1) The sublingual route of administration is not relevant for PN 200—110; however, additional formulation work would be required to improve the capsule. (2) Improvements in the analytical methodology were necessary to accurately and reproducibly measure the low plasma levels encountered. (3) From the plasma level profiles a twice a day or more frequent dosage regimen would be appropriate provided that there is a direct correlation between drug level and activity.

The conduct of this pilot pharmacokinetic study at an early stage of drug development provided valuable information concerning effective drug level, possible dosage regimens, and dosage form performance for PN 200—110. However, it is clear that such exploratory or pilot pharmacokinetic programs must be tailored to the situation and requirements posed by each new drug substance. Therefore, this study can serve only as an illustration of one of many possible approaches toward pharmacokinetic activities in clinical phase I. The approach taken may or may not include pilot studies but should involve at a minimum the single-dose ADME study described below.

2. Single- and Multiple-Dose ADME Studies (Radioactive)

Preclinical pharmacokinetic studies in the rat and dog showed that PN 200—110 is subject to considerable first-pass metabolism. The high variability of bioavailability parameters seen in the pilot pharmacokinetic study in humans is consistent with this. Dose proportionality in the 5—20 mg range established in the pilot study suggested the absence of saturable pharmacokinetic processes for PN 200—110 despite a large first-pass effect. Nevertheless, it is desirable early in clinical development to test for dose proportionality, not only of parent drug but also the metabolite composite, and to be assured that essentially all the administered dose can be recovered in the excreta (material or mass balance). Although, as in the case of PN 200—110, analytical techniques for parent drug may already be available in clinical phase I, it is unlikely that they will permit quantitation of the entire administered dose, as is possible with radiolabeled material. The use of a radioactive drug provides investigators with definitive information on the overall disposition of the compound as well as its potential for accumulation upon chronic administration. Additionally, since preclinical studies in animals are normally performed using tracer techniques (see Chap. 4), the human ADME study can indicate which animal species has the potential to serve as a model for the human.

Biotransformation studies on new drugs are normally performed with radioactive samples. Thus blood, urine, and feces from human ADME studies provide a source of biologic materials for biotransformation work. Using radiolabeled drug greatly facilitates the determination of "metabolite patterns," which are obtained by high-performance liquid chromatography (HPLC) of the biologic fluid, either directly or following extraction or other forms of sample pretreatment and subsequent monitoring of the radioactivity in the eluant.

Although human ADME studies are relatively simple in design, usually employing no more than 6−12 subjects, if performed judiciously they can provide a wide range of useful information. The objectives of such studies should include the following.

Estimation of the rate and extent of absorption of the administered dose: Since total radioactivity is measured, one can be assured that unchanged drug and all metabolites (total dose) are included.

Determination of the rate and amount of elimination from the blood as well as the excretory pathways (e.g., urine and feces): Since various analytical techniques readily allow differentiation of parent drug and metabolites in the radioactive sample, conclusive information on the fate of the drug in humans can be obtained. Knowledge of the contribution of renal and hepatic pathways to the elimination of the drug and its metabolites provides rationales for the use of the drug in certain disease states (e.g., renal or hepatic insufficiency).

Generation of pharmacokinetic parameters for both parent drug and metabolites: This information can be employed to design dosing regimens and sampling times for future clinical trials.

Provide definitive data on material balance: Since this type of study can yield complete accountability of the administered dose, information concerning retention and/or accumulation of drug and metabolites can be obtained.

Provide data that are directly comparable to those generated in the preclinical animal AMDE studies: This allows the development of rational animal models.

Human ADME studies are usually performed in normal, healthy, male volunteers. A single dose of the radioactive drug is administered, and if more than one dose level is to be investigated, then parallel groups are utilized. Since radiolabeled material (usually carbon 14 or tritium) is administered in these studies, it is necessary to evaluate the potential hazard of radiation exposure to the volunteers. Of particular importance is what is referred to as the "absorbed dose" of radioactivity, which is normally determined by estimating the energy (rad or rem) imparted to a specific organ or tissue. This can conveniently be estimated by the equation (18)

$$D = 73.8\bar{E}_B C_{max} T_{eff}$$

where
D = absorbed dose (rad or rem)

$\bar{E}_B$ = average β-particle energy (MeV)

C_{max} = maximum tissue or organ concentration (μCi/g)

T_{eff} = effective biologic half-life (days)

For example, if 250 μCi of a carbon 14-labeled drug with a terminal half-life of 48 hr is administered to a volunteer, the exposure to the liver (based on a 310 g mass in a 70 kg man) would be

$$D = (73.8)(0.05 \text{ MeV}) \frac{250 \text{ }\mu\text{Ci}}{310 \text{ g}} (2 \text{ days}) = 5.95 \text{ rem}$$

This value, almost twice the allowable limit for a single dose (19), is an unrealistic estimation since it assumes that the entire radioactive dose localizes in the liver with none distributing to other organs or tissues of the body. A more realistic approach is the use of in vivo animal distribution data (see Chap. 4) in which actual organ and tissue concentration of radioactivity are determined following administration of the labeled drug.

For PN 200—110, a maximum radioactivity concentration of 2.25 μgEq/g was observed in the liver of rats following a 0.25 mg/kg oral dose of the ^{14}C-labeled drug. Thus the estimated maximum liver concentration following a radioactive dose of 250 μCi in a 70 kg man would be

$$C_{max_{-man}} = \frac{2.25 \text{ }\mu\text{gEq/g}}{0.25 \text{ mg/kg}} \frac{250 \text{ }\mu\text{Ci}}{70,000 \text{ g}}$$

$$= 0.032 \text{ }\mu\text{Ci/g}$$

The projected exposure of radioactivity to liver in humans would be

$$D = 73.8(0.05 \text{ MeV})(0.032 \text{ }\mu\text{Ci/g})(2 \text{ days})$$
$$= 0.236 \text{ rems}$$

This value is approximately 25 times less than that calculated without the benefit of the animal tissue distribution data and is considerably less than the allowable 3 rem limit for organs of this type (19). Similar exposure data should be generated for other critical organs and tissues, since in the absence of animal distribution data an extreme overestimation of radioactivity burden normally occurs.

Although the radioactive dose is often administered orally as a solid dosage form (tablet or capsule), a solution or suspension is preferable. In this manner the pharmacokinetics of the drug itself can be evaluated without the added variable of dosage form. However, appropriate stability data for the solution must be generated prior to the study.

In the usual study the radiolabeled dosage form is administered to volunteers after an overnight fast. Serial blood, urine, and fecal samples are then collected for a sufficient time to assure that essentially all of the radioactive dose can be accounted for. Normally, 120 hr or more may be required since in this type of study the radioactive samples contain not only the parent compound but also all metabolites containing the radiolabel. If it is suspected from preclinical investigations or from the position of the label per se that biologic instability of the label could occur, the study design should include the collection of carbon dioxide (exhaled air) or analysis for tritiated water.

PN 200—110 used in the ADME studies was radiolabeled with carbon 14 in the 2-position, as shown in Figure 1. This position is stable to hydrolytic or biotransformation processes, as demonstrated in preclinical animal studies by the absence of exhaled radiolabeled carbon dioxide and complete recovery of radioactivity from the excreta. Analysis for unchanged [^{14}C]PN 200—110 in blood was done by radioimmunoassay and by HPLC. In the latter, quantitation of the low levels of PN 200—110 was achieved by addition of nonlabeled PN 200—110 to the specimen and counting the radioactivity present in the elution window described by the ultraviolet (UV) trace of the added drug (20). Alternatively, direct quantitation of parent drug in the biologic fluid is possible by addition of large quantities of nonlabeled drug, extraction, and recrystallization to constant specific activity (inverse isotope dilution).

Figure 4 depicts the mean blood levels and the cumulative excretion of [^{14}C]PN 200—110 following a 5 mg oral dose to six male volunteers. Similar results were obtained for the 20 mg dose of [^{14}C]PN 200—110 in six additional subjects. At both doses the recovery of radioactivity was nearly complete. Incomplete recovery of radioactivity can jeopardize the validity of an ADME study, and thus efforts should be expended to determine if this was due to incomplete collection or losses through specimen workup or as volatile radioactivity or was caused by the retention of radioactivity in the body. If the last was found to occur, an investigation of the mechanism of this retention is mandatory. Enterohepatic or other modes of recycling, storage in a deep compartment, or actual covalent linkage to tissue are examples of processes leading to drug or metabolite retention.

The single-dose ADME study with [^{14}C]PN 200—110 confirmed the finding of dose proportionality in the pilot study, as well as the existence of a high first-pass effect, previously seen in animals.

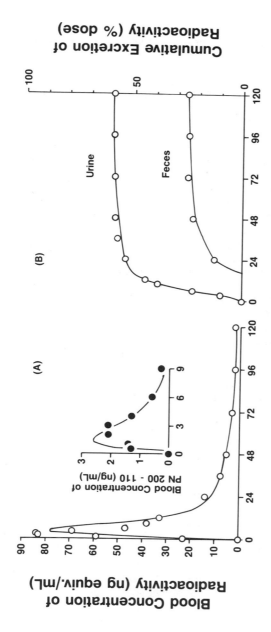

FIGURE 4 Mean blood levels (A) and cumulative excretion (B) following a 5 mg oral dose of [^{14}C]PN 200–110 to six normal, male volunteers. (○) [^{14}C]concentration; (●) PN 200–110 concentration. The curves are computer derived. Excretion of unchanged drug in the urine and feces was <10% of dose.

Through the use of an appropriate model involving simultaneous fitting of all data points from the three compartments (blood, urine, and feces), single-dose pharmacokinetic parameters could be calculated and multiple-dose projections made. This is depicted in Figure 5, where simulated curves based on the single-dose ADME data for PN 200−110 are compared to the actual concentrations of radioactivity and unchanged drug resulting from a multiple-dose study in normal male volunteers performed during clinical phase II of the PN 200−110 development program (also see Table 2).

IV. CLINICAL PHASE II

During this phase of drug development, the first trial of the new drug in patients normally occurs. The primary objectives are to evaluate the efficacy of the drug and to establish its safety under conditions approaching the intended use. This usually involves multiple-dose regimens administered to patients over an extended time period from which sufficient efficacy and safety data are obtained to justify entering the long-term trials of clinical phase III. Pharmacokinetic activities in clinical phase II can be divided into two general areas. (1) Support of clinical studies includes more detailed investigations of drug pharmacokinetics and dosage form performance, especially under conditions of multiple dosing, in normal volunteers but also in patients if there is reason to believe that drug disposition in the latter may be significantly different. (2) Expansion of animal safety data includes a more complete evaluation of animal and human metabolism, such as metabolite characterization through metabolite patterns, isolation of major metabolite(s) from appropriate biologic fluids, and structural characterization and/or identification. A comparison of the type and relative importance of biotransformation pathways in animals and humans validates the choice of the species for long-term toxicity testing, which is normally initiated at this stage.

The multiple-dose radioactive ADME study usually conducted in clinical phase II (see Fig. 5) addresses many of these issues by providing multiple-dose pharmacokinetic data for both parent drug and total radioactivity composite and mass balance data, as well as biologic fluids for metabolism work. It would be very desirable to use the clinical service form (the dosage form chosen for the extended clinical trials in late phase II and in phase III) for the radioactive dose. This is usually not possible, however, because introducing radioactive drug substance into the dosage form production equipment presents a safety hazard. Therefore, finely packed capsules prepared

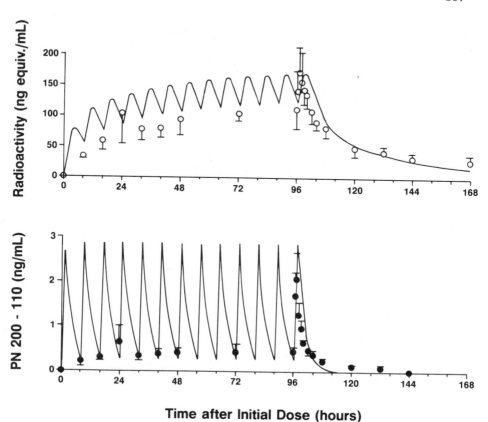

FIGURE 5 Mean blood levels of (○) radioactivity (ng Eq/ml) and
(●) PN 200–110 (ng/ml) during multiple oral administration (5 mg
every 8 hr × 13) of [^{14}C]PN 200–110 to five normal male volunteers.
Bars indicate 1 SD. The curves are simulated based on single-dose
parameters.

by hand in a suitably restricted environment or (preferably) a solution
are normally used for the radioactive ADME study. This unfortunately
precludes an evaluation of dosage form performance of the clinical
service form. Instead such evaluation is usually carried out by
separate studies using normal volunteers or by monitoring phase II
studies in patients. The choice of either approach and the extent
of monitoring is guided by factors similar to those already discussed
for clinical phase I.

Evaluations of the dosage form and dosage strengths to be marketed should also be initiated at this juncture, particularly if the clinical service form is not a likely candidate for marketing. Early scheduling of activities is imperative because of the extended time requirements for development and in particular stability testing of a new dosage form. In the event that bioequivalence testing of clinical service form versus the dosage form proposed for marketing reveals them to be nonequivalent, sufficient time for development of an alternative form should be available prior to the targeted NDA date. Even when the clinical service form is intended for marketing, early bioavailability testing is desirable to ascertain its acceptable performance versus a solution or suspension (the "ideal" formulation). Suboptimal bioavailability increases the potential for higher inter- and intrasubject variability and, as also discussed later, should be avoided. If multiple strengths of the clinical service form are to be marketed, their therapeutic equivalence will have to be demonstrated in a dosage form proportionality study (see Table 2), unless therapeutic equivalence can be established clinically or all dose strengths use the same excipients and have identical ratios of active to inactive ingredients. If the final choice of dosage form to be marketed cannot be made at this stage, prudence dictates that all work necessary for registration be completed as far as possible prior to the ultimate decision point. This may include a dose-proportionality study and intrasubject variability study, examples of which are discussed in the following sections (also see Table 2), as well as attempts to correlate the in vitro dissolution rate with bioavailability in pilot studies.

A. Dose-Proportionality Study

The objective of the dose-proportionality study is to determine the pharmacokinetics of the new drug over the entire dose range employed in clinical use. Specifically, the effect of dose on the rate and extent of the bioavailability of the new drug, as reflected by AUC, C_{max}, and t_{max}, are established. Additional objectives for this study are an assessment of the variability of these parameters and further evaluations of the elimination kinetics of the drug, all of which are useful for the planning of subsequent studies. This study also presents an opportunity for a final critical assessment of the bioanalytical method prior to its use in pivotal bioavailability, bioequivalence, and dosage form proportionality studies. The drug is usually administered to a panel of healthy normal volunteers as a solution or a suspension, since, as with the ADME studies, intrinsic pharmacokinetic properties unobscured by dosage form factors are desirable.

In a 3 × 3 replicated Latin square design, 2.5, 5, and 10 mg solutions of PN 200-110 were administered to 15 normal healthy male volunteers, each administration of drug separated by a 7-day washout period. Blood was obtained at fixed time points between 0 and 12 hr postdose and plasma concentrations of PN 200-110 determined by radioimmunoassay. The derived parameters C_{max} and t_{max} were obtained by inspection and AUC by the trapezoidal rule. Interpolated parameters and AUC $0 - \infty$ were calculated from the best fit equations using a triexponential expression with a lag time to absorption for the curve-fitting process (21). Descriptive statistics were calculated for derived and interpolated parameters and for their logarithmic transforms; the latter is often done to minimize the influence of outlying values. Linear regression analysis was performed for the relationship of parameters with the dose. The appropriateness of a straight line through the origin for this relationship was examined using a test for lack of fit (22). Analysis of variance was performed on the parameters to assess the effects, if any, of study period and dosing sequence. Analysis of variance on dose-corrected parameters represents an alternative approach to test their relationship with the dose. From the error terms in the analysis of variance the number of subjects necessary to discern a given difference in parameter means with an adequate degree of statistical assurance (power calculations) was determined.

As expected from the pilot and ADME studies previously discussed, the dose-proportionality study confirmed a linear dose-bioavailability relationship for PN 200-110. No sequence or period effects were noted. Coefficients of variation of about 40% for AUC, about 50% for C_{max}, and the large error term in the analysis of variance suggest considerable within- and between-subject variability for PN 200-110 bioavailability parameters. Accordingly, the power calculations revealed that to discern 20% differences in parameter means at least 16 subjects would be required for AUC and at least 29 subjects for C_{max}. Any bioavailability difference $\leqslant$ 20% is not considered therapeutically relevant (3).

It is apparent from this study that, except for the quantification of parameter variability and a final comprehensive validation of the bioanalytical method, little additional information on the pharmacokinetics of PN 200-110 was obtained. In retrospect, it may have been possible to combine the study with the "intrasubject variability" study discussed below. In such a combined study, involving four treatment periods, 2.5, 5, and 10 mg PN 200-110 as a solution and a repeat of one of the three dose strengths would be administered in randomized order, providing both dose-bioavailability and more extensive within- and between-subject variability data.

B. Intrasubject Variability Study

A crucial element of the bioavailability regulations is that "a bioequivalence study should have sufficient power statistically to detect
at least a 20% difference in the means of two treatments at α of 0.05
and β of 0.2. A power of 0.8 or better ensures the acceptability of
the study statistically" (2). This means that proof of bioequivalence
is based on average results for the rate and extent of absorption
of reference and test product and appropriate measures of variability.
Thus the number of subjects in the study must be sufficiently large
to ensure a high probability (>0.8) of detecting a 20% difference
between reference and test product if such a difference does indeed
exist. A difference in the means of $<20\%$ is not believed to be clinically
important, as previously mentioned (3).

In addition to the requirement dealing with the average rate and
extent of absorption, rules have been proposed concerning the relative
bioavailability of drugs in individual subjects (4, 23). They relate
to the range of bioavailability within a given study, specifying that
the relative bioavailability of the test product must be $>75\%$ for at
least 75% of the subjects ("75/75 rule") or $>70\%$ for at least 70% of
the subjects in certain cases (24). The statistical power and 75/75
criteria for a study are dependent upon the within- (intrasubject)
and between-subject variability of bioavailability for the drug in
question. Changes in the study design, such as increasing the number
of subjects, alternate choice of reference product with more reproducible pharmacokinetic properties, or utilizing a steady state
rather than single dose-design, have been proposed as a means of
ensuring the statistical acceptability of a study (4). However, drugs
showing a large variability of pharmacokinetic parameters, possibly
associated with a high first-pass effect, may never provide "acceptable"
bioavailability studies even with these changes in study design. For
example, Haynes (6) has calculated empirical probabilities of a study
meeting the 75/75 rule for given within- and between-subject coefficients of variation and intrasubject correlation. He showed that
many studies would not provide sufficient statistical power even when
employing a very large subject panel size.

The FDA BD Code (25) identifies those well-studied drugs that
are known to have "bioequivalence" problems and for which "statistically
acceptable" studies cannot be conducted. In vitro dissolution data may
suffice to demonstrate bioequivalence for these drugs. In the case
of a new drug, however, failure to provide a "statistically acceptable"
study may not be ascribed to a "bioequivalence problem" without
adequate documentation that such a problem indeed exists. Such
documentation would include demonstration of a very large first-pass
effect, the existence of high within- and between-subject variability,

or dissolution problems of the drug substance (4), although it is not quite clear what degree of first-pass effect, variability, and dissolution problems warrants waiver of bioequivalence testing.

The bioavailable fraction of PN 200–110 determined in the single-dose ADME study was 18%. The dose-proportionality study in humans revealed high coefficients of variation for AUC and C_{max}. The panel size projections from the dose-proportionality study suggested using as many as 29 subjects to achieve statistical acceptability for the comparisons of the means, without assurance that individual ratios would be within acceptable limits. It is for all these reasons that the following study on the variability of PN 200–110 bioavailability parameters was undertaken.

A panel of 13 normal healthy male volunteers received a single oral dose of 10 mg PN 200–110 as a solution on three separate occasions, separated by a 7-day washout period. Plasma levels of PN 200–110 were determined between 0 and 12 hr postdose, and derived parameters were obtained as previously described. Analysis of variance was performed on the data, employing a randomized block design as well as nested-design analysis. Power calculations were also performed. Individual bioavailability ratios were determined, and the degree of correlation of individual paramters between the three treatment periods was assessed.

The average bioavailability data for PN 200–110 showed good repeatability. Differences between the three treatment periods for mean AUC and C_{max} were <10% despite considerable within- and between-subject variability. This variability, graphically displayed in Figure 6, was determined from the mean square error and confidence interval of the analysis of variance. Further evidence for high variability was the lack of statistical significance for the intrasubject correlation analysis and failure to meet the 75/75 rule for two of the three pairwise comparisons of AUC and for all three of the pairwise comparisons of C_{max}. It was concluded from this study that the variability inherent in PN 200–100 disposition may on occasion render the bioavailability comparison of a reference and a test formulation of this drug statistically unacceptable, even if the two formulations are indeed identical and a crossover design with 24 subjects (usually viewed to be the practical upper limit for bioavailability testing) is utilized. However, bioavailability assessment of PN 200–110 dosage forms should provide an accurate reflection of their true average rate and extent of absorption.

Upon completion of the clinical phase I and II pharmacokinetic studies described earlier, sufficient pharmacokinetic and bioavailability data should be available to optimize the extended phase III clinical trials, as well as the pharmacokinetic studies performed at that stage of drug development. For certain drugs presenting a bio-

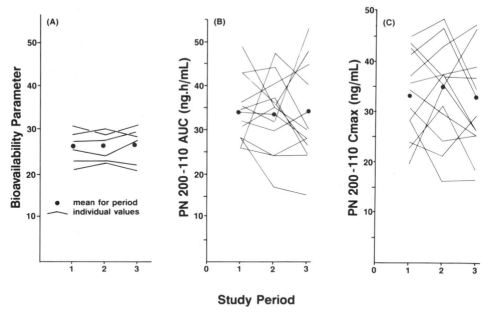

Study Period

FIGURE 6 Individual AUC values for a hypothetical drug possessing
low inter- and intrasubject variability administered to a panel of six
subjects on three separate occasions (A). Individual AUC (B) and
C_{max} (C) values in normal subjects administered a 10 mg solution of
PN 200−110 on three separate occasions. Mean parameter values across
study periods were similar, but the existence of considerable intrasubject variability is apparent.

availability problems, the conduct of an "absolute bioavailability"
study, comparing derived parameters after oral and parenteral administration of drug, may be informative; however, additional toxicity
studies in animals may first have to be performed to demonstrate the
safety of the parenteral route for humans. An amendment to the
original IND containing appropriate manufacturing, biopharmaceutical,
and animal safety data may be filed for this purpose. If both the oral
and parenteral routes of administration are proposed for therapeutic
use, their development usually proceeds under separately filed,
although suitably cross-referenced IND.

The technique of quantitative mass spectroscopy of stable isotope-
labeled drug has been shown to be useful for absolute bioavailability
and other pharmacokinetic studies (26). Coadministration of the nonlabeled drug with the stable isotope-enriched analog(s) as internal
standard(s), followed by mass spectroscopic determination of these

compounds, provides individual drug level profiles and relative bio-availability data from a single set of the biologic sample. The advantages of this approach are therefore a possible consolidation of several administration periods into one and, by reducing the variability inherent in multiple administrations, a smaller subject panel size necessary for statistical acceptability. This technique is therefore particularly useful in studying drugs showing high intrasubject variability. These advantages are offset by the requirement for chemical synthesis of the isotope-labeled standard(s) and the necessary absence of changes in pharmacokinetic and biotransformation processes due to the presence of the stable isotope label, which may have to be verified in an independent study. Another requirement is the presence of linear pharmacokinetics under the doses and conditions of the stable isotope study. In a typical trial, the stable isotope internal standard is administered orally (for bioavailability assessment) or intravenously (determination of absolute bioavailability) followed immediately by an oral dose of the nonlabeled drug formulation to as few as four to six subjects. Various permutations of study design and frequency and sequence of administration of nonlabeled and isotope enriched drug are possible, as discussed by Wolen (27).

V. CLINICAL PHASE III

The scope of pharmacokinetic studies performed in clinical phase III represents not only a continuation and elaboration of previous work on drug biotransformation or dosage form performance but also the initiation and conduct of a new group of studies to determine the effects of such variables as different patient populations, disease states, or environmental conditions on drug disposition. These studies are also referred to as "labeling studies," since they provide information for the appropriate use of the drug in patients, as eventually presented in the package insert. By specifically focusing on a single variable, labeling studies can complement and enhance the projections for general use of a drug made from the clinical data of phase III, irrespective of whether the clinical trials are performed in hundreds or thousands of patients. However, the number of and the protocols for labeling studies usually vary according to drug type, properties, and use. Pharmacokinetic studies of dosage form performance of clinical service forms versus forms proposed for marketing must be completed in phase III, and investigations of possible advantages imparted by the use of novel dosage forms, such as oral controlled-release dosage forms, skin patches, implants, or pumps (see Chaps. 8 and 9) should be seriously considered at this stage. However,

registration activities for these novel forms most often occur under a
separate IND and at a time when the drug, formulated in a standard
dosage form, is already an approved entity.

The extent and complexity of investigations on the biotransformation
of the new drug depend upon drug class and use. In general, however,
phase III activities in this area greatly exceed those performed in
phase II, normally not as a consequence of planning but as a result
of the difficulties inherent in isolating and identifying multiple metabolites that are usually present in minute quantities as complex mixtures
in large volumes of biologic fluid. Frequently a major and time-
consuming program to chemically synthesize the major metabolites
must be undertaken because insufficient quantities of metabolic products can be isolated from the ADME studies. This is especially
critical in the situation in which biotransformation in humans proceeds
to different products than in the animal species used for toxicity
testing. The only alternative is to undertake additional safety assessment of these synthesized products in animals. An approach that is
often utilized is to synthesize "potential" metabolites early in the drug
development process for pharmacological and safety assessment.
Examples of likely candidates for synthesis are products of N-demethylation, de-esterification, and hydroxylation of labile sites.
Computer programs have been devised to assist in evaluating relevant
routes of biotransformation of any chemical structure (28). All these
considerations impacted on the biotransformation work performed for
PN 200—110 in clinical phase III, which included the following:

  Detailed elaboration of the major metabolic pathways in humans
      and all species involved in toxicity testing. These included
      de-esterification, oxidative processes leading to aromatization,
      and glucuronidation and other conjugation reactions. Humans
      and other animals shared similar routes of biotransformation,
      although some quantitative differences were noted.
  Chemical synthesis and evaluation of pharmacological activity of
      metabolites and potential metabolites. None of these compounds
      showed appreciable activity.
  Investigation of the role of metabolites in the accumulation or
      retention of radioactivity in the human ADME studies and
      their presence or absence in the toxicity species.

Since biotransformation of PN 200—110 imparts a loss of pharmacological activity, no other investigations of biotransformation processes
were necessary. If certain PN 200—110 metabolites had been found to
be active, development and validation of bioanalytical methodology
for these metabolites and studies on the dynamics of their generation

and elimination would be desirable. This would have impacted on the conduct of phase III bioavailability and bioequivalence studies (see Table 2). Because of the absence of active metabolites, these studies were analyzed for parent PN 200—110 only.

It is thus clear that knowledge of metabolite activity at the earliest possible opportunity facilitates planning of the entire drug development program. The specific consequences for phase III pharmacokinetic studies resulting from the presence of active metabolites are determined by the precursor or successor relationship of active and inactive species, the time course of conversion, and the relative amounts converted. One extreme is represented by an inactive prodrug that is rapidly converted in vivo to a single pharmacologically active species; the other extreme is the formation of a series of metabolites, each presenting a different spectrum of activity, from an active parent drug. In the former case measurement of the single active compound should suffice to address the requirements posed by scientific and/or regulatory considerations. For the latter, individual monitoring of all or at least the major, active species may be required, since the basis for demonstrating bioavailability according to 21 CFR 320.23 and 320.24 (1) is the measurement of the active drug ingredient or therapeutic moiety or its metabolites in biologic fluids as a function of time, which FDA personnel have interpreted to mean the following: "where there is rapid first pass metabolism, where the metabolite is either present to a much larger extent or has significantly greater pharmacological action the Division of Biopharmaceutics will require that the active metabolites generated also be measured in addition to the parent drug" (29). It can be assumed that the regulatory requirement for appropriate statistical assurance of detecting parameter differences not attributable to subject variability (21 CFR 320.23) holds for metabolite concentration determinations as well as for parent drug.

A. "Regulation" Bioavailability and Bioequivalence Studies

1. Dosage Form Proportionality Study

Guidelines for the basic design and conduct of bioavailability and bioequivalence studies for new drug products or new formulations of active drug ingredients already approved for marketing are provided in 21 CFR 320.25 (1). In accordance with these guidelines, the "regulation" bioavailability study for the PN 200—110 capsules to be marketed was performed in comparison to a reference material, a solution of the drug. The protocol for this study also incorporated relevant findings from the "intrasubject variability" study described previously, in order to increase the likelihood of achieving adequate

statistical sensitivity to detect clinically significant differences (i.e.,
those greater than 20%) in the rate and extent of PN 200—110 absorption
not attributable to subject variability. In addition to establishing the
bioavailability of the capsule versus the solution reference standard,
a further objective was to establish the bioequivalence of equipotent
drug treatments of all capsule strengths to be marketed (2.5, 5, 7.5,
and 10 mg). These capsules, containing the identical ingredients
and showing similar in vitro dissolution profiles, differed in the ratio
of active to inactive ingredients. The ratios ranged from 1:107 for
the 2.5 mg capsule to 1:26 for the 10 mg capsule, with the 5 and 7.5
mg capsules showing ratios within this range. Consequently, if PN
200—110 treatments of 4 × 2.5 mg capsules and 1 × 10 mg capsules
were shown to be bioequivalent, this would also imply equivalence
between equal doses of either of these two capsule strengths and
the intermediate 5 and 7.5 mg strengths.

In a replicated 3 × 3 Latin square design, a panel of 24 normal
healthy male volunteers received single 10 mg oral doses of PN 200—110
as a 10 mg capsule, as 4 × 2.5 mg capsules, or as a 10 mg solution
following an overnight fast. A washout period of 7 days separated
each drug treatment. Plasma levels of PN 200—110 were determined
at fixed time points between 0 and 24 hr postdose. Bioavailability
comparisons were based on the various derived parameters as previously discussed. The mean plasma level data for the 24 subjects
are shown in Figure 7. The capsule formulations demonstrated a
significantly slower rate of absorption, hence lower C_{max}, than the
solution. This observation was similar to that seen with the early
capsule formulation used in the pilot pharmacokinetic study (see
Sec. III.C.1), but unlike the earlier formulation, the new capsule
demonstrated a similar extent of absorption as the solution. Analysis
of variance for the 3 × 3 Latin square design revealed differences in
the mean AUC between the three treatments of <11%, which were
of no statistical significance in the pairwise comparisons. Similarly,
differences between C_{max} values as well as mean t_{max} values of the
capsule treatments were <5% and not statistically significant. It was
concluded that all three formulations show similar extent of absorption,
as reflected by their AUC values, and that equipotent doses of the
2.5 and 10 mg capsules yield similar rates and extent of absorption,
the former reflected by C_{max} and t_{max}. There is "dosage form proportionality" between the 2.5 and 10 mg capsules. As expected, the
large differences in C_{max} between solution and capsule treatments
were highly significant. An alternative approach to evaluate bioavailability parameter differences is to compare confidence intervals
for the mean parameters ratios. These intervals can be obtained
in two ways: (1) employing Fieller's theorem (30), and (2) calculating
the confidence interval for the difference of the means followed by

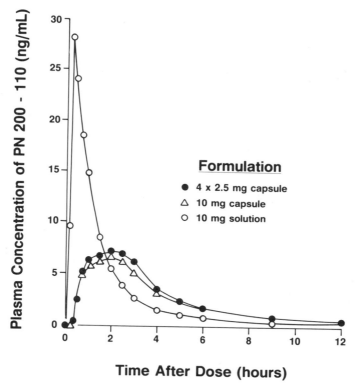

Time After Dose (hours)

FIGURE 7 Mean plasma levels of PN 200—110 in normal volunteers administered the drug as a 1 × 10 mg capsule, 4 × 2.5 mg capsules, and a reference solution containing 10 mg.

arithmetic transformation of the end points as described by Metzler (31). The results obtained by either of the two methods confirmed the preceding bioavailability conclusions from the analysis of variance. Additional useful techniques for parameter comparisons, not employed for the present study but applied to the data of the interaction studies described in Section V.B, are the evaluation of posterior probability that the parameter means differ by less than 20% (Bayesian analysis) (32) and the "two one-side t-test" procedure as proposed by Schuirmann (8).

The intrasubject variability (CV) for AUC, C_{max}, and t_{max} of the solution, as well as the AUC values of the two capsule formulations, ranged from 20 to 28%, which is in excellent agreement with the variability observed for the solution in the phase II intrasubject variability study. In contrast, the intrasubject variability (CV) for

C_{max} and t_{max} of the capsule treatments was considerably higher,
ranging from 38 to 49%. This is not surprising since the absorption
of a solid dosage form is usually more variable than that of a solution,
the "ideal" formulation. Interestingly, though, the between-subject
variability for the solution C_{max} was significantly greater than that
for the capsule C_{max} as established by the Pitman-Morgan test (33).
In agreement with the predictions made from the intrasubject variability
study, the 75/75 rule was not uniformly met for the present dosage
form comparisons. These results also presented several consequences
for the power calculations that were performed to gauge the statistical
acceptability of the study. In accordance with the predictions made
by the intrasubject variability study, acceptable statistical power
was achieved in the present study for the AUC parameter. Owing to
the large difference in the magnitude of the parameter means for
capsule and solution treatments, the very low statistical power for
C_{max} was unexpected. Consequently, and further justified by the
results of the Pitman-Morgan test, the two capsule treatments alone
were compared to each other by analysis of variance using a randomized
block design. Again, there were no statistically significant differences
between the two capsule treatments, confirming that there exists
dosage form proportionality for the 2.5 and 10 mg capsules and, by
inference, for the 5 and 7.5 mg capsules as well. By limiting the
comparison to the two capsule treatments, in which the mean square
error was not inflated by the contribution of the solution data, a
statistical power of >0.8 was achieved to discern C_{max} or t_{max} differences $\geq 30\%$. Statistical acceptability by strict regulatory criteria
was therefore not realized. Since it is unlikely that a 30% difference
in C_{max} or t_{max} would be clinically important for this type of drug,
where a 20% difference by regulatory definition is not, this short-
coming of the study should be irrelevant.

2. Bioequivalence Study (Steady State)

A design frequently encountered in a "regulation bioavailability"
study is that of comparing the dosage form to be marketed with the
clinical service form using a solution of the drug as reference standard
(see Table 2). Such a study is described here, comparing a capsule
form used in clinical trials of the drug HC 20−511 (ketotifen; see
Fig. 1 for structure) with the tablet proposed for marketing, and a
HC 20−511 reference solution. Instead of the usual single-dose administration, this study was performed at steady state, that is,
making the appropriate parameter comparisons after each dosage
form was administered for a sufficiently long period to achieve the
steady-state concentrations. Pharmacokinetic theory indicates that the
area under the curve for a dosing interval equals the AUC $(0 - \infty)$

after a single dose of the drug (21) and provides the rationale for a steady-state study. It is clear that because of the greater complexity and cost of a steady-state study and the underlying principle that subjects should not be unnecessarily exposed to a drug, whether experimental or approved, this design should be reserved for those instances in which a single-dose bioavailability or bioequivalence study would be unsuitable. The steady-state design for the bioequivalence study of HC 20—511 was chosen because the bioanalytical method was not sufficiently sensitive to determine drug levels after a single 2 mg dose over three half-lives (the mean $t_{\frac{1}{2}}$ of HC 20—511 in normal subjects is about 23 hr). The "three half-lives rule" is explicitly stated in the bioavailability regulations (1), although this rule seems overly restrictive in those instances when the terminal half-life of a drug does not appreciably contribute to its AUC. An alternate approach that should be acceptable to the regulatory agency is to accurately and precisely measure drug concentrations to 1/10 of peak. The alternative of increasing the dose of the single-dose administration to achieve measurable drug levels, was not feasible for HC 20—511 owing to possible subject intolerance.

In a three-period randomized crossover design, 21 healthy normal male volunteers received 2 mg doses of HC 20—511 as a tablet, a capsule, and a solution. Subjects received one of the three dosage forms every 12 hr for 7 days, immediately followed by the second dosage form every 12 hr for 7 days and then the third dosage form every 12 hr for 7 days (34). Thus, instead of the usual drug-free washout period in single-dose crossover studies, the present design simultaneously allowed washout of the prior dosage form and achievement of steady state with the next form to be evaluated. Blood samples were collected immediately prior to and for up to 12 hr subsequent to dose 13 (day 7) and dose 27 (day 14) and immediately prior to and for up to 96 hr subsequent to the final dose (day 21). Concentrations of HC 20—511 were determined by radioimmunoassay. Figure 8 shows the mean plasma level data obtained during the three evaluation periods on study days 7, 14, and 21—24. Achievement of steady state by days, 7, 14, and 21 was verified by similarity of 0 and 12 hr C_{min} values and evaluation of drug half-lives during the washout period. With the exception of one subject who was excluded from the bioavailability comparisons for this reason, the terminal half-lives were <36 hr, which implies that steady-state conditions were established for each formulation by dose days 7, 14, and 21. Bioavailability comparisons were based on evaluations of derived parameters (AUC, C_{max}, t_{max}, C_{min}), either observed or interpolated using a three-exponential expression for steady-state levels (21). Concentrations of HC 20—511 from all three 12 hr dosing intervals plus the washout period were curve fit simultaneously. Elimination parameters were fit independently of formulation; however

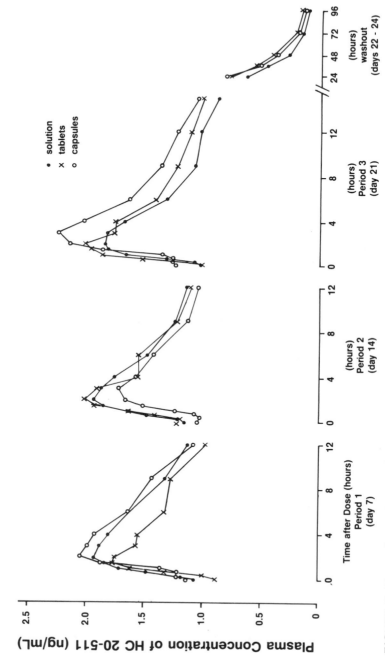

FIGURE 8   Mean plasma levels of HC 20−511 determined on days 7, 14, and 21 in normal volunteers receiving 2 mg twice a day of ketotifen capsules, tablets, and reference solution over a 21-day period.

best fits were sought separately for each of the three formulations with respect to input rates and the fraction of drug bioavailable compared to the reference solution. Statistical analysis of these parameters indicated bioequivalence of the tablet and capsule formulations, showed their acceptable bioavailability compared to the solution reference standard, and also demonstrated adequate statistical power to discern 20% differences, had they existed between the three formulations. All parameters except t_{max} met the 75/75 rule. The regulations specify that a drug product that differs from the reference material in its rate of absorption but not in its extent of absorption may be considered bioavailable if the difference in the rate of absorption is not detrimental to the safety and effectiveness of the drug product (21 CFR 320.23) (1). For drugs that achieve their therapeutic effect upon long-term administration and for which the incidence of acute adverse effects is similar, irrespective of different rates of absorption between dosage forms, variability in the t_{max} should be of no consequence.

The clinical service forms and dosage forms to be marketed for PN 200—110 and HC 20—511 showed bioavailability similar to that of the reference solutions. However, for some drugs, poor aqueous solubility, pK_a, and other physicochemical properties can adversely affect dissolution and hence reduce bioavailability. This occurs particularly for those drugs showing a high first-pass effect in which bioavailability depends upon the absorption flux. Further consequences may be highly variable and unpredictable bioavailability, compounded by environmental factors, such as food intake. For example, it is for these reasons that phenytoin has been identified as a drug with high risk potential for bioavailability failures (35). An evaluation of the bioavailability of various commercial dosage forms of phenytoin has revealed considerable variability between them (36). Therefore, efforts should be made during drug development to formulate a dosage form that produces adequate and reproducible bioavailability compared with a solution reference standard. To obtain clinical experience with a poor dosage form is clearly unacceptable. Pilot pharmacokinetic studies, typically involving four to six normal volunteers and a crossover design, are the most efficient means to evaluate dosage forms of drugs with high risk potential for bioavailability failures, unless a valid animal model has been elaborated. In vitro dissolution data can serve to prescreen dosage form candidates but is usually no substitute for in vivo evaluations.

B. Special Pharmacokinetic Studies (Labeling Studies)

In addition to the regulation bioavailability and bioequivalency studies performed in clinical phase III, special studies are often undertaken to answer specific questions about the disposition of the compound that arise during the development process. At present there are no

federal regulations concerning which special studies are required
in an NDA. It has been suggested, though, that population pharmacokinetic studies will prove useful in identifying specific special studies
that should be undertaken for a particular drug candidate (37).
Special studies are often conducted in selected segments of the population to determine the effects of such variables as demographics
(age, race, and sex), disease state, or environmental factors (drug
interactions and food) on the pharmacokinetics of the drug. This
information allows a sponsor (manufacturer) to support dosage
labeling claims (i.e., "labeling studies") with definitive bioavailability
and pharmacokinetic data. The following examples of special studies
done with PN 200—110 are representative of those most commonly
conducted. Depending on the specific indication of the drug as well
as the intended patient population, additional studies may also be
appropriate. On occasion,labeling studies should be performed in
clinical phase II. For example, with a poorly soluble drug showing
incomplete and/or erratic absorption in early pharmacokinetic trials,
the effect of food on bioavailability may be considerable and the degree
should be known to optimize the conduct of the phase III trials.
Conversely, not all of the studies specified may be required for all
drug candidates, and in a few cases, none may be necessary.

1. Different Populations: Effect of Age

Because of the therapeutic indication for PN 200—110 (hypertension),
it was likely that the target population would consist of a high percentage of elderly patients. Since numerous physiological changes
occur in the elderly that can be relevant to drug disposition (38),
this type of study is essentially mandated for any new chemical
entity undergoing drug development.

In a 2 × 2 replicated Latin square design, PN 200—110 capsules
(5 and 10 mg) were administered as single doses to a group of 26
healthy elderly (mean age 70, range 65—83 years) male volunteers.
Based on potential difficulties in recruiting an adequate number of
subjects at a single clinical site, the study was performed by two
investigators with 13 subjects enrolled at each center. Administration
of the two dose levels of the drug was separated by a 5-day washout
period. Plasma levels of PN 200—110 were determined at fixed time
points between 0 and 24 hr postdose. Bioavailability evaluations were
based on the various derived parameters as previously discussed.
There were no statistically significant differences between the
bioavailability data from either study site. The mean plasma level
data for the 26 elderly subjects following the 10 mg capsule dose in
comparison to the mean plasma levels obtained in pharmacokinetic
studies with young healthy volunteers (see below) are shown in Figure
9. Overall, for the 26 elderly subjects, both AUC and C_{max} exhibited
a linear relationship with dose in the 0—10 mg range, as had been
shown earlier for young normal individuals.

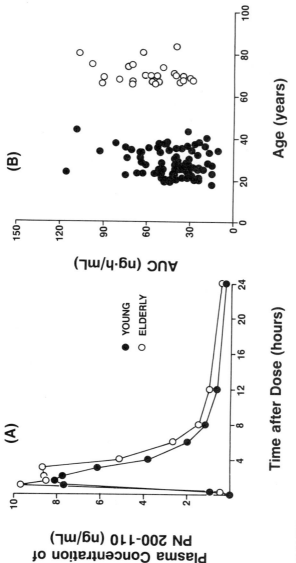

FIGURE 9 Mean plasma levels of PN 200–110 in young (n = 57) and elderly (n = 26) normal subjects following administration of 10 mg capsules (A). Individual AUC values obtained in young and elderly normal subjects (B).

The mean bioavailability data for the 10 mg capsule in the elderly were compared with a database (n = 57 subjects) gathered from three previous PN 200–110 pharmacokinetic studies in which the same 10 mg capsule formulation was administered to young healthy male volunteers (mean age 28 years). On average, the elderly showed statistically significantly higher AUC (by 55%) and C_{max} (by 25%), no change in t_{max}, and statistically significant reductions in the terminal elimination rate (by 40%), clearance (by 9%), and first-pass metabolism (by 41%). Individual AUC data for the young and elderly subjects are also summarized in Figure 9.

The types of changes observed in the elderly in this study compared with those in younger subjects are consistent with reduced drug elimination capacity or lower volume of distribution generally seen in this population. Since PN 200–110, as other dihydropyridines, is subject to considerable intrasubject variability in the young and in the elderly, however, it would be necessary to apply this finding cautiously in any labeling (package insert) statements. A rational approach is to avoid a blanket proposal of dose reduction in the elderly and instead suggest individualized therapeutic regimens of initially low doses with subsequent titration to a safe and efficacious dose level.

2. Disease State: Effect of Renal Insufficiency

Obtaining pharmacokinetic data in patients is particularly useful if the disease can sufficiently alter the disposition profile of the drug so that dosage adjustment is necessary. Of special importance are renal and hepatic dysfunction since they can play a major role in altering drug elimination. The studies become almost mandatory if it has been shown previously that disease state alters the pharmacokinetics of drugs that are structurally similar to the drug under development.

In the case of PN 200–110, it was observed that the pharmacokinetics of the structurally related drugs (dihydropyridines) nifedipine (39) and nitrendipine (40) were variably altered when administered to patients with renal impairment. Also, although elimination of PN 200–110 by the renal route is of little importance, the majority of the administered dose is excreted by this pathway in the form of metabolites. It has also been shown that the effect of renal disease is not only related to excretion, but can have a major effect on drug metabolism (41–43).

In a single-period parallel group design, 23 subjects grouped according to varying degrees of kidney function (creatinine clearance ml/min < 10, n = 6; 11–30, n = 5; 30–80, n = 6; >80, n = 6 each received a single 10 mg capsule of PN 200–110. Serial blood samples were obtained 0–48 hr postdose. During this evaluation period no hemodialysis was performed. Bioavailability comparisons were based on the various derived parameters as described in the previous pharmacokinetic studies in this chapter. The mean data for the 23 subjects are shown in Figure 10. There were no statistically significant differences in the mean critical bioavailability or pharmacokinetic parameters between subjects with normal renal function and patients with mildly or moderately impaired renal function. The trend toward higher PN 200—110 levels in the midly impaired subjects may be a result of their relatively higher age. This illustrates the necessity for closely matching groups when a parallel study design is used. Severely impaired or anuric patients showed a significant reduction ($\simeq 50\%$ of normals) in AUC and C_{max}. These findings for PN 200—110 parallel those reported for other dihydropyridines (39, 40).

From this study it would appear that severe renally impaired or anuric patients may require somewhat higher doses of PN 200—110 to achieve drug levels comparable to those seen in subjects with more normal renal function. Thus, pharmacokinetic studies in the disease state can potentially yield information that plays a major role in drug safety and efficacy. Since hemodialysis may remove circulating drug or metabolites, its use was contraindicated during the evaluation periods of the renal insufficiency study. However, particularly for new drugs with a potential for abuse or those with a small threshold between therapeutic and toxic drug concentrations, the effectiveness of hemodialysis should be evaluated in a separate pharmacokinetic study.

3. Environmental Studies

a. Concomitant Medication It is extremely common for patients to receive two or more drugs concomitantly. There is also the possibility that some of the drug combinations can interact adversely. From a pharmacokinetic standpoint, these interactions may involve an alteration in the absorption, distribution, metabolism, or excretion of one or both compounds. Since it is not possible to study all potential drug interactions for a new drug under development, judicious choices must be made about which particular combinations will be evaluated. Selection is normally limited to drugs that are likely to be prescribed simultaneously by clinicians. Thus for PN 200—110, its potential interaction with hydrochlorothiazide needed to be investigated.

Using a 3 × 3 replicated Latin square design, 21 volunteers were administered 10 mg capsules of PN 200—110 or 50 mg hydrochlorothiazide (HCTZ) tablets, either individually or concomitantly. Each administration was separated by a 5- to 10-day washout period. Serial blood samples were obtained between 0 and 30 hr following each dosing period and plasma concentrations of PN 200—110 and HCTZ were determined. The mean data for the 21 subjects are shown in Figure 11. The bioavailability parameters evaluated for this study were the same as

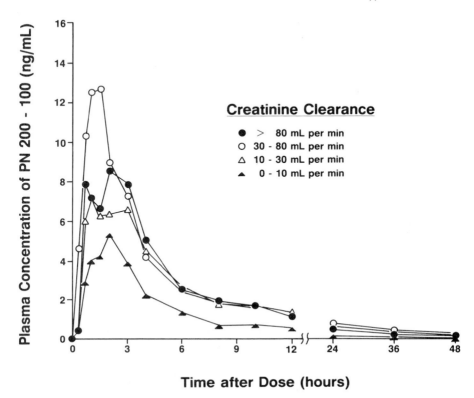

Time after Dose (hours)

FIGURE 10 Mean plasma levels of PN 200–110 in subjects grouped
by varying renal function.

those discussed previously for the other pharmacokinetic studies.
For PN 200–110 there were no statistically significant difference in
the bioavailability parameters on concomitant administration of HCTZ
compared to PN 200–110 alone. Differences in AUC and C_{max} were
< 10%. Similar results were observed with HCTZ, for which differences
for AUC and C_{max} were < 5%.

These results demonstrate that concomitant administration of PN
200–110 and HCTZ does not result in altered pharmacokinetics of
either agent. However, drug interactions may manifest themselves
not only in altered pharmacokinetics. Pharmacological drug-drug
interactions (additive, antagonistic, or synergistic effects) or mis-
cellaneous interactions, such as the effect of acidic urine on methena-
mine (44), are also possible and should be the subject of the investigators' attention during the phase III clinical trials.

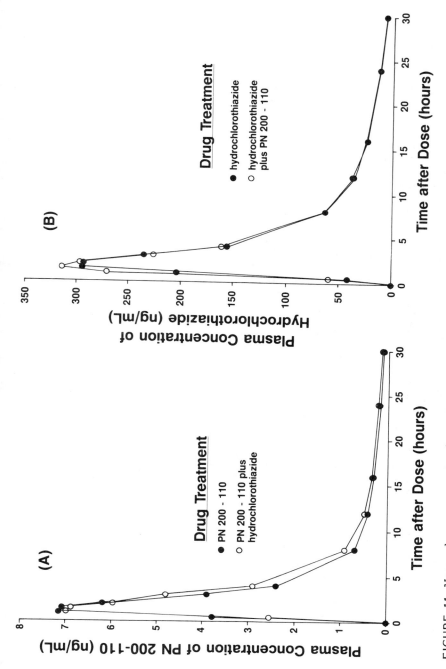

FIGURE 11 Mean plasma concentrations of PN 200—110 following administration of 10 mg PN 200—110 or 10 mg PN 200—110 plus 50 mg hydrochlorothiazide (A). Mean plasma concentrations of hydrochlorothiazide following administration of 50 mg hydrochlorothiazide or 50 mg hydrochlorothiazide plus 10 mg PN 200—110 (B).

b. *Food Interaction* Since it has been well established that meals, especially those containing a high fat content, can have a profound effect on the rate and extent of absorption of drugs (45), food inter- action studies have become an integral part of most NDA submissions. This type of study was of particular importance for PN 200—110, since nifedipine, a drug with a similar structure (dihydropyridine) and pharmacological class (antihypertensive), had previously been shown to have a delayed peak (by 3 hr) and a lower C_{max} (by one-third) when administered with food than in the fasting state (46).

A panel of 15 normal volunteers in a two-period crossover design received single oral doses of PN 200—110 capsules on an empty stomach or with a high-fat breakfast. The two study periods were separated by 6- to 7-day washout period. Serial blood samples were obtained 0—15 hr postdose. Bioavailability parameters were obtained as pre- viously described for other studies in this chapter. The mean data for the 15 subjects are shown in Figure 12. Following administration of PN 200—110 on a fasted stomach, the drug was rapidly absorbed with mean peak plasma levels achieved after 1.4 hr. Administration of the drug with food resulted in a statistically significant increase in the lag time to absorption by about 50 min and consequently a delay in the time to peak of about 50 min. However, the extent of bioavailable PN 200—110, as reflected by the AUC, was unchanged.

Thus, the administration of PN 200—110 with food has no appreci- able effect on bioavailability. This means that dosing restrictions with respect to food intake are unnecessary for this drug.

c. *General Pharmacokinetic Screen* (*"Population Pharmacokinetics"*) In all the previously discussed studies on PN 200—110, average phar- macokinetic parameters were obtained from small, relatively homo- geneous groups of volunteers or patients. The summation of these studies defines a general, though not all encompassing, pharmaco- kinetic profile for PN 200—110. A major, clinically relevant purpose in determining this profile was to develop dosing guidelines for specific populations who may be at particular risk when taking the drug. The disadvantage of this approach is that the overall pharma- cokinetic profile elaborated from specific studies is limited to the various patient characteristics and underlying pathology, which were a priori assumed to be relevant for all future patients taking the drug. In an alternative approach, that of the prospective phar- macokinetic screen, the population, rather than the individual, serves as the unit of pharmacokinetic analysis (47). By evaluating PN 200—110 levels in a large number of patients a more representative sample of the target population was accessible, even though far fewer data points per patient are normally available in such "popu- lation pharmacokinetic" studies compared with the pharmacokinetic

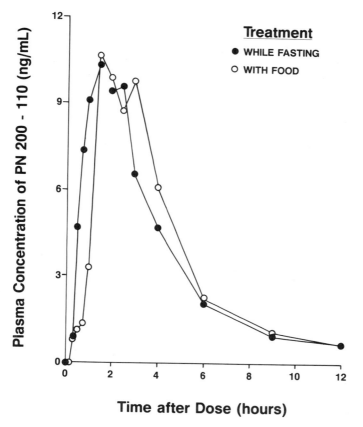

Time after Dose (hours)

FIGURE 12 Mean plasma levels of PN 200–110 following administration of the drug with food or in the fasting state.

studies discussed previously. In the course of seven clinical studies assessing the safety and efficacy of orally administered (5–20 mg/day) PN 200–110, plasma samples were obtained during their routine clinic visits from hypertensive patients taking the medication for blood pressure control. Sampling was performed at any convenient time point after the morning dose but before the second dose of the twice a day regimen of the drug in capsule formulation. No restrictions with respect to sampling frequency, number or type of patients sampled, concomitant medications, or other variables were made. Of the nearly 1500 plasma samples collected in the course of the study, 735 samples from 263 patients who had complied with their assigned dosing regimen were available for evaluation (samples from suspected noncompliers were also evaluated for metabolite concentrations; all subjects showing no measurable parent drug and metabolite concentrations and those on placebo control were excluded). Figure 13 depicts a plot of the dose-normalized PN 200−110 concentrations in these 735 specimens as a function of time after the morning dose.

Several computational techniques have been advocated for the evaluation of population pharmacokinetic data (48, 49). These techniques are discussed in detail in Chapter 10. Since the major focus of the population screen for PN 200−110 levels was to identify subgroups of patients differing from the majority and to identify those factors possibly contributing to the differences in PN 200−110 levels, the approach taken was to group individual data into the classifications low, middle, and high plasma levels using cluster analysis (50). Figure 13 depicts these data groups. The groups were compared with respect to demographic variables, clinical laboratory data, and frequency of adverse reactions encountered in the course of the study. Of the demographic data, only age showed significant differences among groups, a higher age being associated with higher PN 200−110 levels, a finding corroborated in the separately performed labeling study discussed previously. Mean clinical laboratory parameters showed no statistically significant differences between groups. There were no differences in the frequency of adverse reactions between groups.

The collection of large numbers of blood specimens in the course of clinical trials, particularly under conditions that ensure the integrity of analyte, presents great logistical difficulties. Therefore, the advantage of a population pharmacokinetic study over the performance of separate labeling studies is open to question. The intent of a population pharmacokinetic study is to search for the unexpected and unusual response in drug level to a given dose. Therefore, the value of a population pharmacokinetic study over separate labeling studies for a given drug will have been demonstrated only if the search was successful, that is, if the study was able to characterize such subpopulations of patients showing excessive or subtherapeutic drug levels, not readily identifiable in the standard labeling studies described above. Consequently, it is also unclear if the evaluation of 735 plasma samples from 263 patients in the PN 200−110 population pharmacokinetic study was sufficient to identify all groups potentially at risk. Only further experience with this type of study, and with a variety of drugs, can address such questions.

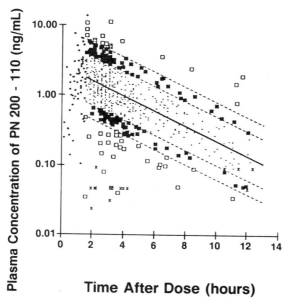

Time After Dose (hours)

Y-axis: Plasma Concentration of PN 200 - 110 (ng/mL)

FIGURE 13 Individual (dose normalized) PN 200—110 levels in 263 hypertensive patients evaluated in a "population pharmacokinetic" screen: values for upper and lower 10th percentile (□), 10—15th percentile (■) and mid-70th percentile (·) of values in the time interval 1.5—12.5 hr postdose; values in the absorption phase (0—1.5 hr) (○) and values below the limit of detection of the analytical method (×) were excluded from subsequent analysis. The solid line represents linear regression of data points 1.5—12.5 hr postdose.

VI. POST-NDA STUDIES

The studies presented as examples in this chapter represent a basic pharmacokinetics package that would meet present FDA requirements for an NDA submission. However, it is often necessary to perform a number of other pharmacokinetic studies during the clinical development process (phases I through III) or even after the drug has been approved for marketing. This postapproval stage is frequently referred to as phase IV. Typical trials may include the evaluation of alternate routes of administration, of improvements in the dosage form described in the original NDA, or of alternate dosage forms that modify the release of the drug compared to the conventional oral form. The evaluation of new indications for drug use may also necessitate further special pharmacokinetic (labeling) studies. As previously discussed, an amendment to the original IND or a new IND submission may be required to conduct such additional pharmacokinetic studies, and upon their completion either a new NDA or an NDA amendment may have to be filed. The scope of the pharmacokinetic studies will depend upon the changes sought from the original NDA. Thus, for example, regulatory approval of a modified-release version of an approved oral form requires a detailed pharmacokinetic evaluation after single oral doses and at steady state in comparison to the approved form, as well as an assessment of the effect of environmental factors, such as food intake, on the performance of the modified-release form. It is unlikely in today's regulatory climate that approval will be obtained solely on the basis of such pharmacokinetic studies, and thus additional clinical studies to evaluate safety and efficacy may be prudent. Chapters 8 and 9 discuss these aspects in more detail and also provide the regulatory point of view. In contrast, for a new formulation of an approved drug that makes no claims of a controlled or modified release, or any other claims not contained in the original NDA, a single-dose bioavailability study should suffice for regulatory approval. In a typical study the experimental form is compared to the marketed form in fasted normal volunteers using the standard two-way crossover design. The previously discussed criteria apply for bioequivalence and statistical acceptability. The data for this study and appropriate revisions to the original drug labeling can be submitted in the form of an abbreviated NDA (ANDA) or a supplement to the original NDA.

VII. CONCLUSIONS

From the discussions in this chapter it is apparent that pharmacokinetic studies play a vital role in the clinical drug development process. Although the suggested "package" of studies outlined in Table 2 is normally adequate for an FDA biopharmaceutics submission based on present federal regulations and guidelines, there is no guaranteed "cookbook" approach that can be utilized for all NDA submisions. Obviously, all drug candidates are different and therefore pharmacokinetics must be used as a flexible tool that can aid the clinical researcher in dealing with the wide range of problems encountered during the NDA process. Approached in this way, pharmacokinetic studies can substantially decrease the risk to subjects (blood level monitoring), isolate subpopulations that should be dosed differently, aid in the design and evaluation of clinical trials, and contribute to the development of more effective dosage forms. Thus, if correctly applied, pharmacokinetics can play an important role in the development of safer and more effective drug therapy. Essential elements for judicious application are carefully planned pharmacokinetic studies. Since these studies are performed throughout the drug development process, which usually takes many years to come to fruition, this poses a major challenge to the individuals responsible for their design, scheduling, and execution. In particular, a changing regulatory climate, as well as ongoing scientific progress, render long-term planning difficult. Continued dialogue between workers in the field of drug development and the regulatory agency, as well as discussions as exemplified in this volume, should assist in facilitating this process.

ACKNOWLEDGMENTS

In concert with the multidisciplinary nature of pharmacokinetic studies, a number of individuals contributed to the studies discussed in this chapter, particularly K. Andriano, E. Abisch, J. Dain, L. Gonasun, A. Hassell, R. Laplanche, R. Lehr, W. Niederberger, H. Schwarz, T. Smith, F. Tse, and R. Voges.

REFERENCES

1. U.S Code of Federal Regulations, Title 21, Bioavailability and Bioequivalence Requirements, Parts 320 1–320.62, Special Edition of Federal Register. U.S. Government Printing Office, Washington, D.C., 1981, pp. 120–138.
2. S. V. Dighe, Current bioavailability and bioequivalence requirements and regulations. Clin. Res. Pract. Drug Reg. Affairs 2: 401–421, 1984.
3. J. P. Skelly. Bioavailability and bioequivalence. J. Clin. Pharmacol. 16: 539–545, 1976.
4. B. E. Cabana. Assessment of 75/75 Rule: FDA viewpoint. J. Pharm. Sci. 72: 98–99, 1983.
5. R. Temple. FDA's new guidelines for NDA submissions. Presented at 5th Annual Arnold Schwartz Memorial Program, New York, November 1, 1984.
6. J. D. Haynes. Statistical simulation study of new proposed uniformity requirements for bioequivalency studies. J. Pharm. Sci. 70: 673–675, 1981.
7. B. E. Rodda and R. L. Davis. Determining the probability of an important difference in bioavailability. Clin. Pharmacol. Ther. 28: 247–252, 1980.

8. D. J. Schuirmann. Approaches to statistical data analysis of bioavailability/bioequivalence studies. Paper presented at the Drug Information Association Meeting, Biopharmaceutics Considerations in NDA/ANDA Submissions, November 1985, Hilton Head Island, South Carolina.

9. C. E. Handler and E. Sowton. Safety, tolerability and efficacy of PN 200—110, a new calcium antagonist in patients with angina and coronary heart disease. Eur. J. Clin. Pharmacol. 27: 415—417, 1984.

10. T. J. Petcher and H. P. Weber. Conformations of some rigid neuroleptic drugs. J. Chem. Soc. Perkin II: 1415, 1976.

11. A. von Wartburg and R. Traber. Chemistry of the natural cyclosporin metabolites. Prog. Allergy 38: 28—45, 1986.

12. C. Vibelli and G. Rudelli. Ketotifen in bronchial asthma: Results of a multicenter study. Med. Torac. 5: 105—119, 1983.

13. N. H. G. Holford and L. B. Sheiner. Understanding the dose-effect relationship: Clinical application of pharmacokinetic-pharmacodynamic models. Clin. Pharmacokinet. 6: 429—453, 1981.

14. V. F. Smolen. Bioavailability and pharmacokinetic analysis of drug responding systems. Annu. Rev. Pharmacol. Toxicol. 18: 495—522, 1978.

15. M. Montagne. Issues in the design and conduct of clinical trials. Clin. Res. Pract. Drug. Reg. Affairs 3: 23—44, 1985.

16. C. M. Metzler and D. C. Huang. Statistical methods for bioavailability and bioequivalence. Clin. Res. Pract. Drug Reg. Affairs 1: 109—132, 1983.

17. B. E. Cabana and J. F. Douglas. Bioavailability-pharmacokinetic guidelines for IND development. Paper presented at the 15th Annual International Pharmacy Conference, Austin, Texas, February 23—27, 1976.

18. W. R. Hendee. Radioactive Isotopes in Biological Research. John Wiley and Sons, New York, 1973, p. 300.

19. U.S. Code of Federal Regulations, Title 21, Drugs Used in Research, Part 361.1. U.S. Government Printing Office, Washington, D.C., 1986, pp. 160—164.

20. F. L. S. Tse, J. M. Jaffe, and J. G. Dain. Pharmacokinetics of compound 58—112, a potential skeletal muscle relaxant, in man. J. Clin. Pharmacol. 24: 47—57, 1984.

21. J. G. Wagner. Fundamentals of Clinical Pharmacokinetics. Drug Intelligence Publications, Hamilton, Illinois, 1975, pp. 102—106.

22. N. R. Draper and H. Smith. Applied Regression Analysis 2nd ed. John Wiley and Sons, New York, 1981, pp. 33—40.

23. Fed. Reg. 43: 6968, 1978, Fed. Reg. 45: 11853, 1980, Fed. Ref. 45: 48160, 1980, and Fed. Reg. 45: 72200, 1980.

24. Fed. Reg. 45: 56832, 1980.

25. Fed. Reg. 42: 1648, 1977.

26. M. Eichelbaum, G. E. von Unruh, and A. Somogyi. Application of stable labelled drugs in clinical pharmacokinetic investigations. Clin. Pharmacokinet. 7: 490−507, 1983.

27. R. L. Wolen. The application of stable isotopes to studies of drug bioavailability and bioequivalence. J. Clin. Pharmacol. 26: 419−424, 1986.

28. R. Voges, B. R. von Wartburg, and H. R. Loosli. Tritiated compounds for in vivo investigations: CAMP and ^{3}H-NMR spectroscopy for synthesis planning and process control. Proceedings of 2nd International Symposium on Synthesis and Applications of Isotopically Labeled Compounds, Kansas City, Missouri, 1985. Elsevier Science Publishers, Amsterdam, 1986, pp. 371−376.

29. S. V. Dighe. Current bioavailability and bioequivalence requirements and regulations. Paper presented at the Educational Seminar sponsored by Regulatory Affairs Professional Society, August 3, 1983, Morristown, New Jersey.

30. D. J. Finney. Statistical Methods in Biological Assay, 2nd ed. Charles Griffin & Co., London, 1971.

31. C. M. Metzler. Bioavailability−a problem in equivalence. Biometrics 30: 309−317, 1974.

32. B. E. Rodda and R. L. Davis. Determining the probability of an important difference in bioavailability. Clin. Pharmacol. Ther. 28: 247−252, 1980.

33. E. Pitman. A note on normal correlation. Biometrica 31: 9−12, 1939.

34. B. Schmidt-Redemann, P. Brenneisen, W. Schmidt-Redemann, and S. Gonda. The determination of pharmacokinetic parameters of ketotifen in steady state in young children. Int. J. Clin. Pharmacol. Ther. Toxicol. 24: 496−498, 1986.

35. Academy of Pharmaceutical Sciences. Report of the Ad Hoc Committee on drug product selection. J. Am. Pharm. Assoc. NS 13: 278, 1973.

36. A. P. Mekikian, A. B. Straughn, G. Slywka, P. L. Whyatt, and M. C. Meyer. Bioavailability of 11 phenytoin products. J. Pharmacokinet. Biopharm. 5: 133−146, 1977.

37. R. Temple. Discussion paper on the testing of drugs in the elderly (memorandum). U.S. Food and Drug Administration, Department of Health and Human Services, Washington, D.C., September 30, 1983.

38. J. G. Outstander. Drug therapy in the elderly. Ann. Intern. Med. 95: 711−722, 1981.

39. C. H. Kleinbloesem, P. Van Brummelen, J. Van Harten, M. Danhof, and D. D. Breimer. Nifedipine: Influence of renal function on pharmacokinetic/hemodynamic relationship. Clin. Pharmacol. Ther. 37: 563−574, 1985.

40. G. R. Aronoff and R. S. Sloan. Nitrendipine kinetics in normal and impaired renal function. Clin. Pharmacol. Ther. 38: 212–218, 1985.

41. M. M. Reidenberg, H. Kostenbauder, and W. Adams. Rate of drug metabolism in obese volunteers before and during starvation and in azotemic patients. Metabolism 18: 209–213, 1969.

42. E. Englest, Jr., H. Brown, D. G. Willardson, S. Wallack, and E. L. Simon. Metabolism of free and conjugated 17-hydroxy-corticoids in subjects with uremia. J. Clin. Endocrinol. Metab. 18: 36–38, 1958.

43. M. M. Reidenberg, M. James, and L. G. Dring. The rate of procaine hydrolysis in serum of normal subjects and diseased patients. Clin. Pharmacol. Ther. 13: 279–284, 1972.

44. P. D. Hansten (ed.). Drug Interactions, 3rd ed. Lea and Febiger, Philadelphia, 1975, p. 2.

45. R. D. Toothaker and P. G. Welling. The effect of food on drug bioavailability. Annu. Rev. Pharmacol. Toxicol. 20: 173–199, 1980.

46. K. Hirasawa, W. F. Shen, D. T. Kelly, G. Roubin, K. Tateda, and J. Shibata. Effect of food ingestion on nifedipine absorption and haemodynamic response. Eur. J. Clin. Pharmacol. 28: 105–107, 1985.

47. B. Whiting, A. W. Kelman, and J. Grevel. Population pharmacokinetics: Theory and clinical application. Clin. Pharmacokinet. 11: 387–401, 1986.

48. L. B. Sheiner and L. Z. Benet. Premarketing observational studies of population pharmacokinetics of new drugs. Clin. Pharmacol. Ther. 38: 481–487, 1985.

49. J. L. Steimer, A. Mallet, and F. Mentre. Estimating the interindividual pharmacokinetic variability. In Variability in Drug Therapy: Description, Estimation and Control. Edited by M. Rowland, L. B. Sheiner, and J. L. Steimer. Raven Press, New York, 1985, pp. 65–111.

50. SAS Institute Inc. The "Fastclus" Procedure, SAS User's Guide, 5th ed. Box 8000, Cary, North Carolina, 1985, pp. 377–401.

6

Simulation of Oral Drug Absorption: Gastric Emptying and Gastrointestinal Motility

GLEN D. LEESMAN, PATRICK J. SINKO,
and GORDON L. AMIDON *College of Pharmacy, The University of Michigan, Ann Arbor, Michigan*

I. INTRODUCTION

The modeling of the gastrointestinal tract for oral absorption may vary in complexity from the treatment of the entire gastrointestinal tract as a one-compartment "black box" to complex physiologically based absorption models. The black box approach is usually adequate only for those drugs whose absorption characteristics are not affected by their position in or the environment of the gastrointestinal tract. This is not usually the case; however, even in the most well "behaved" cases, an absorption lag time may be needed to account for the time the drug resides in the stomach prior to passage to the small intestine. In order to demonstrate the effects of gastric emptying and gastrointestinal motility on oral dosage form performance, a physiological flow model has been chosen as the basis for the simulations.

Based on their absorption properties two classes of drugs have been chosen to demonstrate the use of physiological flow modeling for plasma level simulations. The fundamental step in this type of modeling is to have a thorough knowledge of how the drug passes through the gastrointestinal tract and to understand the drug's mechanism of absorption. Based on transit considerations and the drug's absorption characteristics, variations in plasma level time curves can be explained. This chapter emphasizes the effect of the transit of drugs through the gastrointestinal tract and focuses on the effects of gastric emptying and gastrointestinal motility on oral dosage form performance.

II. REVIEW OF GASTRIC EMPTYING AND GASTROINTESTINAL MOTILITY

A. Physiological Flow Model

Physiological modeling of drug absorption from the gastrointestinal tract must account for the physiological properties of the gut as well as the properties of the drug. One must understand the parameters pertaining to drug absorption and how they are affected by either their location in the gastrointestinal tract or the environment of the gastrointestinal tract.

A schematic diagram of the physiological flow model of the gastrointestinal tract, as proposed by Topp and Amidon (1), is shown in Figure 1. In this model the gastrointestinal tract is represented as a series of well-mixed tanks where the concentration of drug in each compartment is assumed to be uniform throughout and equal to the concentration of drug at the exit stream. The transfer of drug from one compartment to another is represented by first-order rate constants determined from the flow from each compartment divided by the corresponding volume of that compartment and is represented by the first-order rate constant

$$K_i = \frac{Q_i}{V_i} \tag{1}$$

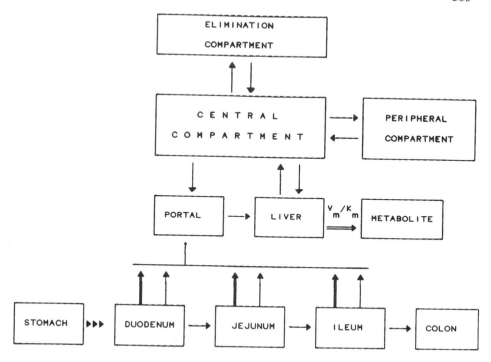

FIGURE 1 Simulation model schematic of physiological flow model.
(From Ref. 1. Reproduced with permission of the publisher.)

where Q_i is the physiological flow rate from that compartment and V_i is equivalent to the physiological volume of that compartment. The compartment volumes and intercompartmental flow rates are reported in Topp and Amidon (1), together with the literature values.

The inclusion of physiological gastrointestinal tract compartments into a pharmacokinetic model allows evaluation of the contribution of gastric emptying and gastrointestinal motility in a manner closely related to the physiological transport of drugs through the gastro-intestinal tract. In this manner the absorptive characteristics in each portion of the intestine as well as the transit of the drug through the gastrointestinal tract can be accounted for in a rational manner.

B. Gastrointestinal Motility

1. Gastric Motility and Gastric Emptying

Drug absorption occurs primarily in the small intestine. The fraction
of dose absorbed from the stomach is small, but gastric emptying
and gastrointestinal motility dramatically influence the absorption
profile of the drug. In order to understand how the transfer of drugs
from the stomach to the duodenum and on to the rest of the small
intestine affects plasma level time curves, gastric motility and gastric
emptying are characterized in both the fasted and in the fed state.
This in turn gives an understanding of the influence of the fasted
and fed states as well as the influence of gastric emptying and motility on oral drug absorption.

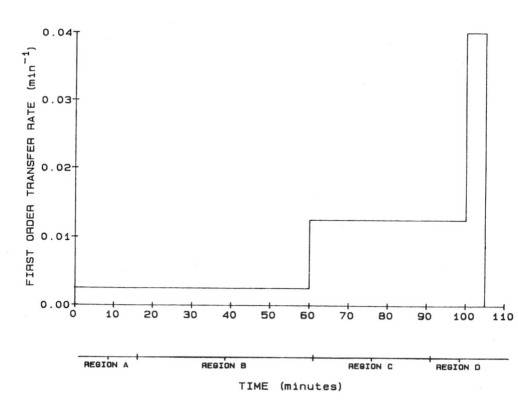

FIGURE 2 Rates of flow from the stomach and illustration of defined
regions A, B, C, and D. (From Ref. 2. Reproduced with permission
of the publisher.)

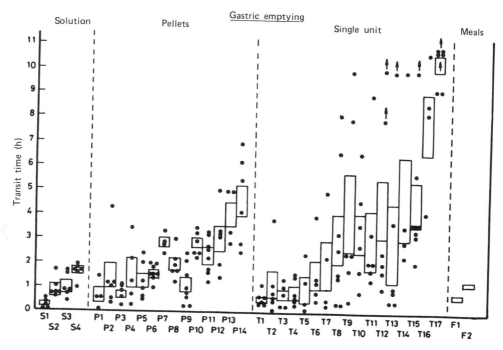

FIGURE 3 Gastric emptying of pharmaceutical dosage forms. Individual data points as filled circles. Mean±SEM. (From Ref. 3. Reproduced with permission of the publisher.)

a. Fasted State Gastrointestinal motility in the fasted state is characterized by four phases. Phase I is considered a quiescent period. Phase II consists of intermittent and irregular contractions. These contractions gradually increase in strength, culminating in a short period of intense contractions called phase III or the housekeeper wave. Phase IV is a brief transition period from phase III to phase I.

The activity associated with gastric motility originates in the distal part of the stomach and/or duodenum and is propagated throughout the rest of the small intestine, referred to as the migrating motor complex (MMC). Shown in Figure 2 is a representation of the cyclic nature of gastric motility in the fasted state in terms of first-order rate constants (2). This motility pattern has been incorporated into the physiological flow model in order to account for the transfer of drug from the stomach to the intestine.

During the fasted state, depending on the size of the dosage form, retention in the stomach varies. The main consequence is that the drug or dosage form is delayed in entering the small intestine and hence there is a lag time for absorption. Shown in Figure 3 are the half-times for gastric emptying of various dosage forms (3). As can be seen from Figure 3, the gastric emptying can vary from a $t_{1/2}$ of 5 min in the case of liquids to a $t_{1/2}$ of greater than 4 hr in the case of nondisintegrating dosage forms.

b. *Fed State* In the fed state, the motility pattern in the gastrointestinal tract resembles the motility that occurs during phase II. This gastric motility pattern continues during the digestion phase after which the motility pattern returns to the pattern of the fasted state.

2. Small Intestinal Transit Time

For most drugs, the primary site of absorption is the small intestine, with minimal absorption occurring in either the stomach or colon. Small

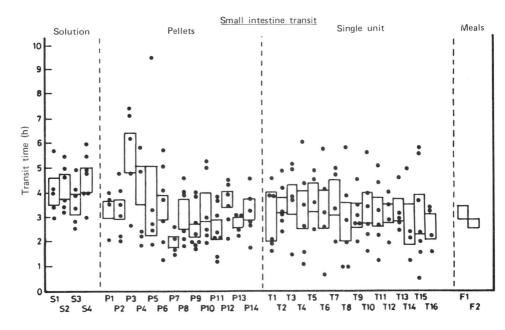

FIGURE 4 Small intestinal transit of pharmaceutical dosage forms. Individual data points as filled circles. Mean±SEM. (From Ref. 3. Reproduced with permission of the publisher.)

intestinal residence time is a function of bulk flow rate and the intestinal length. Ho, Higuchi, and coworkers have developed a physiologically based physical absorption model (4–6) that defines the anatomic reserve length of absorption as the length of intestine remaining after absorption is completed. For humans, the maximum reserve length is about 300 cm, assuming that absorption occurs only from the small intestine. Other factors affecting intestinal absorption include the flow rate, intestinal spreading, drug permeability, and intestinal motility. Using gamma scintigraphy, Davis et al. (3) found that, in contrast to gastric motility, the intestinal transit time was much more consistent than the gastric emptying time. The mean intestinal transit time is about 3 hr (±1 hr) and is independent of the dosage form or digestive state (see Fig. 4) (7). The extent of absorption of those drugs that are absorbed by specialized intestinal carriers is strongly influenced by changes in the intestinal transit time. These effects are examined in the next section.

III. EVALUATING THE EFFECTS OF GASTRIC EMPTYING AND GASTROINTESTINAL MOTILITY THROUGH PHARMACOKINETIC MODELING AND SIMULATIONS

The model of the gastrointestinal tract used in the following simulations is a reduction of the preceding physiological flow model and the gastric motility. The physiological flow model is reduced to three compartments: stomach, small intestine, and colon. The cyclic effect of gastric motility is assumed to be active only in the stomach and is represented as a first-order rate constant. Two aspects of the physiological model are examined; gastric emptying rate-limited absorption for rapidly absorbed drugs and small intestinal transit time-limited absorption for carrier-mediated drugs.

A. Rapidly Absorbed Drugs

In general, drugs with high membrane permeability are rapidly absorbed. The rate at which the drug is presented to the site of absorption is the rate-limiting step to the absorption process. For those drugs with a short plasma level half-life, the resultant effect on the plasma level time curves is more dramatic and the amount of drug in the plasma compartment will closely follow the amount of drug remaining in the intestine (8,9). As the plasma level half-life increases, this phenomenon is less pronounced and the plasma level time curves become less dependent upon the amount of drug remaining in the intestine owing to the increase in the mean residence time of the drug in the plasma. The following discussion is limited to those drugs with half-lives less than 4 hr.

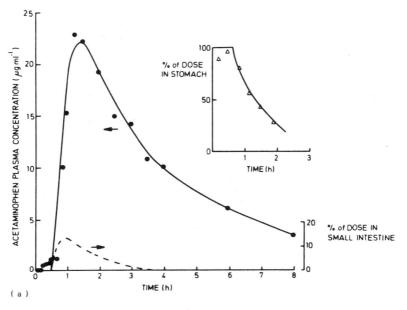

FIGURE 5 Plasma acetaminophen concentration plotted against time.
(●) Data points; (——) calculated curve; (- - -) predicted percentage
of dose in small intestine. (Inset) Gastric emptying pattern. (△) Data
points; (——) calculated curve. a) Type 1 gastric emptying with a
lag period. b) Type 3 gastric emptying. (From Ref. 8. Reproduced
with permission of the publisher.)

A classic study of this phenomena was work done by Clements
et al. (8). In a pharmacokinetic study of acetaminophen, both the
amount of the drug remaining in the stomach and the resultant plasma
levels were measured as a function of time. Shown in Figure 5 are
the results of this study representing two types of gastric emptying
profiles and the resultant amount of drug remaining in the small intestine
and the measured plasma levels, illustrating the correlation between
the amount of drug remaining in the stomach and the resultant plasma
level-time curves.

One of the more pronounced effects is the influence of gastric
emptying on acetaminophen plasma level-time curves illustrated in
Figure 5b. In this example, the gastric motility pattern was of a complex nature, with rapid initial emptying followed by a period of time
with little gastric emptying, and culminating in a rapid emptying of

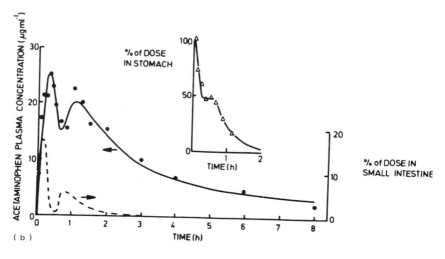

Figure 5 (continued)

the remaining drug from the stomach. This gastric motility pattern resulted in a double peaking in the acetaminophen plasma level-time curves.

Bodemar et al. (10) reported this double-peaking phenomenon for cimetidine in a comparison study of patients in the fasted and fed states. In this study, double peaking occurred in those patients who were in the fasted state. A thorough explanation of the double-peaking phenomenon for cimetidine has been presented by Oberle and Amidon (2). In their analysis of the gastric motility pattern during the fasted state, the shape of the plasma level-time curve is dependent on the time at which the dose is given with respect to the gastric motility cycle.

Shown in Figure 6 are the four types of plasma level-time curves for cimetidine that are dependent on the time at which the dose is given in the gastrointestinal motility cycle (2). As the elimination half-life of the drug increases, there is a smoothing of the plasma level-time curves and a reduction in the variability due to an increased residence time in the plasma. The result of an increase in elimination half-life is shown in Figure 7 for a drug with an elimination half-life four times that of cimetidine. The variability in the plasma level-time curves for cimetidine due to random dosing in relation to the gastric motility cycle (2) is shown in Figure 8, illustrating the expected variation in the plasma level-time curves during the absorptive phase.

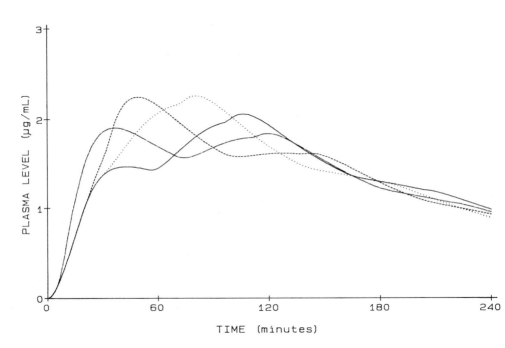

FIGURE 6 Effect of time of dosing in the gastric motility cycle on the
plasma level time curves for cimetidine: (——) type 1 gastric emptying
(region A); (····) type 2 gastric emptying (region B); (---) type 3
gastric emptying (region C); (—·—) type 4 gastric emptying (region
D). (From Ref. 2. Reproduced with permission of the publisher.

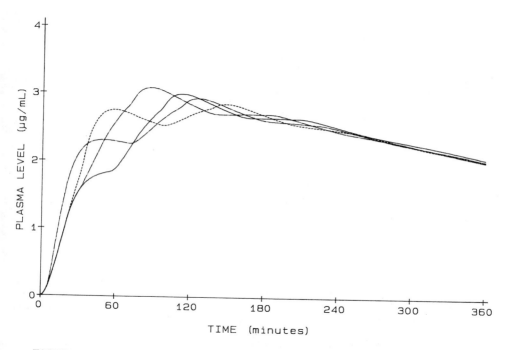

FIGURE 7 Effect of time of dosing in the gastric motility cycle on plasma level-time curves for longer half-life drug: (———) region A; (····) region B; (---) region C; (—·—) region D.

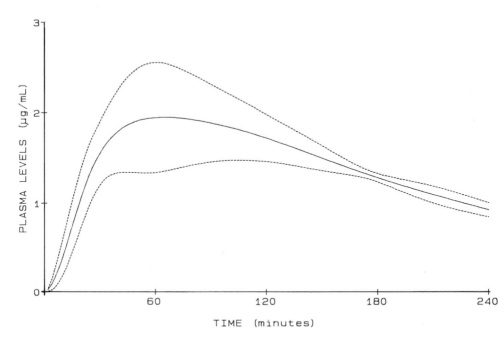

FIGURE 8 Effect of random dosing on plasma level time curves of cimetidine. Mean ± 2 SD.

The simulated data for cimetidine was further utilized to illustrate the difficulty in analyzing plasma level-time curves with a simple first-order gastric emptying rate constant. Nonlinear regression was performed on the simulated data for a selected plasma level-time curve from Figure 6. In the regressions, all parameters were fixed to the simulation values, except the gastric emptying rate constant. The results are shown in Figure 9 illustrating the lack of fit using a first-order gastric emptying rate constant.

B. Carrier-Mediated Absorption

The amino β-lactams are efficiently absorbed from the small intestine even though they are fully ionized at the physiological pH of the small intestine. The apparent deviation from the pH-partition hypothesis, which states that drugs are absorbed in their unionized form, is accounted for because absorption occurs by specialized intestinal carriers. Several investigators (11–13) have reported concentration-de-

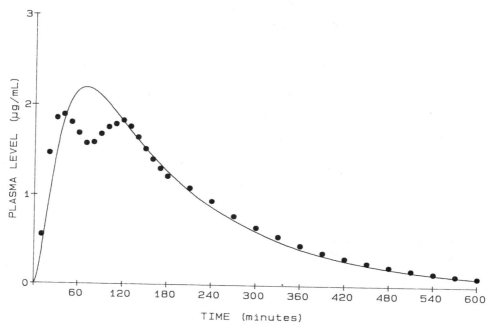

FIGURE 9 Results of fitting simulated cimetidine plasma level time
curves from region D with first-order gastric emptying rate constant:
(●) simulated data; (———) fitted curve.

pendent absorption for almost all the β-lactams in rats; others (14–
15) have also reported it in humans. The amino β-lactams possess di-
or tri-peptidelike structures and have been shown to share this absorption pathway in rats (12,16).

Recent studies of the intestinal membrane permeability of the orally
absorbed cephalosporins have lead to the definition of a concentration-
dependent absorption rate constant (17),

$$k_a = \frac{A}{V} \frac{R}{D} \frac{V}{D_0} J^*_{max} \ln \frac{1}{(1 + \frac{D_0}{V})/K_m} \tag{2}$$

where A/V is the surface area to volume ratio of the intestine, R is
the radius, D is the aqueous diffusion coefficient, V is the volume of
the lumen, D_0 is the dose given, J^*_{max} is the maximal flux, and K_m
is the Michaelis constant. Using the measured parameters from rat

TABLE 1 Comparison of Reported[a] (Actual) k_a (hr −1) and Calculated Mean k_a for Cefatrizine

Dose	Mean k_a (eq 2,)	Reported k_a
250	0.34	0.77
500	0.26	0.63
1000	0.20	0.53

[a]From Reference 18.

intestinal perfusions, the dose-dependent absorption rate constants are given in Table 1. These parameters combined with the known intravenous kinetic parameters allows one to simulate the expected plasma level-time curves.

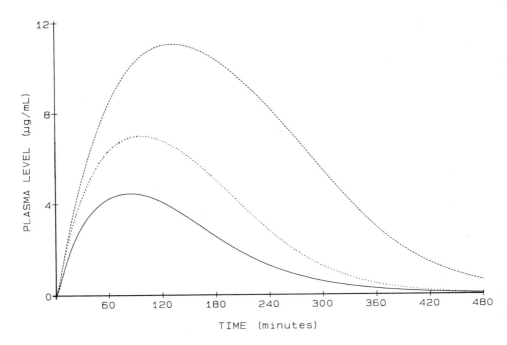

FIGURE 10 Effect of dose on plasma level-time curves of cefatrizine. Doses given were (——) 250, (···) 500, and (---) 1000 mg.

TABLE 2 Summary of Pharmacokinetic Parameters for Cefatrizine

Dose	F^U (%)	F^{AUC} (%)	C_{max} ($\mu g/ml$)	t_{max} (min)
		Reported[a]		
252.5	71.8 (12.1)	76.8 (6.8)	4.9 (1.2)	84 (24)
505	76.8 (29.1)	75.0 (10.2)	8.6 (1.0)	96 (12)
1010	55.2 (19.4)	46.8 (10.2)	10.2 (2.1)	120 (36)
		Simulated		
252.5		77.4	4.55	85
505		71.7	7.14	97
1010		65.0	11.22	133

[a]From Reference 18.

Specifically, for the antibiotics presented here the rat absorption parameters are used along with human intravenous pharmacokinetic parameters to simulate the plasma levels. Shown in Figure 10 is the effect of dose on the plasma level-time curves of cefatrizine. Three doses, 250, 500, and 1000 mg, were given to humans on an empty stomach. The dose-dependent absorption behavior was reflected by an increase in t_{max}, a less than linear increase in C_{max}, and a reduction in the bioavailability with increasing dose. The simulated parameters are in agreement with the actual parameters reported by Pfeffer et al. (18) (see Table 2). Studies in rats suggest that β-lactam absorption does not occur in the colon (17). Therefore, the reduction in cefatrizine's bioavailability is most likely due to intestinal transit effects combined with a low Michaelis constant. A low Michaelis constant per se means that the intestinal drug concentration will probably be in the zero-order region for a longer period of time, resulting in slower absorption. Practically this implies that the cefatrizine has a negative "reserve length" of absorption indicating incomplete absorption.

The effects of food on cephradine absorption have been studied by Harvengt et al. (19) and Mischler et al. (20). In the first study, the dose (500 mg as capsules) was given 30 min after light breakfast. In the second study, the dose (also 500 mg as capsules) was given immediately after the meal (890 calories). The effect of dosing 30 min after the light breakfast were minimal. Apparently the gastric emptying was slightly delayed. In the second study, however, the peak levels

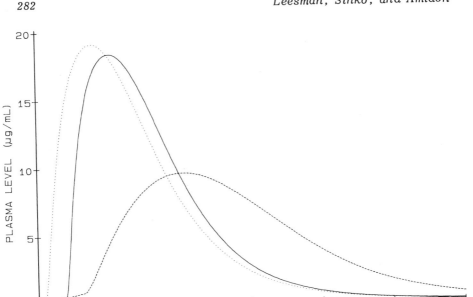

FIGURE 11 Effect of time of administration of dose with respect to the meal on plasma level-time curves of cephradine. Dose given: (···) fasted, (——) 30 min after meal, (---) with meal.

were halved and the time to peak was doubled, but the AUC was essentially unchanged. Utilizing a small intestinal (absorbing) compartment and a nonabsorbing colon compartment, the effect of food can be modeled. One approach is simply to delay gastric emptying. This approach may be appropriate when given near the end of the digestive phase. When the dose is given immediately after the meal there may be retarded disintegration and/or dissolution of the dosage form resulting in the drug being metered out of the stomach at a slow rate. The presence of the peptides in the intestine may also inhibit absorption, possibly through a competitive process as seen in rats (16). Both the fasting and fed simulations are shown in Figure 11. The simulations were performed using a slight gastric emptying delay for the first study and a slower gastric emptying rate combined with a slightly lower absorption rate for the second study. The results are in agreement with the published data.

IV. SUMMARY

The results of simulating plasma level-time curves for oral dosage forms, given the intravenous kinetic parameters and a physiological flow model for the gastrointestinal tract, are quite encouraging. Although many of the gastrointestinal parameters need to be better defined, refinement of this approach will make it possible to estimate oral plasma level-time curves given intravenous kinetic data (in humans) and absorption rate constants estimated from intestinal perfusion studies in rats. This approach will then be useful in the design of drugs and dosage forms for effective oral therapy.

REFERENCES

1. E. M. Topp and G. L. Amidon. Physiological flow modeling of the gastrointestinal tract and its use in dosage form design and evaluation. In Interrelationships Between GI Physiology and Dosage Form Design. Edited by E. G. Rippie and J. R. Cardinal. American Pharmaceutical Association, Washington, D.C., In Press (1988).
2. R. L. Oberle and G. L. Amidon. The influence of variable gastric emptying and intestinal transit rates on the plasma levels of cimetidine: An explanation for the double peak phenomenon. J. Pharm. Biopharm., 15: 529−544, 1987.
3. S. S. Davis, J. G. Hardy, and J. W. Fara. Transit of pharmaceutical dosage forms through the small intestine. Gut 27: 886−892, 1986.
4. W. I. Higuchi, N. F. H. Ho, J. Y. Park, and I. Komiya. Rate limiting steps and factors in drug absorption. In Drug Absorption. Edited by L. F. Prescott and W. S. Nimmo. Adis Press, Australia, 35−60, 1981.
5. N. F. H. Ho, J. Y. Park, W. Morozowich, and W. I. Higuchi. Physical model approach to the design of drugs with improved intestinal absorption. In Design of Biopharmaceutical Properties Through Prodrugs and Analogs. Edited by E. B. Roche. American Pharmaceutical Association, Washington, D.C., 1977, pp. 136−227.
6. N. F. H. Ho, J. Y. Park, P. F. Ni, and W. I. Higuchi. Advancing quantitative and mechanistic approaches in interfacing gastrointestinal drug absorption studies in animals and humans. In Animal Models for Oral Drug Delivery in Man: In Situ and In Vivo Approaches. Edited by W. Crouthamel and A. C. Serapu. American Pharmaceutical Association, Washington, D.C., 1983, pp. 27−106.

7. S. S. Davis, J. G. Hardy, M. J. Taylor, D. R. Whalley, and
C. G. Wilson. The effect of food on the gastrointestinal transit
of pellets and an osmotic device (Osmet). Int. J. Pharm. 21: 331–
340, 1984.
8. J. A. Clements, R. C. Heading, W. S. Nimmo, and L. F. Prescott.
Kinetics of acetaminophen absorption and gastric emptying in
man. Clin. Pharmacol. Ther. 24: 420–431, 1978.
9. W. S. Nimmo. Gastric emptying and drug absorption. Pharm.
Int. 1: 221–223, 1980.
10. G. Bodemar, B. Norlander, L. Fransson, and A. Walan. The
absorption of cimetidine before and during maintenance treatment
with cimetidine and the influence of a meal on the absorption of
cimetidine—studies in patients with peptic ulcer disease. Br.
J. Clin. Pharmacol. 7: 23–31, 1979.
11. T. Kimura, H. Endo, M. Yoshikawa, S. Muranishi, and H.
Sezaki. Carrier mediated transport systems for aminopenicillins
in rat small intestine. J. Pharm. Dyn. 1: 262–267, 1978.
12. E. Nakashima, A. Tsuji, S. Kagatani, and T. Yamana. Intestinal
absorption mechanism of amino-β-lactam antibiotics. III. Kinetics
of carrier-mediated transport across the rat small intestine in
situ. J. Pharm. Dyn. 7: 452–464, 1984.
13. T. Kimura, T. Yamamoto, M. Mizuno, Y. Suga, S. Kitade, and
H. Sezaki. Characterization of aminocephalosporin transport
across rat small intestine. J. Pharm. Dyn. 6: 246–253, 1983.
14. D. A. Spyker, R. J. Rugloski, R. L. Vann, and W. M. O'Brien.
Pharmacokinetics of amoxicillin: Dose dependence after intravenous,
oral, and intramuscular administration. Antimicrob. Agents
Chemother. 11: 132–141, 1977.
15. M. Chow, R. Quintiliani, B. A. Cunha, M. Thompson, E.
Finkelstein, and C. H. Nightingale. Pharmacokinetics of high-
dose oral cephalosporins. J. Clin. Pharmacol. 19: 185–194, 1979.
16. P. J. Sinko, M. Hu, and G. L. Amidon. Carrier mediated transport of amino acids, small peptides, and their drug analogs. J.
Controlled Release. 6: 115–121, 1987.
17. P. J. Sinko and G. L. Amidon, Characterization of the oral absorption of β-lactam antibiotics. I. Cephalosporins. Determination
of intrinsic membrane absorption parameters in the rat intestine.
insitu, Pharm. Res, submitted (October 1987).
18. M. Pfeffer, R. C. Gaver, and J. Ximenez. Human intravenous
pharmacokinetics and absolute oral bioavailability of cefatrizine.
Antimicrob. Agents Chemother. 24: 915–920, 1983.
19. C. Harvengt, P. De-Schepper, F. Lamy, and J. Hansen. Cephradine absorption and excretion in fasting and nonfasting volunteers.
J. Clin. Pharmacol. 13: 36–40, 1973.
20. T. W. Mischler, A. A. Sugerman, D. A. Willard, L. J. Brannick,
and E. S. Neiss. Influence of probenecid and food on the bioavailability of cephradine in normal male subjects. J. Clin.
Pharmacol. 14: 604–611, 1974.

7

Central Role of Pharmacokinetics in Determining the Feasibility of Targeting Drug Delivery

C. ANTHONY HUNT, RODERICK D. MACGREGOR, and RONALD A. SIEGEL   *University of California at San Francisco, San Francisco, California*

I. INTRODUCTION

The future of pharmacokinetics lies with its application and use in solving an expanding sphere of complex problems. In this chapter, we focus on how pharmacokinetic concepts can be used to identify the opportunities and limitations governing targeted in vivo drug delivery.

Targeted drug delivery is a goal of basic pharmacokinetic and drug design research. Being able to direct a drug to its target site while avoiding any undesirable sites is an ultimate achievement currently reserved for the next generation of scientists. Building a drug that binds both specifically and tightly to some macromolecular receptor is not enough. The drug must be given the ability to find the target tissue while ignoring nontarget tissues. Further, the drug must be given the ability to avoid a variety of interception and removal systems. It must have both "cloaking" and "guidance" systems. Designers of prodrugs have had these goals in mind (1). Combining a drug with a monoclonal antibody and putting a drug in a uniquely designed liposome are two different ways one might approach achieving these goals.

It is widely believed that if one were able to deliver almost any drug directly to its target sites, then the clinical and therapeutic results would be dramatically superior. This is true only under specifiable conditions (2). It is also widely believed that if one avoids delivery of a drug to a site that originates toxicity, then larger doses can be given without concern for the toxic side effects. This too is true only under specifiable conditions, and in both cases pharmacokinetics is central to determining those conditions. In the following pages we develop several relatively new pharmacokinetic tools that allow one to quickly and easily decide these issues.

II. DELIVERY SYSTEM

Before we go any further we must define several terms to ensure that we are using a common language. First let us restrict our attention to therapeutic molecules — drugs — that demonstrate activity when administered to other humans or animals by any one of several conventional means. These molecules are *the drug*. The drug can then be attached to another inactive (or minimally active) molecule to give either a *prodrug* or a *drug-carrier combination*. Neither should be active, but both should release the active drug. If the attached molecule is no more than about 10 times the molecular weight of the drug, then the combination is a *prodrug*. If the attached molecule is more than ten times the weight of the drug, then the combination is usually a *drug-carrier* combination. Drug carriers are not restricted to being large single molecules. They can also be a supramolecular complex, such as liposome; in this case the drug need not be attached to the carrier. It can be simply entrapped. A targeted drug delivery system is one that is designated to be administered (parenterally) at a point distant from the target tissue but finds its way preferentially to the site of action and, once there, release the drug (3). To what extent can an in vivo drug carrier, such as a liposome or antibody, function as a targeted drug delivery system to improve an agent's therapeutic effectiveness through site-specific, targeted delivery?

The drug as just defined can fall into one of two sets. Set 1 includes all drugs that if released in vivo distant from the target site can still generate the desired pharmacological response. Drugs in this set can partition or be transported across cell membranes, given time, and so can reach intracellular target sites. Set 2 includes all drugs that if released as before will be inactive because they cannot reach the target site unaided because of some physical barrier, such as a cell membrane the drug cannot cross. An organic cation that needs to act intracellularly is one example; a peptide for which there is no transport system is another example. Drugs in this second set could be active in a variety of in vitro systems but would be inactive if given to animals or humans by any typical route and so must be excluded from this discussion. However, it is often possible to chemically modify the set 2 drug to produce a set 1 drug, and the products of this chemical modification are also called prodrugs. Stella and Himmelstein (1, 4) provide an excellent discussion of favorable and unfavorable situations for molecular modification or prodrugs overcoming such barriers and improving site-specific drug delivery. In many instances the use of a drug-carrier combination and molecular modification to produce a prodrug are simply different means to the same end.

If we know something about the pharmacokinetic properties of a drug, can we then predict the magnitude of an improved therapeutic effect or the increased apparent potency or the reduced toxicity when either a targeted drug carrier or prodrug is administered? First, before we answer this question, what is it that we are after? We want to improve therapeutic effectiveness. How will we accomplish this improvement? A targeted in vivo drug carrier must accomplish two things: it must get the therapeutic agent to the target tissue and then release the agent at a reproducible rate. The design of the carrier should allow one a degree of control over the release rate profile, and there should be a reduction in the relative amount of drug reaching the *toxicity sites*. Developing a useful model to make predictions about which drugs benefit most by combination with a targeted drug carrier is relatively simple if we assume that targeted carriers can be engineered with built-in rate control and that they will be capable of delivery up to 100% of an agent to any given set of target sites. We then employ a pharmacokinetic model to generate equations for calculating two new parameters: *therapeutic availability* and *drug targeting index*. These parameters allow predictions of the magnitude of the improved therapeutic efficacy or increased apparent potency that result when the drug is administered as a drug-carrier combination. They allow one to identify specific physicochemical, pharmacokinetic, and physiological attributes that a drug and its corresponding target must meet for either to be a rational candidate for targeted drug delivery.

III. USEFUL PHARMACOKINETIC MODEL

Assume that the species of interest is the human. However, if one is actually interested in another species, then interspecies pharmacokinetic scaling can be used to obtain the appropriate parameters (5). An adequate model for this discussion is Scheme 1. It can describe the pharmacokinetic properties of a range of real and hypothetical drugs. Compartment II represents all tissues containing the target therapeutic sites for the desired response and has an effective blood flow of Q_R, which is measured in terms of percentage of cardiac output (6). It is subsequently referred to as the response compartment. The effective drug concentration at these therapeutic sites that is available to initiate the pharmacological cascade is designated C_R when the drug is administered in its free form and C_r when the drug is administered as a drug-carrier combination. To facilitate building a theoretical foundation, we assume that the effective concentration at the action site is a function of the measurable concentration in that tissue's exiting venous blood or plasma (whichever is the reference fluid). Situations in which partitioning between the response sites and blood is rate limiting or there is poor partitioning between the blood and response sites are addressed in a later section.

Compartment IV, the toxicity compartment, represents tissues containing toxicity sites, where the cascade of events leading to a toxic response is initiated, and has an effective blood flow Q_T. The effective concentration of drug at these sites is designated C_T when the drug is administered in its free form and C_t when the drug is administered as the drug-carrier combination. It is understood that if these toxicity sites are located in the same tissue as target sites, then a drug carrier is unlikely to provide the desired improvement in therapeutic efficacy.

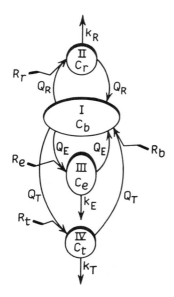

SCHEME 1

Both the drug-carrier combination and the drug alone are eliminated by separate mechanisms. In Scheme 1, compartment III is designated the elimination compartment for drug only. It represents both liver and kidney and has a blood flow Q_E. Drug elimination is controlled by k_E in the elimination compartment. Additional elimination processes associated with the response and toxicity compartments are shown. They combine elimination and metabolism. For convenience, apparent elimination rate constants are subsequently replaced by clearances. All metabolites are assumed to be inactive. Compartment I represents blood and all other tissues not accounted for by the other three compartments. Blood flow within this compartment is limited to 100% of cardiac output minus $Q_R + Q_T + Q_E$. Compartment I is not the traditional pharmacokinetic central compartment. Nevertheless, it is subsequently referred to as the blood compartment. The blood level of drug in this compartment is designated either C_B or C_b when free drug or a drug-carrier combination, respectively, is administered.

For each of the four compartments, delivery of drug is designated by one of two different input rate functions: R_B is the intravenous input function for free drug; R_b, R_r, R_e, and R_t are the release rates (and also input functions) of free drug from the carrier, as illustrated in Scheme 1, into each of the corresponding compartments when the drug is actually administered as a drug-carrier combination. In the special case when $R_b = R_t = R_e = 0$, the drug carrier is an

ideal target-specific drug carrier. It is important to note that as long
as drug remains associated with the carrier, regardless of its location
in vivo, it is assumed to be inactive. Note that neither the blood nor
the tissue level of the drug-carrier combination is referred to in
Scheme 1 or in any of the subsequent equations. Any drug tht remains
with the carrier (or as a prodrug), even though it may be near the
target site, has not yet been *administered*.

IV. THERAPEUTIC INDEX

Regardless of the amount of sophisticated pharmacokinetic data that
may have been collected for a drug, the pharmacological end point
for an individual in a phase III clinical trial is often simply yes or no.
Did it work or not? Sometimes effectiveness is crudely quantified.
This situation is governed by U.S. Food and Drug Administration
(FDA) considerations. The same is often true of toxicities and side
effects. Thus, for an individual there will be a minimum effective
dose (MED) and a maximally tolerated toxic dose (MTTD). The ratio
of these doses is an individual's therapeutic index (TI). For the
population, the therapeutic index is a statistical measurement defined
as the average of the individual ratios:

$$TI = \frac{MTTD}{MED} \tag{1}$$

There are many ways to quantify both clinical response and toxicity.
Temporal measurements that allow quantitation of the duration of
effect, the magnitude of the effect, and its occurrence relative to
dosing are preferred, because we know that if drug is administered
either at a different site, at a different rate, or both, then MED
and MTTD can change. With this consideration in mind we define the
total response (or toxicity) as the area under the response (or toxicity)
versus time curve. In order to relate therapeutic index more easily
to Scheme 1, attention is restricted to drugs that meet two additional
conditions. When the drug is adminstered as a targeted drug-carrier
combination, a new dose, the carrier-derived minimum effective dose
(MED'), is expected to generate the same response as is produced
by the free-drug MED. Also, another dose, the carrier-derived
maximum tolerated toxic dose (MTTD'), is expected to be required
to generate the same toxicity as is produced by the MTTD. The
therapeutic index for the drug-carrier combination TI' thus becomes
the ratio of these new carrier-derived values:

$$TI' = \frac{MTTD'}{MED'} \tag{2}$$

The relationships between these two measures of therapeutic index are illustrated in Figure 1 for a hypothetical drug in a typical individual.

V. DRUG TARGETING INDEX

The ratio of therapeutic index obtained when a targeted drug carrier is used, Equation (2), to that for the free drug given by a standard route, in this case intravenously, is an ideal measure of how much the targeted drug carrier has helped. We define this ratio as the drug targeting index (DTI).

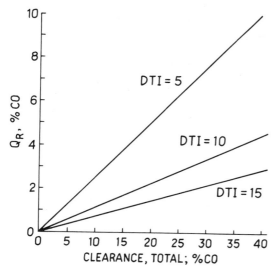

FIGURE 1 The required values of blood flow Q_R to the response site are plotted versus total clearance as percentage cardiac output (CO) when DTI is fixed at 15, 10, or 5. For DTI = 15 and a high total clearance, 40.5% of CO, $Q_R \leqslant 2.9\%$ of CO. For DTI = 10 and a medium clearance, 27% of CO, $Q_R \leqslant 3\%$ of CO. For DTI = 5 and a low clearance, 13.5% of CO, $Q_R \leqslant 3.38\%$ of CO.

$$DTI = \frac{TI'}{TI} \tag{3}$$

Equation (3) states that for the typical individual the ratio of the therapeutic inex value obtained from a drug-carrier combination to that obtained from an equal dose of the free drug will be a constant that is independent of the total dose (or dose rate) for a specified drug carrier but uniquely dependent on the fraction of the dose delivered by the carrier to the various tissues.

VI. TARGET AVAILABILITY AND TOXIC AVAILABILITY

If the therapeutic index for the free drug is large, then improving it further by using an in vivo drug carrier is unlikely to yield a significant clinical advantage. It could in theory, however, considerably reduce the actual dose needed to get the desired effect. To quantify this property we define a new term: *target or therapeutic availability* (TA). Analogous to the definition of the drug targeting index, the therapeutic availability can be defined as a ratio of either area values or steady-state drug levels (6). Here the area values are areas under drug level versus time curves and are designed AUC. We assume that response is proportional to the time course of drug at the target site; this AUC value is designated AUC_r when the drug-carrier combination is given and AUC_R when free drug is given. Thus,

$$TA = \frac{AUC_r}{AUC_R} = \left(\frac{C_r}{C_R}\right)_{ss} \tag{4}$$

We also define an analogous term, *toxic availability* (TXA), which is the ratio of AUC values at the site where toxicity originates from drug release from a targeted drug carrier to that which occurs when the free drug is administered by the reference route:

$$TXA = \frac{AUC_t}{AUC_T} = \left(\frac{C_t}{CT}\right)_{ss} \tag{5}$$

The ratio of TA to TXA gives DTI. Clearly, DTI, TA, and TXA are conceptually useful terms. The more important need is to relate these concepts directly to parameters in Scheme 1.

VII. EXTENDING DEFINITIONS TO NONIDEAL CASES

Each compartment in Scheme 1 is depicted as "well-stirred"; that is, equilibration of drug within the compartment is fast relative to blood blow. Because of this assumption, the preceding AUC and C values can refer to both the concentration at the action site and the compartment's exiting venous concentration. However, in most cases these two concentrations are likely to be quite different. There may also be a considerable time lag before a change in the tissue's blood level concentration is reflected at the action site. Yet, in most such instances, as the following discussion shows, Equations (4) and (5) are still valid.

Let the concentration at a target site be S and the organ's exiting venous concentration be C. Assume that S is related to C by a sequence of transfer that can be described by a set of linear differential equations

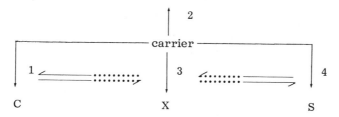

The time course of drug at the two extreme sites will be $C(t)$ and $S(t)$. The Laplace transforms of these two functions are $\tilde{C}(s)$ and $\tilde{S}(s)$, where $\tilde{S}(s) = \tilde{T}(s)\tilde{C}(s)$. $\tilde{T}(s)$ is the Laplace transform of the function describing transfer between C and S, $T(t)$. When $s = 0$, $\tilde{S}(0) = \tilde{T}(0)\tilde{C}(0)$, which can be rewritten as

$$\int_0^\infty S(t)\ dt = \tilde{T}(0) \int_0^\infty C(t)\ dt \tag{6}$$

or

$$AUSC_i = \tilde{T}_i(0)AUC_i \tag{7}$$

Consider four examples of drug release from the carrier: (1) drug is released from the carrier into blood in the target tissue; (2) drug is released from the carrier into blood at some site distant from both C and S; (3) drug is released at a site X between C and S; and (4) drug is released directly to the action site. When AUSC values are used in place of AUC values to define DTI,

$$
DTI = \frac{\tilde{T}_r(O)}{\tilde{T}_R(O)} \frac{\tilde{T}_T(O)}{\tilde{T}_t(O)} \frac{AUC_r/AUC_t}{AUC_R/AUC_T} \tag{8}
$$

In many situations one would expect the product of the two transfer function ratios to be approximately 1, and so Equation (8) reduces to

$$
DTI = \frac{AUC_r/AUC_t}{AUC_R/AUC_T} \tag{9}
$$

The corresponding expression for TA reduces to Equation (4). We recognize that there may be situations in which the drug release properties of the carrier may alter $\tilde{T}_i(O)$ and that, for some drugs or physiological situations, a nonlinear set of differential equations may be needed to describe $T(t)$, and so these exceptions are excluded from this discussion.

VIII. DEVELOPING SPECIFIC EQUATIONS

Equations (10) through (13) are the set of differential equations that describe the model in Scheme 1 when free drug is given intravenously, consistent with the definitions and limitations already given:

$$
V_B \frac{dC_B}{dt} = -(Q_R + Q_E + Q_T)C_B + Q_R C_R
$$

$$
+ Q_E C_E + Q_T C_T + R_B \tag{10}
$$

$$
V_R \frac{dC_R}{dt} = Q_R C_B - Q_R C_R - \frac{Q_R E_R C_R}{1 - E_R} \tag{11}
$$

$$
V_E \frac{dC_E}{dt} = Q_E C_B - Q_E C_E - \frac{Q_E E_E C_E}{1 - E_E} \tag{12}
$$

$$
V_T \frac{d c_T}{dt} = Q_T C_T - \frac{Q_T E_T C_T}{1 - E_T} \tag{13}
$$

The constants V_B, V_R, and V_T are the apparent volumes of distribution of the corresponding compartments. The constants E_i are extraction ratios defined as the ratio $(C_{in} - C_{out})/C_{in}$, where C_{in} is the arterial drug concentration and C_{out} is the venous concentration. The term R_B is the rate of intravenous drug input, and $\int_0^\infty R_B\, dt = D$ where D is the dose. When drug is administered intravenously as the drug-carrier combination, the alternate set of differential equations is given by Equations (14) through (17):

$$V_B \frac{dC_b}{dt} = -(Q_R + Q_E + Q_T)C_b + Q_R C_r + Q_E C_e$$
$$+ Q_T C_t + R_b \tag{14}$$

$$V_R \frac{dC_r}{dt} = Q_R C_b - Q_R C_r - \frac{Q_R E_R C_r}{1 - E_R} + R_r \tag{15}$$

$$V_e \frac{dC_e}{dt} = Q_E C_b - Q_E C_e - \frac{Q_E E_E C_e}{1 - E_E} + R_e \tag{16}$$

$$V_T \frac{dC_t}{dt} = Q_T C_b - Q_T C_t - \frac{Q_T E_T C_t}{1 - E_T} + R_t \tag{17}$$

This set of equations includes four drug input functions, R_r, R_t, R_e, and R_b, such that $\Sigma \int_0^\infty (R_i)\, dt = D'$, where D' is the total amount of drug released from the drug carrier. For convenience, we set $D' = D$. A reasonable assumption is that the various mechanisms governing drug release are similar at the response and other tissue sites. Under these conditions the rates of drug release can be combined and rewritten as

$$R_b + R_r + R_e + R_t = (F_b + F_r + F_e + F_t)R_0 = R_B \tag{18}$$

where R_0 is the average in vivo drug release rate from the total carrier dose, and the F_i terms are the fractions of drug release occurring in each of the four compartments, so that $R_t = F_t R_0$, and so on. One or more F_i values can equal zero. Further, to compare the relative benefit derived from the drug-carrier combination to that resulting from intravenous administration of free drug, we set $R_B = R_0$.

The most frequently reported pharmacokinetic property of a drug is its total-body clearance. For Scheme 1 total clearance is $Q_E E_E + Q_R E_R + Q_T E_T = Cl_E + Cl_R + Cl_T = Cl_{tot}$. Finally, we define the relative blood flow parameters n and m by the relations

$$Q_E + nQ_R \quad \text{and} \quad Q_T = mQ_R \tag{19}$$

For the vast majority of drugs, both the response and the toxicity are a function of the time course of drug at the target and toxicity sites, respectively. Single measurement descriptions include the area under the site concentration-time curve, the steady-state drug level, the peak drug level, and the duration above some minimum effective level. We limit attention to drugs for which either the area measurements or the steady-state levels provide sufficient information for reasonably estimating the drug effect and toxicity.

The expression for DTI can be derived considering steady states and AUC values. We focus here on the latter. The area under the target and toxicity site drug concentration curves can be obtained by integrating Equations (10) through (17) from time zero to infinity. When this is done, the left-hand side of each equation vanishes, and each concentration C_i is replaced by $\int_0^\infty C_i \, dt = AUC_i$. Each compartment's drug input rate R_i in Equations (14) through (17) is replaced by $\int_0^\infty R_i \, dt = F_i D$, where F_i is the fraction of the drug delivered by the carrier directly to the ith compartment and D is the dose as defined previously. The results for Equations (10) through (12) and (14) through (16) are

$$D - Q_R[(1 + n + m)AUC_B - AUC_R - nAUC_E$$
$$- mAUC_T] = 0 \tag{20}$$

$$Q_R\left(AUC_B - \frac{AUC_R}{1 - E_R}\right) = 0 \tag{21}$$

$$Q_R\left(mAUC_B - \frac{mAUC_T}{1 - E_T}\right) = 0 \tag{22}$$

$$F_b D - Q_R[(1 + n + m)AUC_b - AUC_r - nAUC_e$$
$$- mAUC_t] = 0 \tag{23}$$

$$Q_R\left(AUC_b - \frac{AUC_r}{1 - E_R}\right) + F_r D = 0 \tag{24}$$

$$Q_R\left(mAUC_b - \frac{mAUC_t}{1 - E_T}\right) + F_t D = 0 \tag{25}$$

Equations (20), (21), and (22) correspond to Equations (10), (11), and (13), respectively. The equation corresponding to Equation (12) is not shown. Equations (23), (24), and (25) correspond to Equations (14), (15), and (17), respectively. The equation corresponding to Equation (7) is not needed and so is not shown. Solving these two new sets of equations for the two sets of four AUC terms leads to Equations (26) through (29):

$$AUC_R = \frac{D(1 - E_R)}{Q_R \Phi} \tag{26}$$

$$AUC_T = \frac{D(1 - E_T)}{Q_R \Phi} \tag{27}$$

$$AUC_r = \frac{D(1 - E_R)\Gamma_F}{Q_R \Phi} \tag{28}$$

$$AUC_t = \frac{D(1 - E_T)\Lambda_F}{Q_R \Phi} \tag{29}$$

Equations for AUC_B, AUC_b, AUC_E, and AUC_e are not needed and so are not listed. In Equations (26) through (29),

$$\Gamma_F = F_b + (1 + nE_E + mE_T)F_r + (1 - E_E)F_e + (1 - E_T)F_t \tag{30}$$

$$\Lambda_F = F_b + (1 - E_R)F_r + (1 - E_E)F_e + \left(\frac{E_R}{m} + \frac{nE_E}{m} + 1\right)F_t \tag{31}$$

and

$$\Phi = E_r + nE_E + mE_T \tag{32}$$

Substitution of these AUC values into the definition of DTI gives

$$DTI = \frac{F_b + (1 + nE_E + mE_T)F_r + (1 - E_E)F_e + (1 - E_T)F_t}{F_b + (1 - E_R)F_r + (1 - E_E)F_e + (E_R/m + nE_E/m + 1)F_t} \tag{33}$$

When the input rate of free drug and the release of drug from the drug-carrier combination are matched, TA is given by Equation (30) and TXA by Equation (31). Note that when the drug carrier behaves ideally, then $F_b \simeq F_t \simeq F_e \simeq 0$ and Equation (30) reduces to

$$TA = 1 + nE_E + mE_E = 1 + \frac{Q_E E_E}{Q_R} + \frac{Q_T E_T}{Q_R} \qquad (34)$$

Even if E_E and E_T are small, large values of TA are possible when Q_E/Q_R and Q_T/Q_R are large. When the drug carrier behaves ideally,

$$TXA = -E_R$$

which is not sensitive to relative changes in blood flow. Again, for the ideal carrier,

$$DTI = \frac{1 + nE_E + mE_T}{1 - E_R} \qquad (35)$$

which rearranges to

$$DTI - 1 = \frac{\text{total clearance}}{Q_R(1 - E_R)} \qquad (36)$$

IX. DRUGS THAT BENEFIT FROM TARGETED DRUG DELIVERY

It is convenient to base this discussion on several fixed reference points. Here we consider three sets of drugs having either high (H), medium (M), or low (L) total clearance values. Values of Q_R are arbitrarily limited to less than 20% of the cardiac output. Blood flow to the eliminating organs Q_E is often fixed at 54% of the cardiac output (i.e., 2.7 liters/min in humans: 1.5 liters/min for liver plus 1.2 liters/min for kidney), which in turn limits the range for n values (i.e., Q_E/Q_R). The value of m (Q_T/Q_R) is limited to 0.33, 1.0, or 3.0. The high, medium, or low total clearance values are set at 75, 50, or 25% of the combined liver and kidney blood flow, that is, 40.5, 27, or 13.5% of the cardiac output, respectively.

Clearance values are available for 178 drugs currently used in humans (7). These values yield useful statistics that add perspective to this discussion. The range representing approximately 68% of the tabulated drugs is 81–1873 ml/min for a 70–kg person or 1.6–37.5% of the cardiac output; the average drug's clearance is 7.8% of the cardiac output. Assuming that the tabulated values are representative of all currently used drugs, then 14% of them have total clearance values greater than 40.5% of the cardiac output (our high-clearance value), 79.4% have clearance values less than 27% of the cardiac output, and 63.7% have clearance values less than 13.5% of the cardiac output (our low-clearance value).

Clearly, if the drug is not significantly cleared at or near the target site ($E_R \doteq 0$), the DTI $- 1 \doteq$ total clearance/Q_R and we see that only the higher clearance drugs are likely to have large DTI values, but even that conclusion is conditioned on the magnitude of Q_R. If, however, the drug is cleared at the target site, then the possible range of DTI values can increase dramatically.

What is a desirable DTI value? As long as we are assuming an ideal carrier ($F_r = 1$), we propose that a minimal acceptable value (to warrant use of a targeted drug carrier) would be 15; if the carrier is actually only 20% efficient, then the maximum obtainable DTI value would be approximately 3, which to use seems marginally acceptable. Figure 1 is a graph of Q_R versus total clearance for the

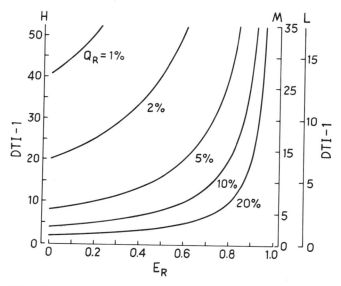

FIGURE 2 The dependence of the drug-targeting index [Eq. (30)] on the extraction ratio E_R of the response compartment is shown. Each curve is for a fixed value of Q_R ranging from 20 to 1% of the cardiac output. Ordinate H designates DTI values for the set of drugs with a high total clearance value, ordinate M is the set with a medium total clearance, and ordinate L is the set with a low total clearance.

unique set of values that allow DTI to reach or exceed a value of
5, 10, or 15 when $E_R = 0$. A high-clearance drug is thus a good
candidate for combination with a targeted carrier if the target site
has an effective blood flow of 2.9% of cardiac output or less; for a
low-clearance drug it would have to be less than 1%. Figure 2 shows
how the stringent requirements depicted in Figure 1 can be relaxed
when the drug is cleared at or near the target site.

X. INCREASING APPARENT POTENCY

Therapeutic availability, unlike the classic term "bioavailability,"
can have values either greater than or less than 1. An increase in
therapeutic availability is effectively equivalent to an increase in
potency. If, for example, a drug-carrier combination has a therapeutic
availability value of 6.0, then one-sixth of the dose D_i, when administered as the drug-carrier combination, will have the same effect
as giving that free drug dose intravenously at the same rate it is

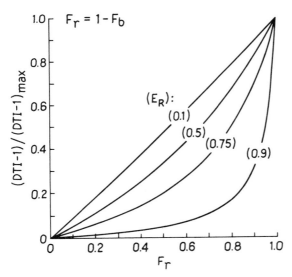

FIGURE 3 The expected value of DTI $-$ 1 as a fraction of its maximum
possible value $(DTI - 1)_{max}$ for a fixed set of clearance and blood
flow values is plotted versus F_r when $F_r = 1 - F_b$ and Eq. (30)
reduces to Eq. (31). The four curves show values for four different
values of E_R ranging from 0.1 to 0.9.

released from the drug carrier. Note that if $E_R \doteq 0$ then $TA - 1 \doteq$
$DTI-1$ and Figure 1 can be used to approximate when $TA = 15$. However, even if $E_R \neq 0$, $TA - 1 =$ total clearance$/Q_R$.

Values of $DTI - 1$ are graphed in Figure 2 as a function of E_R.
It is clear that large DTI values are possible only under specific
conditions. The maximum value of DTI is directly proportional to the
total clearance and can be dramatically influenced by E_R. Smaller
values of Q_R allow larger maximum DTI values. Figure 3 shows that a
low-clearance drug will have a maximum DTI value of 2.35 ($DTI - 1 =$
1.35) when $Q_R = 10\%$ of the caridac output and there is no significant
elimination of drug at the response site, whereas another compound
acting at the same target and having the same total clearance will
have a maximum DTI value of 9.0 if it has a 0.85 response-site
extraction ratio. If Q_R is smaller, 1.25% of cardiac output, and $E_R =$
0.85, then the DTI value rockets to 216.

XI. DRUG TARGETING INDEX VALUE WITH LESS THAN PERFECT CARRIER

No carrier in practice is likely to provide optimally efficient delivery
to targets. Inspection of Equation (33) shows that simple trends are
not evident when F_r decreases below 1. Here we consider a limited
number of instructive examples. We can simulate suboptimum targeting
by setting $1 - F_r$ equal to F_b, F_e, or F_t. First consider $1 - F_r = F_b$,
that is, drug release from the carrier that does not occur at the target
occurs in blood; Equation (33) then reduces to

$$DTI - 1 = \frac{\text{total clearance} \times F_r}{Q_R(1 - F_r E_R)} \qquad (37)$$

Note that if we define $(DTI - 1)_{max} =$ total clearance$/Q_R(1 - E_R)$
then the fraction of the maximum value that results because $(1 - F_r) =$
F_b is

$$\frac{DTI - 1}{(DTI - 1)_{max}} = \frac{(1 - E_R)F_r}{(1 - E_R F_r)} \qquad (38)$$

Vaules of this ratio are plotted in Figure 3 as a function of F_r. If
we are talking about changing the site and/or rate of drug release
from a carrier, then the drug and subject are constant. It is therefore
not surprising that this ratio reduces to an expression with only two
variables, F_r and E_R. The fraction of the maximum $DTI - 1$ value

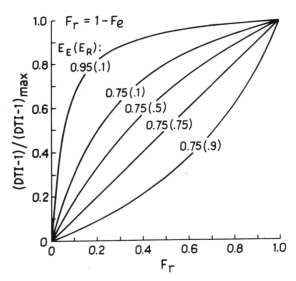

FIGURE 4 The expected value of DTI $-$ 1 as a fraction of its maximum possible value for a fixed set of clearance and blood flow values is plotted versus F_r when $F_r = 1 - F_e$ and Eq. (30) reduces to Eq. (32). Of the five curves, four are for high-clearance drugs where $E_E = 0.075$. One curve has $E_E = 0.95$, and E_R ranges from 0.1 to 0.9.

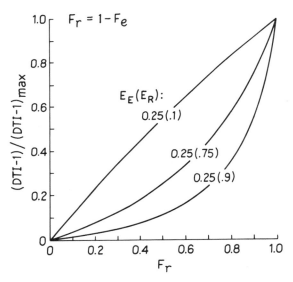

FIGURE 5 The expected value of DTI $-$ 1 as a fraction of its maximum possible value for a fixed set of clearance and blood flow is plotted versus F_r when $F_r = 1 - F_e$ and Eq. (30) reduces to Eq. (32). The three curves are for low-clearance drugs where $E_E = 0.25$; E_R ranges from 0,1 to 0.9.

that is obtainable when $(1 - F_r) = F_e$ is

$$\frac{DTI - 1}{(DTI - 1)_{max}} = \frac{(1 - E_R)F_r}{1 - E_R F_r - E_E(1 - F_r)} \leqslant 1 \tag{39}$$

Values of this ratio are plotted in Figures 4 and 5 as a function of F_r. Because $F_e = (1 - F_r)$, this ratio must include E_E, but not Q_E, as a variable.

The extraction ratio of the response site is clearly a key variable in each of these equations. However, compounds that are cleared to some extent at the response site are rare. Antimetabolites for cancer chemotherapy exemplify such drugs. One reason that such compounds are rare is that our entire drug selection process is biased against such compounds. In fact, drugs that are good candidates for combination with a targeted drug carrier are unlikely to survive the current drug-screening system. Few currently used drugs have significant target-organ extraction ratio or clearance values, and this is a necessary consequence of current drug-screening practices. The best candidate drug for clinical use is often selected from a set of active molecules having similar mechanisms of action. The most potent member of that set having the least toxicity is preferred. A molecule that has even a modest target-organ extraction ratio will appear to be less potent when it is administered intravenously and compared to a sister molecule having the same inherent potency but no target organ clearance. As a consequence, the current drug-screening system is biased against drugs that would be good candidates for use as drug-carrier combinations. Therapeutic proteins and peptides generally have not been a product of these screens. As a set they tend to have high total clearance values and so may represent better candidates.

Inspection of Figure 2 shows that large values of $DTI - 1$ are possible when Q_R is small and E_R is >0. The downside of this situation is illustrated in Figure 3: the larger the E_R value, the greater the negative consequences of having a suboptimally performing drug carrier. Interestingly, very high clearance drugs with nonzero but small E_R values, for example the far-left curve in Figure 4, are relatively insensitive to drops in F_r (from 1) as long as extra target drug release occurs within the eliminating organs.

The utility of Figures 1 through 5 is that they can be used to predict how much a given drug will benefit from combination with an optimum or even suboptimum targeted drug carrier, and they require only limited pharmacokinetic data.

XII. COMPOUNDS THAT HAVE DIFFICULTY GAINING ACCESS TO THE TARGET SITE

Movement of some drugs from blood to the target site can be relatively slow, such that there is a considerable time lag before a change in blood or extracellular fluid drug levels is reflected in a change in corresponding levels at the target site, and vice versa. Under such conditions one would expect $\tilde{T}_t(0) \neq \tilde{T}_T(0)$. Yet even in such situations one may find that $\tilde{T}_R(0) \simeq \tilde{T}_T(0)$ and $\tilde{T}_r(0) \simeq \tilde{T}_t(0)$ is a reasonable approximation. If these approximations are reasonable, then there is therefore no net impact on the final equations for DTI.

There may also be situations in which this approach simply cannot provide useful predictions. Consider an immunotoxin, a toxic molecule attached to all or part of a monoclonal antibody; the system is intended to be a cancer chemotherapeutic agent. We specify that the toxin along cannot enter cells and so is not toxic or active. Only when it is delivered into the cell's cytoplasm does one observe toxicity. How can the DTI approach help to decide how well such a therapeutic system could work? It cannot. That is, one cannot calculate a DTI value because there is no parent or reference compound. The immunotoxin must be treated and evaluated as a new chemical entity; it does not fit our definition of a drug-carrier combination. An active agent encapsulated in liposome does fit the definition.

XIII. FREE DRUG CONTROL STUDIES

It is generally recognized that changing the route of administration or the dosing rate can alter the therapeutic availability and the therapeutic index. In order to quantify the additional advantage resulting from targeting, as contrasted with an advantage resulting from sustained release, the intravenous free-drug input rate must match the release, rates of drug from the drug carrier. Unfortunately, release rates from drug carriers in vivo are difficult to determine. The problem could be overcome by comparing relative effectiveness after infusing both the free drug (in one study) and the drug-carrier combination (in another study) until steady state is reached. Because such experimental designs are expensive and technically demanding when feasible, investigators have chosen to compare the pharmacological results following a bolus dose of the drug-carrier combination to the results following a bolus intravenous dose of free drug (e.g., Refs. 7–10). This approach has been seen as a means to approximate experimentally the therapeutic advantage of using the drug carrier. Unfortunately, the benefits cannot be assigned solely to the carrier's target site delivery properties when the control study is simply an intravenous dose of free drug, because the intravenous dose rate of free drug would not match the overall drug release rate from the carrier as required by Equation (18). Given the multiple variables being assessed, experimental strategies that lack such controls may generate little useful information relative to the indirect, theoretical approach described here.

REFERENCES

1. V. J. Stella and K. J. Himmelstein. J. Med. Chem. 23: 1275–1282, 1980.
2. G. Levy. Pharmacol. Res. 4: 3–4, 1987.
3. A. T. Florence. In Rate Control in Drug Therapy. Edited by L. F. Prescott and W. S. Nimmo. Churchill Livingstone, Edinburgh, 1985, p. 103.
4. V. J. Stella and K. J. Himmelstein. In Optimization of Drug Delivery, Alfred Benson Symposium 17. Edited by H. Bundgaard, A. B. Hansen, and H. Kofod. Munksgaard, Copenhagen, 1982, pp. 134–155.
5. J. Mordenti. J. Pharm. Sci. 75: 1028–1040, 1986.
6. C. A. Hunt, R. D. MacGregor, and R. S. Siegel. Pharmacol. Res. 3: 333–344, 1986.
7. Goodman, T. W. Dall, and F. Murad (eds.). The Pharmacological Basis of Therapeutics, 7th ed. Macmillan, New York, 1985, p. 1668.
8. I. J. Fidler, A. Raz, W. E. Fogler, R. Kirsch, P. Bugelski, and G. Poste. Cancer Res. 40: 4460–4466, 1980.
9. M. B. Yatvin, J. N. Weinstein, W. H. Dennis, and R. Blumenthal. Science 202: 1290–1292, 1978.
10. E. Mayhew, Y. M. Rustum, F. Szoka, and D. Papahadjopoulos. Cancer Treat. Rep. 63: 1923–1928, 1979.
11. F. Olsen, E. Mayhew, D. Moslow, Y. M. Rustum, and F. Szoka. Eur. J. Cancer Clin. Oncol. 18: 167–176, 1982.

8

Bioavailability and Bioequivalence of Oral Controlled-Release Products: A Regulatory Perspective

SHRIKANT V. DIGHE and WALLACE P. ADAMS   *U. S. Food and Drug Administration, Rockville, Maryland*

307

I. INTRODUCTION

An increasing number of drugs previously available in conventional-release dosage forms only are being formulated and marketed in controlled-release dosage forms. This is the result of the well-recognized therapeutic and patient convenience benefits of controlled-release dosage forms for many drugs. The rapid growth of many pioneer controlled-release brands has inspired generic manufacturers to develop controlled-release product copies of brand-name drug products. Current regulations require that the bioavailability or bioequivalence of a controlled-release drug product intended for oral administration be demonstrated in comparison to a suitable and appropriate reference standard.

The U.S. Food and Drug Administration (FDA) has established bioavailability and bioequivalence requirements for controlled-release products. At the present time, specific requirements are in a state of transition, as exemplified by the report of Skelly et al. (1). The issues and controversies involve questions centering partly around appropriate study design. However, questions also exist regarding the most appropriate means of pharmacokinetic analysis once a study has been performed. Determination of extent of absorption is generally straightforward. However, many methods for the determination of rate of absorption and particularly of fluctuation have been presented in the past, representing conflicting opinion about the most appropriate means of quantifying these parameters.

This chapter describes the requirements established by the FDA to assure the bioavailability or bioequivalence of controlled-release products. It also surveys several methods that have been used to quantify controlled-release performance and discusses both strengths and weaknesses, where apparent. The survey is not exhaustive; rather, it presents some methods that may be of value in assessing controlled-release performance. In addition, the chapter describes the FDA dissolution requirements for controlled-release products. For insight into other aspects of controlled-release products, many excellent review articles and monographs are available.

II. TYPES OF PRODUCTS

There is no single standard terminology to describe the oral dosage forms designed to provide long-acting therapy. However, the products have recently been described as sustained release, controlled release, repeat action, and delayed release (2−4). The sustained-release products are often designed with an initial loading dose intended to establish rapidly therapeutic drug blood levels and additional drug intended to maintain those levels for a prolonged period. Those products providing only the slow-release component and lacking the immediate-release component have sometimes been termed prolonged release. Prolonged-release products are therefore of use when an immediate therapeutic effect is not required. Controlled-release products are essentially sustained release products that are capable of maintaining a constant and predictable drug blood level for a specified time period. Repeat action products generally contain two doses of the drug. The first dose is for immediate release; the second dose is generally contained within an enteric coated (but not a slow-release) core intended for release at a later time. The delayed-release products, similar to the repeat action products, do not contain a slow-release core; rather, the product is enteric coated for release in the intestines.

The terminology suggests that significantly different in vivo performance characteristics can occur among these dosage forms, emphasized by Table 1, which describes some of the more common physicochemical mechanisms used in the design of these products. Other means of obtaining controlled release, such as orally administered prodrugs (e.g., chloramphenicol palmitate; valpromide, or valproic acid amide) or a hydrocolloid system that floats on the gastric fluid and slowly releases drug into the gastrointestinal tract (Valrelease, Roche), are also utilized. It is apparent that the many mechanisms of controlled drug release may have significantly different release profiles, as well as different degrees of sensitivity toward such factors as gastrointestinal pH, food content, fluid volume, and electrolyte composition. These factors may profoundly influence the rate and/or extent of drug absorption of conventional-release products as well as sustained-release products manufactured by different firms. It is essential, therefore, that in vivo studies be conducted to assure the bioavailbility or bioequivalence of these products. For convenience, all these products except the delayed-release (enteric coated) products are referred to as controlled-release products.

III. REGULATORY ASPECTS

The Food and Drug Administration considers most controlled-release dosage forms new drugs requiring scientific data to ensure their safety and efficacy (5). A controlled-release product thus requires a full new drug application (NDA) or abbreviated new drug application (ANDA), depending upon whether it is a new controlled-release dosage form or a generic version of the already marketed controlled-release drug product. A controlled-release dosage form for a drug

TABLE 1 Selected Physicochemical Mechanisms of Controlled Release of Oral Dosage Forms

I. Diffusion: The rate-limiting step is diffusion of drug across a membrane or out of a matrix.

A. Reservoir devices: Drug core is surrounded by a porous or nonporous polymeric membrane. Commercial examples: 8-Hour Bayer Timed-Release Aspirin Tablets (Glenbrook); Nitro-Bid Plateau Caps (Marion).

B. Matrix devices: Drug is dispersed throughout a matrix composed of an inert plastic, an erodible wax or fat, or a hydrophilic polymer. Commercial examples: Desoxyn Gradumet tablets (Abbott); Procan SR tablets (Parke-Davis).

II. Dissolution: Drug release is determined by the dissolution rate of a polymer or wax coating or by the dissolution or hydrolysis rate of a matrix.

A. Polymer- or wax-encapsulated drug: Drug core is surrounded by a coating that, when dissolved, releases all drug contained within the particle. Commercial examples: Compazine Spansule capsules (SK&F); Bellergal-S tablets (Sandoz).

B. Matrix devices: Drug is dispersed throughout a matrix that slowly erodes and releases drug. Commercial example: Tenuate Dospan tablets (Merrell Dow).

III. Complexation: Insoluble complexes are formed between ionic drugs and either an ion-exchange resin or certain organic acids.

A. Ion-exchange resin complexes: Rate of drug release is governed by such factors as the degree of resin cross-linking and particle size, which alter the rate of drug diffusion, as well as the gastrointestinal tract ionic concentration. The resin beads may be surrounded by a polymeric membrane that functions as a diffusion barrier. Commercial example: Ionamin capsules (Pennwalt).

B. Organic acid complexes: Poorly soluble and slowly dissolving complexes of basic drugs have been prepared with tannic acid or polygalacturonic acid. Commercial examples: Rynatan tablets and pediatric suspension (Wallace); Cardioquin tablets (Purdue Frederick).

IV. Osmotic pressure: The elementary osmotic pump design consists of a tablet core surrounded by a semipermeable membrane through which water passes by osmosis. As a hydrostatic pressure difference is established across the membrane, drug solution is forced out of a small hole in the membrane at a constant rate. Commercial example: Acutrim tablets (Ciba).

that was originally approved in a conventional-release dosage form as a full NDA on the basis of safety and effectiveness data may require controlled clinical studies to demonstrate safety and effectiveness. However, when the relationship between clinical response (therapeutic and toxic) and plasma concentration of the drug and/or its active metabolite(s) is well defined, the FDA may accept bioavailability study data in lieu of clinical trials for approval of the controlled-release product. Under these conditions the blood levels and/or urinary excretion rates of the controlled-release dosage form should be comparable to those of multiple doses of the appropriate conventional-release dosage formulation; the labeling must clearly state the recommended dosing regimen and must be identical to that of the conventional-release dosage formulation in terms of indications (except those covered by exclusivity).

The Report of the Workshop on Controlled Release Dosage Forms: Issues and Controversies (1) identifies circumstances under which clinical studies may be required. Thus with drugs for which (1) therapeutic effect is indirect, (2) there is evidence of development of pharmacodynamic tolerance, (3) there is possibility of occurrence of irreversible toxicity, (4) the peak to trough differences of the controlled-release dosage form are large, or (5) there is reasonable uncertainty with regard to the relationship between drug plasma concentration and pharmacodynamic effects, it will probably be necessary to conduct clinical studies for approval of the first controlled-release dosage form. Claims of clinical advantages (e.g., decrease in incidence of side effects) for a controlled-release drug product over a conventional-release dosage form must be substantiated by adequate, well-controlled clinical trials.

A. Safety and Efficacy of Controlled-Release Drug Products

The general regulatory requirements for controlled-release dosage forms may be outlined as follows.

I. For all pre- and post-1962 drugs approved on the basis of safety and effectiveness in conventional-release dosage forms and for which there is no approved listed* controlled-release drug product on the market:

---

*A "listed drug" means a new drug product that has been approved for safety and effectiveness under 21 USC355(c) or approved under 21 USC355(j) of the Federal Food, Drug and Cosmetic Act. The listed drug status is evidenced by the drug product's inclusion in the current edition of the FDA "Approved Drug Products with Therapeutic Equivalence Evaluations" (the List, also called the "Orange Book") and any current supplement to the List.

a. Controlled and adequate clinical studies may be required to demonstrate safety and effectiveness of the controlled-release formulation.

b. Bioavailability and pharmacokinetic data for the controlled-release formulation are also required and may be acceptable in lieu of clinical studies when the relationship between clinical response and plasma concentration of the drug and/or its metabolite(s) is well defined.

II. For all pre- and post-1962 drugs approved on the basis of safety and effectiveness in controlled-release dosage forms and for which there is an approved listed controlled-release drug product on the market:

a. Bioequivalence data are required and acceptable when the data for the test controlled-release product are comparable to those for the listed controlled-release drug product.

b. The labeling for the test controlled-release product must be identical to that of the reference listed controlled-release product with regard to indications (except those indications covered by exclusivity).

Bioavailability data are required in support of a new drug application for a controlled-release drug product. FDA's Bioavailability and Bioequivalence Regulations describe the purpose of an in vivo bioavailability study involving a drug product for which a controlled-release claim is made (6). The provisions of these regulations address themselves to the rate and extent of absorption, dose dumping, appropriate reference material for such a bioavailability study, and labeling. Thus a firm seeking approval for its controlled-release drug formulation should provide information from in vivo bioavailability study to demonstrate that all the following conditions are met:

1. The drug product meets the controlled release claims made for it.

2. The bioavailability profile established for the drug product rules out the occurrence of any dose dumping.

3. The drug product's steady-state performance is equivalent to that of a currently marketed noncontrolled release or controlled-release drug product that contains the same active drug ingredient or therapeutic moiety and that is subject to an approved full new drug application.

4. The drug product's formulation provides consistent pharmacokinetic performance between individual dosage units.

The in vivo data on a controlled-release test product in comparison to an approved noncontrolled release or controlled-release product provide information on the pharmacokinetic profiles of the test and reference drug products and the rate and extent of bioavailability of the controlled-release test product. The data so generated are important in assuring the controlled-release nature of the test drug product, absence of dose dumping, absorption of an acceptable percentage of the dose in the controlled-release formulation, and acceptably low subject-to-subject variability for the test controlled-release formulation.

In addition to in vivo bioavailability and bioequivalence data, the firm needs to submit in vitro dissolution data in order to obtain approval of the controlled-release drug product. The dissolution data should provide drug release rate profiles generated by a well-designed, reproducible testing method. The apparatus normally used for solid oral dosage forms should be employed. The dissolution media should be aqueous acidic, basic, and buffer solutions of different pH. The test medium and methodology should be sensitive enough to detect any changes in formulations and lot-to-lot variations. Cabana and Chien (7) observed that the key elements of a successful test are

1. Reproducibility of the method
2. Proper choice of medium
3. Maintenance of perfect sink conditions
4. Control of solution hydrodynamics

Skelly and Barr (8) noted that the dissolution testing should assure

1. Lack of dose dumping, indicated by a narrow limit on the 1-hr dissolution specification
2. Controlled-release characteristics by employing additional sampling windows over time
3. Complete drug release indicated by 75-80% minimum release specification at the last sampling interval.

B. Bioavailability Studies for a Controlled-Release Version of an Approved Conventional-Release Drug Product

The type of pharmacokinetic studies needed to be performed is dependent upon our knowledge of the drug and its clinical pharmacokinetics and biopharmaceutics. When this information is limited and inadequate, clinical studies are required. For a controlled-release oral dosage form of a marketed conventional-release drug product for which an extensive data base of pharmacokinetic and pharmacodynamic information exists, the pharmacokinetic studies delineated below may suffice as the basis of approval of the drug product. It it recommended that appropriate divisions of the FDA Center for Drugs Evaluation and Research should be consulted prior to initiation of studies to determine that an adequate data base does exist for approval.

I. A single-dose, three-way crossover study (described elsewhere in the chapter as a modified single-dose study)
   employing the following treatments:
a. The controlled-release dosage form administered under fasting
   conditions.
b. A rapidly available dosage form (an oral solution or a well-
   characterized FDA-approved conventional-release drug product
   containing the same drug entity or therapeutic moiety as
   the controlled-release product) administered under fasting
   conditions according to its regimen.
c. The controlled-release dosage form administered immediately
   after a high fat content meal.

   If no significant differences in area under the concentration-
time curve (AUC) and peak concentration C_{max} as a function of meal
are observed in the study, further food effect studies are not necessary. If significant food effect is found, the applicant should carry
out studies to determine whether the observed food effect is a result of
(1) problems with the dosage form or (2) problems unrelated to the
dosage form, such as changes in the absorption of the drug in the
gastrointestinal tract and/or changes in the disposition of the drug.
Such studies should be conducted as single-dose crossover studies
comparing the test controlled-release product to an oral solution (or
conventional-release dosage form) under fasting and nonfasting conditions.
   In addition, studies should be conducted to determine the effect
of the interval between dosing and a meal. The controlled-release
drug product should be tested in a four-way crossover with the
following treatment conditions: fasting, drug product administered
immediately after a high fat content meal, drug product administered
1 hr before a high fat content meal, and drug product administered
2 hr after a high fat content meal.

II. Multiple-dose, steady-state studies
a. When the pharmacokinetics of the conventional-release product
   is known to be linear, a multiple-dose steady-state crossover
   study using the highest strength of the controlled-release
   formulation as the test product and a conventional-release
   drug product as the reference product should be conducted.
   At least three consecutive trough concentrations C_{min} should
   be measured to ensure that the subjects are at steady state.
   Concentrations of the drug and/or its metabolite(s) at steady
   state over at least one dosing interval of the controlled-
   release product should be measured in each leg of the study.
   It may be desirable, in the case of a drug undergoing diurnal
   variation in its absorption or disposition, to measure concen-

tration of the drug over an entire day in each leg of the crossover. The controlled-release product should produce an area under the concentration-time curve equivalent to that of the conventional-release product and the degree of fluctuation for the controlled-release product should be less than or similar to that for the conventional-release product.

b.   When the conventional-release product is known to follow nonlinear pharmacokinetics or data to establish linear pharmacokinetics are not available, two separate multiple-dose steady-state studies should be conducted: (1) on the high end of dose strengths of the controlled-release formulation and (2) on the low end of dose strengths of the controlled-release formulation. The same considerations with regard to AUC and fluctuation as described previously apply for acceptability of data.

C. Bioequivalence Studies for a Generic Version of an Approved Controlled-Release Product

The Federal Food, Drug and Cosmetic Act of 1984 (9) describes a bioequivalent drug as follows:

A Drug shall be considered to be bioequivalent to a listed drug if—(i) the rate and extent of absorption of the drug do not show a significant difference from the rate and extent of absorption of the listed drug when administered at the same molar dose of the therapeutic ingredient under similar experimental conditions in either a single dose or multiple doses; or

(ii) the extent of absorption of the drug does not show a significant difference from the extent of absorption of the listed drug when administered at the same molar dose of the therapeutic ingredient under similar experimental conditions in either a single dose or multiple doses and the difference from the listed drug in rate of absorption of the drug is intentional, is reflected in its proposed labeling, is not essential to the attainment of effective body drug concentrations on chronic use, and is considered medically insignificant for the drug.

These two nonexclusive descriptions of bioequivalent drugs hold for conventional-release dosage forms as well as controlled-release dosage forms.

The current approach to the evaluation of generic controlled-release products is as follows. A single-dose two-way crossover study comparing the generic formulation with the approved (listed) controlled-release drug product under fasting conditions is conducted to ensure the controlled-release nature of the generic formulation as well as the absence of dose dumping. For controlled-release products ad-

ministered once a day, a three-way crossover study comparing the
generic version under fasting and nonfasting conditions with the
approved controlled-release product administered under fasting
conditions is performed. A single-dose crossover study under fasting
and nonfasting conditions is also conducted when the approved
controlled-release product has a label claim that it can be administered
regardless of meal and is administered more often than once a day
(twice to four times a day regimen).

In addition, a multiple-dose steady-state study comparing the
generic formulation with the approved controlled-release product is
also required (10). Such a study must demonstrate that the generic
product is comparable to the approved controlled-release product
with respect to AUC, C_{max}, and C_{min} on the basis of the FDA
statistical criteria for equivalence.

In vitro dissolution testing for controlled-release drug products
has already been described. Dissolution testing should be conducted
on lots of the test controlled-release product employed in in vivo
bioavailability and bioequivalence testing.

IV. CODING FOR CONTROLLED-RELEASE DRUG
PRODUCTS IN AN FDA PUBLICATION

The FDA issues an annual publication (updated by monthly cumulative
supplements), *Approved Drug Products with Therapeutic Equivalence
Evaluations* (11). This publication identifies drug products approved
by the FDA as safe and effective. The main criterion for inclusion
of any product is that it is the subject of an approved application
(NDA or ANDA). The list also contains therapeutic equivalence
evaluations for approved multisource prescription drug products.
The two-letter coding system for therapeutic equivalence evaluation
is employed so that users can determine quickly whether the FDA
has evaluated a particular approved product as therapeutically equivalent to other pharmaceutically equivalent products. Controlled-release
products are usually coded AB or BC. Controlled-release products
containing the same active ingredient in equal strengths and for which
acceptable bioequivalence data are submitted are coded AB. The controlled-release products that have not been shown to be bioequivalent
to the listed controlled-release drug product are coded BC. The controlled-release products for a specific drug entity coded AB in the
List are considered by the FDA to be therapeutically equivalent.

V. DISSOLUTION REQUIREMENTS

Both the FDA and the U.S. Pharmacopeia (USP) require dissolution
data for controlled-release products. The current requirements for
a specific product may be the same or may differ between these two
regulatory bodies. An overview of the current status indicates the
differences.

The USP currently recognizes (12) two types of modified-release
dosage forms: (1) extended-release dosage forms, which allow at
least a twofold reduction in dosing frequency compared with that for
the drug in a conventional dosage form, and (2) delayed-release
dosage forms, which release the drug(s) at a time other than promptly
after administration (e.g., enteric coated products). The oral controlled-release tablets and capsules are thus extended-release dosage
forms. The USP proposes in its *Pharmacopeial Forum* (13–15) to
subdivide the extended-release dosage forms into Cases 1,2, and 3
for USP monograph purposes. The dissolution requirements for Case
1 products involve sampling at three times, expressed as fractions
of the normal dosing interval D:

Sampling time	% Labeled drug dissolved
0.25D	20–50
0.50D	45–75
>0.50–1.0D	≥ 75

When two or more dosing intervals are stated in the product labeling,
the shortest D value is used.

The purpose of the 0.25D specification is to assure there is no
dose dumping from the dosage form, yet to allow the inclusion of a
loading dose. The purpose of the last specification is to assure the
nearly complete dissolution of drug; the range extends as low as 75%
to allow the inclusion of a reservoir of excess drug that is not released within the sampling time. The intermediate specification assures
that drug release over the 0.25–0.50D period occurs neither too
slowly nor too rapidly.

Skelly and Barr (8) have pointed out that the 0.25D (6 hr) proposed USP specification for a controlled-release product dosed once
daily would in a few instances fail to provide assurance against dose
dumping. They indicate that the dissolution specifications developed
for each controlled-release product should include a 1 hr specification

to detect possible dose dumping. The acceptance table for the extended-release dosage forms (16) involves testing through three successive levels (sets of criteria) L1, L2, and L3, unless the product conforms to the criterion at either L1 or L2. Each level establishes a criterion for the percentage dissolved ranges at each of the three sampling times. At level 1, only 6 dosage units are tested. At level 2, another 6 units are tested, and at level 3 another 12 units are tested. Thus, 6, 12, or 24 units are tested depending upon the outcome at each level. This three-level acceptance criterion differs from the FDA procedure, which employs 12 dosage units.

The USP proposal envisions many of the extended-release products falling into the Case 1 group. However, many other products are expected to be designed with different release profiles that would not fit Case 1 specifications. These may include innovator products as well as multisource products. Cases 2 and 3 are proposed for such products. Case 2 would apply when the chemical or physical properties of the drug or formulation did not allow application of Case 1. The individual monograph sets forth sampling times, percentage dissolved specifications, and experimental conditions. Case 3 would apply when the chemical or physical properties of the drug formulations among multisource products differ to such an extent that a single set of sampling times, percentage dissolved specifications, and experimental conditions would not be appropriate. In this group of products, the USP monograph would include more than one set of dissolution test conditions with a suitable designation of the formulation type to which each applies. The USP proposes that the product labeling include a graphic or tabular portrayal of the release profile using the dissolution conditions specified in the monograph.

Cases 1 and 2 dissolution requirements, if established, would apply to all drug products for that particular monograph. The FDA dissolution specifications for controlled-release products, however, are generally unique to each firm's product, as explained below.

The potential for pH dependence of drug release from controlled-release formulations is well recognized. Accordingly, the FDA now requires firms in their NDA or ANDA submissions to present dissolution data conducted in several different media. For an NDA, the FDA requires that dissolution profiles in water, simulated gastric fluid TS (SGF) without enzyme (pH 1.2), simulated intestinal fluid TS (SIF) without enzyme (pH 7.5), and appropriate buffer be determined (8). For an ANDA, the FDA requires a similar set of dissolution profiles to be submitted. Profiles are generally based on media in each of the following pH ranges: 1—1.5, 4—4.5, 6—6.5, and 7—7.5. In the past, in an effort to simulate physiologic conditions more closely, the FDA commonly utilized a dissolution medium that consisted of SGF (without enzyme) for 1 hr, followed by SIF (without enzyme) from 1 hr on.

Although this medium is still employed, the FDA is moving toward the use of the constant pH media already mentioned. Dissolution data over the entire approximate pH range of the gastrointestinal tract is obtained, including the pH range intermediate between the pH 1.2 and 7.5 dual-medium system. This intermediate range may be more discriminating for certain drug products. In addition, from an experimental standpoint, the dissolution study is easier to perform if the medium is not changed at 1 hr.

Dissolution conditions frequently specified by FDA for controlled-release tablets and capsules are shown in Table 2. For the 12 tablets or capsules, the FDA usually asks applicants to tabulate at each sampling time the individual dissolution data, the mean percentage

TABLE 2 Dissolution Conditions for Controlled-Release Tablets and Capsules

Apparatus	USP XXI Apparatus 1 (rotating basket)[a] for capsules USP XXI Apparatus 2 (paddle) for tablets
Rotational speed	100 RPM (capsules) 50 RPM (tablets)
Temperature	37 ± 0.5°C
Number of dosage units	12
Dissolution medium	Various
Sampling schedule	Various sampling times to not less than 75–80% drug release
% Dissolved specifications	As established

[a]Although the rotating basket is frequently used for capsule and the paddle for tablet dissolution studies, either apparatus may be used for either dosage form, as specified by the FDA or USP. The attempt to standardize the basket speed at 100 RPM or the paddle speed at 50 RPM for a particular drug product arose from the observation (primarily for conventional-release dosage forms) that dissolution results using either of these sets of conditions were frequently similar. Other speeds may be specified, however. Sampling that continues until not less than 75–80% of the labeled amount of drug in the dosage form is released is generally preferred.

dissolved, the standard deviation, the percentage CV, and the range. The range is important in determining adherence to the acceptance table. With certain exceptions, the FDA requires at least single-dose bioavailability or bioequivalence studies to be performed on all strengths of the controlled-release product. It also requires dissolution data on all strengths of the controlled-release product. When applicable, the dissolution profiles are determined on the same lots of the test and reference products used in the in vivo study or studies. The lot of the test product used in both the in vivo study and the in vitro dissolution studies should be a production lot or a lot produced under production conditions.

Skelly and coworkers have recently described a topographical dissolution technique (17) in which the percentage dissolved versus time profile is plotted as a function of pH in a three-dimensional plot. Intra- and interproduct differences in sensitivity to pH and changes in aqueous buffer type (should they exist) are readily apparent in these plots. Therefore, in addition to the tabular presentation of data, the firm may, if it wishes, utilize either the topographical dissolution technique or two-dimensional plots to display its data. Of primary concern is the determination of pH dependence or independence of drug release from the product. In the event of pH-dependent release, generally the most discriminating dissolution medium is the most appropriate. This medium should be the most effective as a quality control tool for the assurance of lot uniformity.

Owing to the variety of physicochemical mechanisms that may be used in multisource controlled-release products, in vitro-in vivo correlations may be difficult to obtain. In the event that a correlation is established, it is quite possible that a subsequent controlled-release product, perhaps utilizing a different release mechanism, does not fit the observed correlation. Dissolution data therefore serve only as a quality control measure for a firm's specific product; they are not directly related to the in vivo release of the drug. Nevertheless, intuitively, it would appear desirable that in vitro release continue over a prolonged time period, ideally resulting in complete drug release over a sampling interval equal to the labeled dosing interval of the product. (An exception would be a once daily controlled-release product in which complete drug release over a shorter time period is intended because of the long biologic half-life of the drug.) This approach is realistic for a product dosed two or more times daily. For a 24 hr product, such an approach would be inconvenient from an experimental standpoint. From a practical standpoint, sampling through 8 hr for a twice daily product and through 12 hr for a once daily product may be adequate provided no less than 75-80% of drug has been released. If lesser release occurs, further sampling or a change in dissolution conditions (apparatus, speed, and/or medium) to accelerate dissolution is recommended.

The establishment of FDA dissolution standards for controlled-release products is a joint effort between the individual pharmaceutical firms and the FDA and occurs as follows. The firm is requested, as part of the NDA or ANDA approval process, to provide dissolution data utilizing the conditions described previously. It is also requested to propose a specification and tolerances for its product at three or more sampling times, generally including 1, 3 or 4, and 8 hr for a twice daily product. Specifications at one or more additional sampling times may be included for a once daily product. The data, specification, and tolerances are reviewed by the FDA and accepted or alternative specifications are proposed. The final specifications apply to the test product only, not to the reference product. This procedure is repeated for each firm. Thus, each approved multisource controlled release product of a particular drug may have its own unique set of dissolution conditions and specifications. Since the specifications are intended for quality control purposes, a uniform set of dissolution conditions and specifications for all controlled-release products of a given drug, although desirable, may be impractical. This product-specific approach to establishing dissolution conditions is somewhat similar to the USP proposed Case 3 approach in which more than one set of dissolution conditions may be specified.

We emphasize that the bioavailability or bioequivalence of each approved controlled-release product must be established through in vivo studies. Dissolution data are utilized by the firm as a quality control tool and by the FDA in the evaluation of minor formulation changes or minor process changes. In the case of conventional-release products in which an acceptable bioavailability or bioequivalence study has been conducted, acceptable dissolution data (along with formula proportionality) serve as the basis for waiver of in vivo bioequivalence study of a lower strength product (18). This is not the case for controlled-release products. Bioavailability or bioequivalence studies are generally required for all strengths of the product, the main exception being beaded tablets or capsules in which the lower strength product contains smaller numbers of the identical bead used in the high-strength product upon which the in vivo study was conducted.

VI. METHODS TO EVALUATE CONTROLLED-RELEASE CHARACTER

Parameters used to evaluate the bioavailability or bioequivalence of controlled-release dosage forms are the conventional AUC, C_{max}, and T_{max} terms. Additional parameters that may be used to characterize these products include drug concentrations at each sampling time, apparent rate constant for elimination, apparent biologic half-life, urinary excretion rate, and amount excreted in the urine at infinity. Controlled-release products are designed to provide a controlled rate of absorption of the drug. The slow release of drug from the formulation over a prolonged period of time is the rate-limiting step in the overall absorption process, producing plasma concentrations with decreased fluctuation (relative to a corresponding conventional-release product) over an 8-hr, 12-hr, or in some cases over a 24-hr period. Therefore, it is desirable that absorption rate and fluctuation be determined. This section examines several bioavailability and bioequivalence parameters that may be utilized to characterize controlled-release products.

A. Absorption Rate Profile

Controlled-release character may be established (in part) by demonstrating that absorption is prolonged. Controlled-release products may release drugs by zero, first, or mixed order. Therefore, a method of determining the rate of drug release that is independent of order, such as the Wagner-Nelson method (19), is of particular value. The utility of the Wagner-Nelson method as part of the bioavailability profile for NDA and ANDA controlled-release submissions has been discussed (20, 21). Although for multicompartment drugs the method yields only estimates of the absorption rate constant and the time period for absorption (22), it does not require intravenous data. Treatment of the body as a one-compartment model in the absorption of controlled-release products has been justified on the basis of difficulty in defining distribution rate constants in the presence of slow drug absorption (23). For multicompartment models in which intravenous data are available, the Loo-Riegelman (24) or other methods are preferable.

Cumulative fraction absorbed or fraction remaining to be absorbed plots based on the Wagner-Nelson method provide valuable information regarding the performance of controlled-release products:

1. The plots, obtained from single-dose studies, may indicate that the drug release and absorption process is occurring by either an apparent first-order or zero-order process. This information provides insight into the steady-state plasma concentration-time profile of the drug. Once pseudo-steady-state conditions have been attained in the body, a zero-order process should in theory maintain a constant blood level of drug throughout the period of absorption. A first-order process results in a sawtooth pattern, although the fluctuations will be low the longer the biologic half-life of the drug (25).

2. The apparent rate constants may be used to estimate the fraction of the drug eventually absorbed from the product that is available for absorption over any particular time period. Although drug absorption does occur from the large intestine (26), absorption from the colon is thought to be poor and/or unpredictable for many drugs (27). Therefore, for these drugs efficient drug absorption can only occur within the limited time period that the dosage form is within the upper regions of the gastrointestinal tract. As an approximation, this time period is assumed to be 9–12 hr (22).

3. The plots may be used to compute "gut residual," the amount of drug remaining unabsorbed from the previous dose(s). Since absorption from the colon may be poor and/or unpredictable, drug remaining in the gastrointestinal tract at the time of the subsequent dose has the potential of increasing variability in steady-state levels (28).

4. Individual plots of fraction absorbed versus time enable the estimation of intersubject variability in drug absorption. Owing to the much slower rate of drug release over a longer region of the gastrointestinal tract, the controlled-release dosage form is potentially subject to a much wider range in physiologic variables than is a conventional-release product. Subject variables influencing the drug in the dosage form include pH and gastrointestinal motility; those influencing the drug after release from the product include gastrointestinal transit times, differing rates of absorption throughout the gastrointestinal tract, and various food effects. Many other variables can be cited (26). These variables may result in excessively slow or rapid release of drug from the product (29).

5. The plots may be used to establish an in vitro-in vivo correlation or association. A correlation has been shown between the fraction of drug released with time in vitro from an Oros (Alza) product and the fraction of the drug absorbed (30).

B. Fluctuation

The absorption rate profiles are based upon single-dose studies and provide evidence that the product is in fact a controlled-release dosage form, that is, that the desired rate and duration of drug release were designed into the product. Single-dose studies cannot assure that the plasma levels at steady state will actually be within the therapeutic range. Although multiple-dose projections may be made, these require the assumption of linear kinetics. Multiple-dose steady-state studies permit mean plasma levels and fluctuation to be

determined under conditions of dosing used in the study with no
assumptions made of the kinetic models involved. Thus, optimal
dosing regimens may be devised. They also allow determination of the
extent of absorption and verification of the absence of dose dumping,
although these can also be determined from single-dose studies. This
section describes various measures of fluctuation that have been used
to characterize controlled-release products.

1. Dosage Form Index and Fluctuation Index

The therapeutic index of a drug may be defined in terms of either
drug dose sizes or plasma concentrations. In the latter case, the
therapeutic index is defined as the ratio of the maximum tolerated
drug plasma concentration to the minimum effective drug plasma
concentration (31). The dosage form index is defined as the ratio
C_{max}/C_{min} within a dosage interval at steady state (32). Because of
the similarity in definitions, the dosage form index may be compared
directly to the drug's therapeutic index. A drug product's dosage
form index should not exceed the therapeutic index. The slower the
apparent half-life of the drug, the smaller is the dosage form index.
The result is that a small dosage form index allows a longer dosing
interval τ while maintaining drug levels within the therapeutic range.

The dosage form index has limitations. It does not use all the
available data. Rather, only concentrations at two sampling times
are used per subject. The accuracy of the dosage form index is a
function of the blood sampling schedule, particularly in the region,
of C_{max}; the greater the number of sampling times in this region,
the better will be the estimate of the dosage form index. Since only
the extremes of the data are utilized, this parameter is very sensitive
to aberrant high or low values of C_{max} and/or C_{min}. In addition,
the dosage form index does not provide information regarding the
overall profile.

Fluctuation may also be stated in terms of percentage fluctuation
or fluctuation index. Percentage fluctuation may be expressed as the
percentage increase in drug levels (peak minus trough levels) relative
to trough levels (33):

$$\% \text{ fluctuation} = \frac{C_{max} - C_{min}}{C_{min}} \, 100$$

Owing to the possibility of significant intersubject variability in
trough levels when these levels are low, high variability in percentage
fluctuation may result. Caldwell et al. (34) have therefore proposed
a fluctuation index (FI):

$$FI = \frac{C_{max} - C_{min}}{\bar{C}}$$

where

$$\bar{C} = \frac{AUC(0 - \tau)}{\tau}$$

and τ is the dosing interval. The fluctuation index would be anticipated to be more stable than either the dosage form index or the percentage fluctuation (as defined above). Fluctuation index utilizes all the available data, in that $\bar{C}$ is computed from the plasma concentration-time profile. Therefore, the denominator of the fluctuation index should possess lower variability than the denominators of the other two expressions.

Alternatively, fluctuation index may be calculated utilizing the arithmetic mean of the peak and trough levels as the denominator:

$$FI = \frac{C_{max} - C_{min}}{(C_{max} + C_{min})/2}$$

In common with the dosage form index, fluctuation index provides no information regarding the overall profile. Fluctuation index data, expressed as either a fraction or a percentage, should be included in the bioavailability and bioequivalence submissions (1, 8). FI is also referred to as the degree of fluctuation.

2. Method of Area Deviation

The fluctuation index measures the maximum deviation observed during a dosing interval at steady state, relative to the mean plasma concentration. For the reasons already cited, a parameter that would express the mean deviation observed throughout the dosing interval would be advantageous. Boxenbaum (25) has proposed just such a parameter, the area deviation.

Mean deviation about $\bar{C}$ is determined by measuring the area between $\bar{C}$ and that portion of the plasma concentration-time curve above $\bar{C}$, as well as the area between $\bar{C}$ and that portion of the curve below $\bar{C}$. The sum of these areas (which are equal) is calculated. Areas are determined over a common dosing interval τ for the test product (controlled- or conventional-release) and for the reference product (controlled- or conventional-release). Areas are determined only after plasma concentrations for test or reference products are adjusted to yield the same $\bar{C}$. [Since τ is the same for all products, this is equivalent to normalizing to an identical AUC $(0 - \tau)$].* Since most controlled-release products ideally have a flat plasma concentration-time profile, the area deviation should be small. The method allows the mean deviation of the test product to be compared to that of the reference product. Owing to the normalization process, the method does not yield bioavailability information. Rather, it yields a measure of fluctuation, assuming that the test product produces the same mean plasma concentration as does the reference product. Figure 1 illustrates an application of the method to an elixir and two sustained-release theophylline products.

The method of area deviation has been further discussed by Nimmerfall and Rosenthaler (37), with special reference to intra-muscular injection. It is possible that their approach is applicable to oral controlled-release dosage forms when steady-state plasma level data are considered.

The advantage of the method of area deviation is that it is not defined in terms of the extremes of the data. Rather, it utilizes the data over the entire dosing interval and compares the mean deviation of the plasma concentrations from the mean concentration of that same product if it behaved ideally, that is, produced a perfectly flat drug level $\bar{C}$ throughout the dosing interval. The method provides an indicator of the mean closeness of the plasma levels to $\bar{C}$.

C. Duration of Drug Levels in Plasma

Several investigators have proposed parameters that may be used to quantify the length of time that plasma levels remain above or within certain arbitary limits or remain within the therapeutic range. These parameters may apply only to single-dose studies or to steady-state studies, or may be applicable to both study designs.

---

*When used as a measure of relative product performance, area deviations should only be compared between treatments after all data are adjusted to the same $\bar{C}$, i.e., after adjusting for differences in dose and/or bioavailability. This is readily seen in the case of a one versus two tablet treatment of a specific product exhibiting linear pharmacokinetics. The absolute area deviation due to the two-tablet dose would be twice that due to the one-tablet dose of the same product. If all the data were normalized to the same AUC$(0 - \tau)$, the area deviations would be identical for both treatments, as must be the case. Accordingly, a comparison of absolute area deviations (i.e., without prior adjustment to a common $\bar{C}$) between products is inappropriate (35).

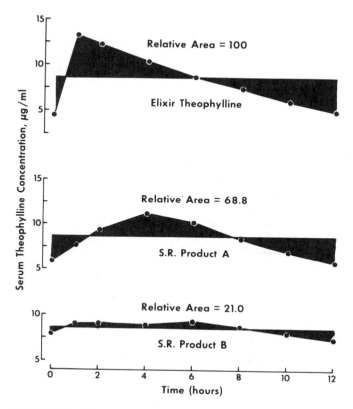

FIGURE 1 Averaged steady-state serum theophylline levels following oral administration every 12 hr of three dosage forms: (top) 250 mg elixir; (center) 250 mg SR capsule; (bottom) 300 mg SR tablet. Serum levels in the top and center segments were multiplied by appropriate factors to produce values of $\overline{C}$ equivalent to the bottom figure, that is, 8.63 μg/ml. Shaded regions are area deviations from the horizontal ideal. (From Ref. 25, reproduced with permission of the copyright owner, Plenum Publishing Corporation; original data from Ref. 36.)

1. Retard Quotients

Meier et al. (38) have defined a retard quotient $R_\triangle$ that measures the width of the plasma concentration-time profile (single-dose study) of a test controlled-release product relative to the corresponding width due to a conventional-release reference product. The width of the curve at a plasma concentration equal to one-half C_{max} serves as the basis for measurement. The HVD (half-value duration) is defined as as the time span for which the plasma concentration exceeds one-half C_{max}. Thus, R_Δ is determined from the ratio of the HVD valves of the controlled-release and conventional (regular)-release products, HVD_{CR} and HVD_{RR}, respectively. The equation

$$R_\Delta = \frac{HVD_{CR}}{HVD_{RR}}$$

quantifies the factor by which the HVD is prolonged for the controlled-release product relative to the conventional-release product.

R_Δ is independent of dose and is applicable whether the controlled-release product exhibits first- or zero-order input. As long as distribution and elimination kinetics are first order, the single-dose conventional-release treatment may consist of a single tablet or capsule or of the number of dosage units equal to the dose of the controlled-release product and the same result is obtained. The authors also proposed a second retard quotient R_c, which is the ratio of C_{max} of the controlled-release product to the C_{max} of the conventional-release product. This ratio is dose dependent. It may be used to quantify the decrease in the peak levels due to the controlled-release formulation. In Figure 2, plasma concentrations based upon single doses of the conventional-release and controlled-release forms of a drug product are plotted. For these plots, $R_\Delta = 3.6 \pm 0.1$ and $R_c = 1.0 \pm 0.1$ (mean $\pm$ SD).

R_Δ is based upon single-dose studies and does not provide information regarding the duration of drug levels within the therapeutic range. It does not provide any indication of the duration of action. Meier et al. intended both retard quotients to be used as a screening tool for comparison of various controlled-release formulations relative to a conventional-release product. The retard quotients could also be used to compare two controlled-release products.

2. Controlled-Release Effectiveness

Vallner et al. (39) have proposed a bioequivalence method for the evaluation of controlled-release products that utilizes area measurements. The method is based upon the assumption that a controlled-release product should yield plasma levels that lie within the minimum and maximum levels produced by sequential doses of the conventional-release product. Controlled-release effectiveness (CRE) is determined from a modified single-dose study or from a steady-state study. In a modified single-dose study, the controlled-release product is administered once; the conventional-release product is dosed in two or three sequential doses according to the normal regimen. Typically, one dose is given every 4 or 6 hr (total dose equal to the controlled-

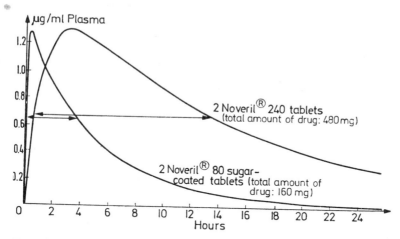

FIGURE 2 Human plasma concentrations of dibenzepin HCl simulated with the averaged pharmacokinetic constants of Noveril and Noveril 240. (From Ref. 38, reproduced with permission of the copyright owner, Springer-Verlag.)

release, product dose) to provide drug levels through one labeled dosing interval of the controlled-release product. C_{min} is defined as the initial plasma trough level in the sequential regimen; C_{max} is defined as the peak level following the last (second or third) dose. For steady-state studies, C_{max} and C_{min} may be taken as the observed peak and trough levels of the conventional-release product dosed sequentially (generally once every 4 or 6 hr) to the steady state. Alternate values for C_{min} were also proposed. The areas within the C_{min} and C_{max} limits are determined over the dosage interval τ for both the conventional and controlled-release products. CRE is defined as the ratio of this area for the controlled-release product to that of the conventional-release product. Treatment equivalence is demonstrated by ratios near unity.

The authors have also proposed the term "absorption rate effectiveness" (ARE), which is the ratio of the apparent absorption rate at which the controlled-release product reaches C_{min} to that at which the conventional-release product reaches C_{min}. Thus, ARE equals the ratio of the time required for the conventional-release product to reach C_{min} to the time required for the controlled-release product to reach C_{min}. ARE is expected to be less than unity but to approach this limit as the rate of absorption of the controlled-release product approaches that of the conventional-release product. ARE is computed only from single-dose data and may provide an indication of the rate of attainment of therapeutic levels.

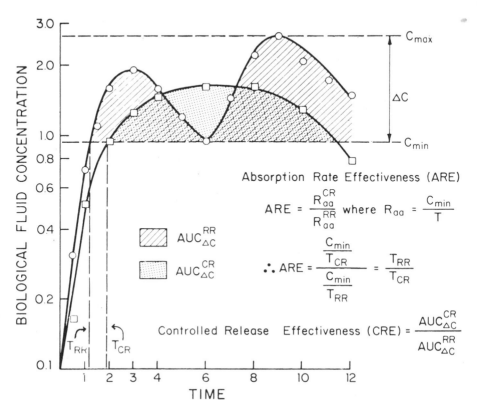

Absorption Rate Effectiveness (ARE)

$$ARE = \frac{R_{aa}^{CR}}{R_{aa}^{RR}} \text{ where } R_{aa} = \frac{C_{min}}{T}$$

$$\therefore ARE = \frac{\frac{C_{min}}{T_{CR}}}{\frac{C_{min}}{T_{RR}}} = \frac{T_{RR}}{T_{CR}}$$

$$\text{Controlled Release Effectiveness (CRE)} = \frac{AUC_{\Delta C}^{CR}}{AUC_{\Delta C}^{RR}}$$

FIGURE 3 Comparative curves for regular release drug product (administered at 0 and 6 hr) and controlled-release product (administered at 0 hr) showing the respective areas under the curves above and below C_{min} and C_{max}, respectively. The C_{min} and C_{max} are obtained from the regular release product administered twice; see text. The times the two products reach C_{min}, involved in determination of absorption rate effectiveness, are also shown. [From Ref. 39, reproduced with permission of the copyright owner, Elsevier Science Publishers B.V. (Biomedical Division).]

Figure 3 illustrates the areas and times utilized in the computation of CRE and ARE in a hypothetical modified single-dose study. Figure 4 illustrates mean profiles obtained in a modified single-dose chlorpheniramine study comparing a single dose of an 8 mg repeat action tablet to a 4 mg conventional-release tablet given at 0 and 6 hr (40). Based upon the mean data, the calculated values of CRE and ARE were 0.65 and 0.38, respectively (39). The authors indicate that values

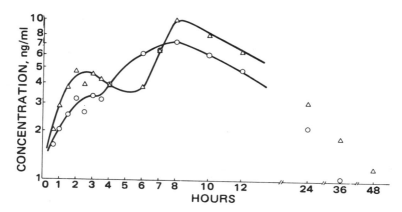

FIGURE 4 Mean plasma chlorpheniramine concentration-time curves for 4 mg conventional-release drug product (administered at 0 and 6 hr) and 8 mg repeat action product (administered at 0 hr): 4 mg tablet (△); 8 mg tablet (○). (From Ref. 40, reproduced with permission of the copyright owner, the American Pharmaceutical Association.)

near unity are optimum for both CRE and ARE. The decreased values of both parameters in the chlorpheniramine study were due to a delay in the initial release of drug from the repeat action product and a significantly lower extent of absorption from the repeat action tablet. In a situation such as this, in which the modified single-dose study revealed low values of CRE and ARE, a steady-state study is instructive (41).

3. Therapeutic Occupancy Time

Therapeutic occupancy time refers to the length of time that a controlled-release product produces drug levels within the therapeutic range at steady state (28), as shown in Figure 5. For those drugs with a known therapeutic range, clearly the controlled-release product should maintain levels within the therapeutic range over as great a fraction of the dosing interval as possible. A caveat in the application of therapeutic occupancy times is necessary since for a particular product and dosing frequency it is dependent upon dose and bioavailability. Therapeutic occupancy time is also dependent upon other factors, including such patient variables as clearance. Thus, a low therapeutic occupancy time cannot necessarily be construed as indicative of poor product performance; it may represent only an inappropriate dosing regimen for therapy.

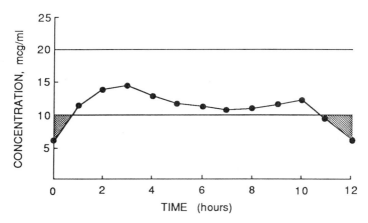

FIGURE 5 Steady-state drug plasma levels during a dosing interval
for a product dosed every 12 hr with a therapeutic range of 10–20
μg/ml. In this example, drug levels are below the minimum effective
level for 2 hr; the therapeutic occupancy time is 10 hr.

VII. DOSE DUMPING

Controlled-release products generally contain two to four times the
amount of drug present in the comparable conventional-release product. In many of the products, a fraction of the total drug is formulated
with an immediate-release component, with the remainder formulated
as a slow-release component, that is, a maintenance dose. The immediate-release component functions as a loading dose to establish
therapeutic drug levels rapidly. If the product's design or manufacture
is faulty, however, or susceptible to the influence of food, a large
amount of drug may be released rapidly from the product, resulting
in excessive drug levels. The bioavailability or bioequivalence profile
of the drug product must rule out such premature release (dose
dumping) (6).

Dose dumping from a controlled-release product has been defined
as the release of more than the usual fraction of drug or as the release
of drug at a greater rate than the customary amount of drug per
dosing interval, such that potentially adverse plasma levels may be
reached (8). It has also been defined as the release of more drug
per unit time than specified in the labeling (28). For some drug
products, labeling may state the amount of drug released initially and
over the entire dosing interval. However, for other products, labeling
may be much less specific, indicating, for example, a gradual release

over a certain time interval or attainment of drug levels equivalent to
the conventional-release product given at the normal dosing interval.
In addition, there are many drugs whose therapeutic range is not
known; in these cases, the relationship between relatively high drug
levels and adverse effects cannot be accurately assessed. Except for
those controlled-release products that are labeled with the amount of
drug released initially, the definitions of dose dumping already stated
are not specific in defining a "customary amount" of drug released
per dosing interval. Nevertheless, these definitions do serve to define
dose dumping qualitatively. A general quantitative definition of dose
dumping must await further work.

An evaluation of dose dumping may be made based either upon a
relative comparison of the test product with the reference product or
upon an absolute basis. Upon a relative basis, possible dose dumping
from the first controlled-release version of a drug previously available
only as conventional-release product(s) may be based upon a comparison
of its single-dose plasma concentration-time profile with the profile
due to the normal dosing regimen of the conventional-release innovator
product. The comparison should be made over one dosing interval
τ of the controlled-release product. The profile for the controlled-
release product should generally remain within the successively increasing peak and trough levels of the conventional-release product
over the interval τ of the test controlled-release product, as shown
in Figure 4. Alternatively, in controlled-release products containing
a substantial immediate-release component as a loading dose, the peak
due to the controlled-release product should generally not exceed
the C_{max} of the last dose of the conventional-release product in a
modified single-dose study. The appropriate listed product with which
to compare the bioequivalence of generic controlled-release products
is the innovator controlled-release product. Possible dose dumping
may be based on a comparison of the test and reference controlled-
release plasma concentration-time profiles. Upon an absolute basis,
determination of dose dumping could be based upon deviation from
theoretically desirable rates of release and absorption or by comparison
of the peak with the overall plasma concentration-time profile for the
test product, for instance by the method of area deviation (37).

Unless otherwise indicated, there is no attempt to suggest that
any of the specific methods described to evaluate controlled-release
character are endorsed and recommended by the FDA as part of a NDA
or ANDA submission. Rather, these methods represent a variety of
approaches to evaluation of the controlled-release product performance
that have been proposed and appear to have potential merit. These
methods or modifications thereof may be appropriate in the evaluation
of controlled-release dosage forms of drugs previously marketed only
in conventional-release forms, or in the evaluation of generic versions

of previously marketed controlled-release forms. This survey is not
exhaustive. Mean residence time, for instance, has not been discussed.
In the absence of a critical evaluation of these methods with various
drug products, their practical advantages and disadvantages cannot
be evaluated. Nevertheless, they provide a basis for the evaluation
of these products.

REFERENCES

1. J. P. Skelly, W. H. Barr, L. Z. Benet, J. T. Doluisio, A. H.
   Goldberg, G. Levy, D. T. Lowenthal, J. R. Robinson, V. P.
   Shah, R. J. Temple, and A. Yacobi. Report of the workshop
   on controlled-release dosage forms: Issues and controversies.
   Pharm. Res. 4: 75–77, 1987.
2. P. L. Madan. Sustained-release drug delivery systems. Part I.
   An overview. Pharm. Manuf. 2(2): 22–27, 1985.
3. R. E. Notari. Basic concepts in biopharmaceutics. In Pharmaceutics and Pharmacy Practice. Edited by G. S. Banker and
   R. K. Chalmers. J. B. Lippincott, Philadelphia, 1982, Chap. 4.
4. M. A. Longer and J. R. Robinson. Sustained-release drug
   delivery systems. In Remington's Pharmaceutical Sciences, 17th
   ed. Edited by A. R. Gennaro. Mack, Easton, Pennsylvania,
   1985, Chap. 92.
5. Timed release dosage forms. 21 CFR (Code of Federal Regulations)
   200.31
6. Guidelines for the conduct of an in vivo bioavailability study. 21
   CFR 320.25 (f).
7. B. E. Cabana and Y. W. Chien. Regulatory considerations in
   controlled-release medication. In Novel Drug Delivery Systems.
   Edited by Y. W. Chien. Marcel Dekker, New York, 1982, Chap.
   10.
8. J. P. Skelly and W. H. Barr. Regulatory assessment. In Controlled
   Drug Delivery: Fundamentals and Applications. Edited by J. R.
   Robinson and V. H. L. Lee. Marcel Dekker, New York, 1987,
   Chap. 7.
9. U.S. Department of Health and Human Services, Food and Drug
   Administration. Federal Food, Drug, and Cosmetic Act, as
   Amended, and Related Laws, 86–1051, Section 505 (j) (7) (B);
   codified as 21 USC (U.S. Code) 355 (j) (7) (B). U.S. Government
   Printing Office, Washington, D.C., 1986, p.66.
10. Guidelines on the design of a multiple-dose in vivo bioavailability
    study. 21 CFR 320.27 (a) (3) (iv).
11. U.S. Department of Health and Human Services, Food and Drug
    Administration. Approved Drug Products with Therapeutic

Equivalence Evaluations, 7th ed., U.S. Government Printing Office, Washington, D.C., 1987.

12. U.S. Pharmacopeia, 21st rev. U.S. Pharmacopeial Convention, Rockville, Maryland, 1985, p. xlvi.

13. Pharm. Forum. Modified-release dosage forms. 8: 2262–2263, 1982.

14. Pharm. Forum. Proposed USP policy on modified-release dosage forms. 8: 2383, 1982.

15. Pharm. Forum. USP policy on modified-release dosage forms. 9: 2999–3000, 1983.

16. Pharm. Forum. Physical tests and determinations. 12: 1769–1770. 1986.

17. J. P. Skelly, L. A. Yamamoto, V. P. Shah, M. K. Yau, and W. H. Barr. Topographical dissolution characterization for controlled release products—a new technique. Drug Dev. Ind. Pharm. 12: 1159–1175, 1986.

18. Criteria for waiver of evidence of in vivo bioavailability. 21 CFR 320.22 (d) (2).

19. J. G. Wagner and E. Nelson. Kinetic analysis of blood levels and urinary excretion in the absorptive phase after single doses of drug. J. Pharm. Sci. 53: 1392–1403, 1964.

20. J. P. Skelly. Division guidelines for the evaluation of controlled release drug products. Division of Biopharmaceutics, FDA, Rockville, Maryland, April 1984.

21. J. P. Skelly and W. H. Barr. Biopharmaceutic considerations in designing and evaluating novel drug delivery systems. Clin. Res. Pract. Drug Regul. Affairs 3: 501–539, 1985.

22. M. Gibaldi and D. Perrier. Pharmacokinetics, 2nd ed. Marcel Dekker, New York, 1982, pp. 155, 189.

23. P. G. Welling and M. R. Dobrinska. Multiple dosing of sustained release systems. In Sustained and Controlled Release Drug Delivery Systems. Edited by J. R. Robinson. Marcel Dekker, New York, 1978, pp. 632–633.

24. J. C. K. Loo and S. Riegelman. New method for calculating the intrinsic absorption rate of drugs. J. Pharm. Sci. 57: 918–928, 1968.

25. H. Boxenbaum. Pharmacokinetic determinants in the design and evaluation of sustained-release dosage forms. Pharm. Res.1: 82–88, 1984.

26. H. G. Boxenbaum. Physiological and pharmacokinetic factors affecting performance of sustained release dosage forms. Drug Dev. Ind. Pharm. 8: 1–25, 1982.

27. M. Gibaldi. Biopharmaceutics and Clinical Pharmacokinetics, 3rd ed. Lea and Febiger, Philadelphia, 1984, pp. 123–124.

28. J. P. Skelly. Issues and controversies involving controlled-release drug product studies. Pharm. Int. 7: 280–286, 1986.

29. J. L. Colaizzi and W. H. Pitlick. Oral drug-delivery systems for prescription pharmacy. In Pharmaceutics and Pharmacy Practice. Edited by G. S. Banker and R. K. Chalmers. J. B. Lippincott, Philadelphia, 1982, p. 229.

30. J. Hirtz. Problems of bioavailability with new drug delivery systems. Pharm. Int. 7: 21—25, 1986.

31. K. R. Heimlich. The evolution of precision drug delivery. Curr. Med. Res. Opin. 8(Suppl. 2): 28—37, 1983.

32. F. Theeuwes and W. Bayne. Dosage form index. An objective criterion for evaluation of controlled-release drug delivery systems. J. Pharm. Sci. 66: 1388—1392, 1977.

33. M. Gibaldi. Prolonged-release medication II. Perspect. Clin. Pharmacol. 2: 25—27, 1984.

34. H. C. Caldwell, W. J. Westlake, R. C. Schriver, and E. E. Bumbier. Steady-state lithium blood level fluctuations in man following administration of a lithium carbonate conventional and controlled-release dosage form. J. Clin. Pharmacol. 21: 106—109, 1981.

35. H. G. Boxenbaum. Merrell Dow Research Institute, Cincinnati, Ohio, personal communication, May 1987.

36. A. B. Straughn and L. J. North. Presented at the 14th Annual Midyear Clinical Meeting, American Society of Hospital Pharmacists, December 2—6, 1979, Las Vegas (data on file, Key Pharmaceuticals, Inc., Miami, Florida).

37. F. Nimmerfall and J. Rosenthaler. Modified release of drug: A way to its quantification. Int. J. Pharm. 32: 1—6, 1986.

38. J. Meier, E. Nüesch, and R. Schmidt. Pharmacokinetic criteria for the evaluation of retard formulations. Eur. J. Clin. Pharmacol. 7: 429—432, 1974.

39. J. J. Vallner, I. L. Honigberg, J. A. Kotzan, and J. T. Stewart. A proposed general protocol for testing bioequivalence of controlled-release drug products. Int. J. Pharm. 16: 47—55, 1983.

40. J. A. Kotzan, J. J. Vallner, J. T. Stewart, W. J. Brown, C. T. Viswanathan, T. E. Needham, S. V. Dighe, and R. Malinowski. Bioavailability of regular and controlled-released chlorpheniramine products. J. Pharm. Sci. 71: 919—923, 1982.

41. J. J. Vallner, J. A. Kotzan, J. T. Stewart, W. J. Brown, I. L. Honigberg, T. E. Needham, and S. V. Dighe. Blood levels following multiple oral dosing of chlorpheniramine conventional and controlled release preparations. Biopharm. Drug Dispos. 3: 95—104, 1982.

9

Classic and Population Pharmacokinetics

WAYNE A. COLBURN and STEPHEN C. OLSON *Parke-Davis Pharmaceutical Research Division, Warner-Lambert Company, Ann Arbor, Michigan*

I. INTRODUCTION

Classic pharmacokinetic methods are widely accepted owing to their
extensive use over the past 30–40 years. In contrast, population
pharmacokinetic methods currently suffer from a variety of problems,
including newness, misconceptions, and generalizations as well as
a general lack of understanding of their appropriate application and
use. A confounding problem is that the terms "population pharmacokinetics," "pharmacokinetic screen," and "NONMEM" are often used
interchangeably---they are *not* the same. This chapter is not a comparison of NONLIN and NONMEM.

To compare classic pharmacokinetic and population pharmacokinetic methods is to compare the old and the new, that is, the time-
proven and the untested, but more important it is to compare an
intensive method to an extensive method, that is, the individual to
the population.

Classic pharmacokinetic methods include manual parameter
estimation through graphics, noncompartmental modeling using statistical
moments and/or polyexponential equations, and compartmental modeling
using sophisticated curve-fitting techniques. The literature abounds
with these methods (1–8). In the simplest case, we can estimate
C_{max}, T_{max}, and AUC (area under the concentration time curve)
to determine relative or absolute bioavailability. In a more complex
case, we can develop an elaborate physiologically based pharmacokinetic model in an attempt to extrapolate animal data to humans.
Classic pharmacokinetic data are generally obtained in a small group
of animals or in a small group of healthy or patient volunteers. The
protocol design is generally rigorous and sampling is intense. A
pharmacokinetic profile is developed for a few individuals.

In contrast, population pharmacokinetic methods use structural
and statistical models to unify a few samples from many individuals
into a population pharmacokinetic profile. Although the protocol
design will be extensive rather than intensive, the protocol design
and its subsequent implementation should be no less rigorous than
those employed to develop a classic pharmacokinetic profile. The
investigator will need to obtain a few precisely timed samples from
many patients to develop an adequate population profile. The emphasis
here is extensive rather than intensive, not imprecise rather than
precise. The importance of this premise to the appropriate use of
population pharmacokinetics is developed. With this in mind, we
attempt to show the advantages and limitations of both methods, to
give relevant examples from our experience, and finally, to emphasize
how the two methods can complement each other to develop a better
understanding of the pharmacokinetics of a drug and how this can
be used to improve drug development as well as the biopharmaceutic
portions of a new drug application (NDA).

II. CLASSIC METHODS

Although the methods described here are applicable to, and presented in the context of, pharmaceutical industrial drug development, the concepts are also applicable to more academic comparisons. The respective positions of classic and population pharmacokinetics as well as the methodologies are the same irrespective of industrial, academic, or regulatory application.

A. Basic Concepts

Clearance, volume of distribution, and half-life comprise the basic concepts of pharmacokinetics. Similarly, absorption, distribution, metabolism, and excretion make up ADME, the basic processes that constitute pharmacokinetics. In theory, these processes and parameters can be determined by intensive classic methods or by the new extensive population methods.

1. Classic Study Designs

Classic pharmacokinetic study designs are generally intensive in that they are conducted in a reasonably small group of subjects, are rigorous in nature, require extensive biofluid sampling from each volunteer, and have concise study objectives. Within this design structure, there are two types of pharmacokinetic studies: baseline and comparative. The specific study group may consist of healthy volunteers or patients with the disease state for which the drug is intended (9). In both cases, the results of the study allow the investigator to estimate various pharmacokinetic parameters for these volunteers with reasonable certainty.

Baseline studies are generally used to define the pharmacokinetic profile of a drug in a specific group of healthy patient volunteers. These studies are not designed to be comparative in nature, although subsequent comparison of one study group to another may occur. Because of this objective, baseline studies may not be quite as rigorous as comparative studies. Examples of this type of study include the pharmacokinetics of the drug in early tolerance studies, renal failure, hepatic failure, heart failure, or the various disease processes for which the drug is indicated.

Comparative studies are used to determine the influence of treatment variables on the pharmacokinetics of the drug. These studies are generally designed to isolate a specific variable, such as absorption or elimination, and its influence on the pharmacokinetics of the drug under various conditions, such as different formulations or dose sizes. In most cases, these studies are crossover designs so that

statistical comparisons can be made among the treatment variables.
The study designs are extremely rigorous to minimize the influence
of extraneous variables on the study outcome. The rigor is reflected
in the inclusion and exclusion criteria as well as in the clinical conduct
of the study, which includes *specific* dosing and sampling times as
well as *specific* mealtimes and composition of meals. The precision
of the results from this type of study is increased, but the study
design may also limit extrapolation of the results to the entire patient
population. Does the patient population behave like the small study
group with respect to the parameter of interest? For example, does
a decrease in absorption with increasing dose in the small study
group indicate that there will be a decrease in absorption in the
patient population of interest? Does a difference in absorption between
two formulations of the same drug product in the small study group
indicate that there will be a difference between the two formulations
in the patient population of interest? To the classic pharmacokineticist,
the answer is "Yes. I am quite confident that it does." To the population
pharmacokineticist, the answer is "I am not sure."

2. Compartmental Models

In classic pharmacokinetics, compartmental models are the first type
of model to come to mind. From the original works of Teorell (10, 11)
to the present, they have gained both widespread acceptance and use.
Even though their utility, in certain circumstances, has been questioned,
they continue to be applied to a wide variety of problems. Compartmental models are useful in classic pharmacokinetics and are commonly
applied in population pharmacokinetics (12, 13). The meaning of
peripheral compartmental concentrations has been questioned and
has lead to the more commonly used polyexponential equations (3)
that are discussed in the next section. Today, the principal use of
compartmental models is to understand the mechanisms that may be
involved in specific pharmacokinetic changes or differences. Curve
fitting to identify mechanisms is not generally accepted. However,
simulation to investigate potential mechanisms is still a viable pharmacokinetic technique. It allows the pharmacokineticist to vary one or
more parameters to see how they impact on the pharmacokinetic
profile. These simulations can be used to support or negate various
mechanisms that may be implicated from classic pharmacokinetic studies.
Examples of this process are contained in References 14—16.

Compartment models are not generally used in the current drug
development process. The inforamtion that is needed and useful in
the NDA process can be gained from a variety of noncompartmental
methods. A noteworthy area of investigation in which this may be
the case is that of pharmacokinetic and pharmacodynamic (PK-PD)

modeling (17-19). The concentration-effect relationship may prove
to be wave of the future that will allow the pharmaceutical industry
to streamline the IND to the NDA process. To achieve this goal, it
will be necessary to construct a model that will allow concentration-
effect relationships to be predicted for a variety of *rates* and *routes*
of administration (18). Goal achievement may require simplistic compartmental models or the more complex physiologic models. Examples
of these are shown in Figure 1. As a case in point, for a central
nervous system (CNS) active drug, the PK-PD model must be able
to predict the effects observed after oral, intravenous, peridural,
and epidural administration. It is not likely that the central effect
model shown in Figure 1a can accomplish this task. On the other
hand, the peripheral effect model showin in Figure 1b or the CNS
effect model showin in Figure 1c should be able to predict the observed
effects from all routes of administration. If the central effect model
cannot be used to predict the effect, then the current nonparametric
models (20, 21) will suffer the same fate, since they are based on
the concept of a central effect. These problems and their possible
solutions have been discussed previously (18).

3. Noncompartmental Models

As noted in the preceding section, most pharmacokinetic and biopharmaceutic drug development needs can be accomplished using
noncompartmental methods. The only question that remains is which
to use. The most common do not involve curve fitting. However,
in some cases polyexponential curve fitting may be required to achieve
the goal if the study design did not allow precise parameter estimation
or if deconvolution techniques will be used to isolate pharmacokinetic
differences between treatments (22).

  a. Observed Parameters Probably the most commonly used method
for determining biopharmaceutical parameters is to read them directly
from the observed individual plasma concentration-time (C−T) data
or urinary excretion (UER) data. The parameters of interest from
plasma are the maximum observed plasma concentration C_{max}, the time
of the maximum observed plasma concentration T_{max}, the area under
the plasma concentration-time curve, and the apparent elimination
half-life $t_{\frac{1}{2}}$. C_{max} and T_{max} are read directly from the C−T data.
AUC is calculated by linear trapezoidal or log trapezoidal summation,
and the half-life is determined by log-linear regression of the terminal
concentrations. The parameters of interest from urine are similar
to those from plasma and include the maximum urinary excretion rate
UER_{max}, the time of the maximum excretion rate T_{max}, total cumulative
amount excreted A_e, and the apparent elimination half-life $t_{\frac{1}{2}}$. These
parameter values are also determined directly from the experimental
data (1).

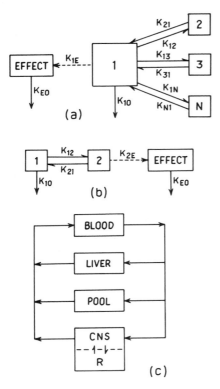

FIGURE 1 Schematic representation of various pharmacokinetic and pharmacodynamic models: (a) a central effect model, (b) a peripheral effect model, and (c) a physiologic CNS model.

These descriptive pharmacokinetic parameters can be determined following a single dose in a bioequivalence trial or within a dosing interval at various points during multiple dosing to evaluate accumulation in various patient populations. A direct comparison of these parameters can be used to establish absolute and relative bioavailability or to compare multiple-dose pharmacokinetics between two patient populations. No assumptions need to be made to compare these parameters because no compartmental model is employed. They are generally the simplest to obtain and the easiest to understand. The only difficulty arises from inadequate sampling times or, in the case of intravenous bolus dosing, an imprecise measure of C_0 (23,24).

b. Moment Analysis Another noncompartmental method that has gained popularity in pharmacokinetic literature during the past few years is moment analysis (2). Although this procedure is relatively new to pharmacokinetics, it has been used for several years in the fields of biochemistry, endocrinology, and physiology. In pharmacokinetics, the zeroth, first, and second moments can be used to evaluate bioavailability, accumulation, and the influence of dose level (2). An advantage of moment analysis over the C_{max} and T_{max} approach in pharmacokinetic and biopharmaceutical analysis is that it can be used to identify an apparent absorption rate constant. A schematic representation of its potential applications are shown in Figure 2. The amount of flexibility offered by this method for bioavailability testing is limited only by the amount of data available, for example, intravenous, oral solution, and oral dosage form(s). Whereas C_{max}, T_{max}, AUC, and $t_{\frac{1}{2}}$ can be compared directly, moment analysis allows these comparisons as well as the calculation of other parameters, such as mean absorption time and mean dissolution time. The disadvantage is the imprecision of some of these estimates as a function of sampling time and extrapolation error (25–27).

c. Curve-Fitting Methods Curve-fitting concentration-time data with polyexponential equations can lead to parameters for comparisons by a variety of procedures, including the Loo-Riegelman method (28), the Wagner-Nelson method (29,30), or deconvolution methods (22). There are pros and cons to each of these methods. The Loo-Riegelman method is noncompartmental in nature but requires intravenous data to determine the absorption characteristics. The Wagner-Nelson method is dependent on one-compartment characteristics to be totally accurate (30). Deconvolution methods require only that there is a common disposition function that can be used as a point of reference of which to overlay the absorption function(s). For example, absolute absorption characteristics can be overlaid on an intravenous profile or relative absorption characteristics can be overlaid on a reference oral formulation. Examples of this type of approach are common in the current literature (31–33) and can be obtained through simultaneous fitting procedures (26).

The common elements for classic pharmacokinetic studies, whether they are evaluated by compartmental or noncompartmental methods, are (1) relatively small, homogeneous study groups; (2) intense, rigorous study designs; and (3) precise dosing and sampling schedules.

B. Classic Studies

Both animal and human pharmacokinetic studies are included in the classic development plan. The animal pharmacokinetic studies employ the same design theory that the human studies employ, including small study groups and rigorous sampling. However, for the purpose of this

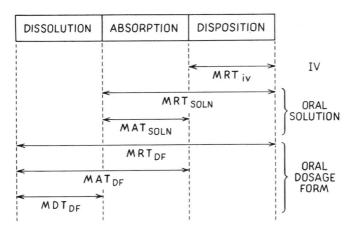

FIGURE 2 Schematic representation of the residence processes involved in the determination of mean residence time (MRT) for various routes and modes of administration.

chapter we do not develop the animal studies. The classic pharmaco-kinetic studies that are considered for inclusion in the clinical develop-ment process are shown in Table 1. Each of these studies has certain common elements as well as certain unique elements. Whether they are ultimately included in the development plan depends on the specific drug and the patient population for which it will be indicated. Similarly, whether healthy patients or volunteers will be used in each study is dependent on the specific drug entity being studies (9).

1. Single- and Multiple-Dose Tolerance and Pharmacokinetics

First time in humans tolerance and pharmacokinetic studies are often conducted in healthy volunteers (34,35) to minimize the influence of other medications on the observed tolerance of the new agent. How-ever, with certain drugs, such as cytotoxic and cardiotonic agents, this study as well as all others is conducted in the intended patient population. The tolerance and pharmacokinetic studies are generally conducted as a placebo-controlled study with two to three volunteers receiving placebo and four to six volunteers receiving active agent at each dose level. The primary objective of this study is to evaluate human tolerance, whereas the secondary objective is to obtain pre-liminary human pharmacokinetic data. For this reason, the pharma-cokinetic sampling schedule may be limited so as not to influence the

TABLE 1 Studies Considered for the Classic Pharmacokinetic Drug Development Plan

1. Single- and multiple-dose tolerance and pharmacokinetics
2. Pilot bioavailability
3. Single-dose proportionality
4. Human metabolism and mass balance
5. Effect of food
6. Effect of age
7. Effect of gender
8. Multiple-dosing regimens
9. Effect of disease states
10. Pharmacokinetic drug-drug interactions
11. Pharmacokinetics and pharmacodynamics
12. Final bioavailability

observed tolerance. The pharmacokinetic characteristics observed in these volunteers allow the pharmacokineticst to refine the sampling schedule for subsequent studies.

The second time in humans multiple-dose tolerance study is conducted in the same way with the same sequential objectives: tolerance first and pharmacokinetics second. However, these single- and multiple-dose studies should provide preliminary information on dose proportionality, time dependence, and, possibly, human metabolism. Examples of these types of studies are published in a variety of journals (36–40).

2. Pilot Bioavailability

Pilot bioavailability studies can be conducted throughout the development process and are generally conducted in healthy subjects. By definition, this study is generally conducted in a limited number (n = 6–8) of volunteers with the intent of evaluating new or modified dosage forms. Volunteers are generally studied in a crossover design. This study is comparative in nature and requires a rigorous dosing and sampling schedule to assure that the characteristics of one formulation can be compared to another or to a reference liquid or intravenous dose. Statistical analysis may or may not be conducted on the results from this study. The results may be used to reformulate, to make a go or no go decision on clinical trials, or to pursue a modified dosage form, such as controlled or sustained release or a transdermal patch. Generally, these data are not published in total, although portins of the data may be published to formalize the pharmacokinetic profile or absolute bioavailability (41,42).

3. *Single-Dose Proportionality*

An integral part of establishing the pharmacokinetic characteristics of a new chemical entity is to determine whether its absorption and disposition characteristics are linear. This too is a comparative study that is generally conducted as a crossover design in healthy volunteers; 8–12 volunteers receive three to four doses that extend across the anticipated therapeutic dose range. Plasma concentration-time data and/or urinary excretion data are statistically evaluated to determine if absorption, distribution, and elimination processes remain linear across the therapeutic dose range. A statistical comparison of C_{max}, T_{max}, AUC, and $t_{\frac{1}{2}}$ values across dose levels leads to a determination of linearity or nonlinearity for the various processes. Examples of this type of study are contained in References 43–46, and the difference results that can be obtained are shown in Figure 3 and 4. The data presented in Figure 3 indicated that cibenzoline exhibits linear, dose-proportional pharmacokinetics over the oral dose range 65–260 mg (44). In contrast, the data presented in Figure 4 indicate that oral isotretinoin is not adequately absorbed from oral doses in excess of 240 mg (45). In an opposing manner, oral doses of midazolan are not cleared linearly in excess of 15 mg (46), resulting in a disproportionate increase in AUC.

4. *Human Metabolism and Mass Balance*

This study is generally conducted in a small number (n = 4–6) of subjects using radiolabeled drug but is extremely important to the overall development process. The metabolic profile determined in humans is compared to that observed in various animal models that are used for the toxicology and pharmacology studies. In addition, this study may identify active metabolites that may help to characterize the clinical pharmacology profile, such as the concentration effect-time relationships. As with the other classic studies, a precise dosing and sampling schedule is required to optimize use of the data. Examples of this type of study are contained in References 47–49.

In two of the examples drugs were extensively metabolized and may have been excreted in the bile. In one case (47), active metabolites of isotretinoin could account for less than 20% of the [^{14}C]AUC

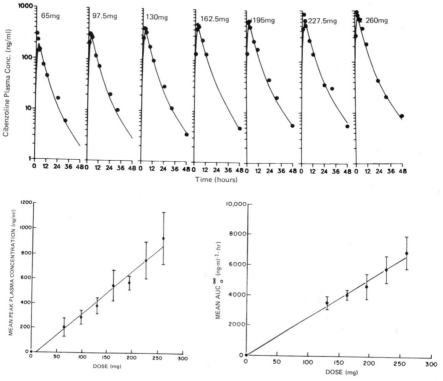

FIGURE 3 Composite of data used to establish that 6.5–260 mg IV doses of cibenzoline displayed linear dose-proportional pharmacokinetics. The upper segment displays the concentration-time profiles from one subject together with the lines predicted with one equation. The lower segment displays mean C_{max} values (left) and mean AUC values (right) for the four healthy volunteers. (With permission from Ref. 44.)

(Figure 5). Subsequent metabolic workup yielded other inactive metabolites. In addition, the ^{14}C and parent drug profiles implicated biliary excretion and enterohepatic cycling as mechanisms for drug disposition.

In the second case (48), etretinate was extensively metabolized to two major active metabolites as well as other unknown metabolites. In contrast to the first example, the data in patients with biliary T-tube damage indicated that the absence of bile precluded significant absorption of the drug, but other qualitative comparisons of the profiles were similar. Metabolic workup identified two major conjugated

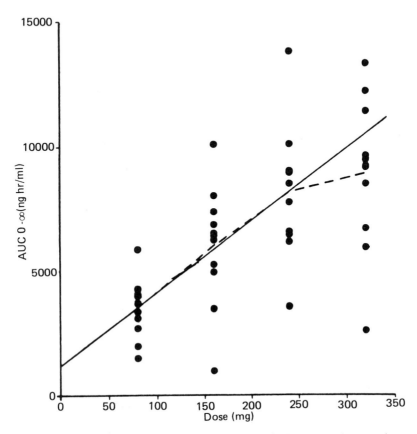

FIGURE 4 Scattergram of the relationship between increasing oral doses of isotretinoin and resulting AUC values. AUC values are linear from 80 to 240 mg but indicate decreased absorption at the 320 mg dose. (With permission from Ref. 45.)

oxidative metabolites in bile. Although implicated in the preclinical work, unlike isotretinoin, enterohepatic cycling did not play a major role in the human pharmacokinetic profile of etretinate.

In the final case (49), cibenzoline was excreted 60% intact in the urine with the remaining nonrenal clearance by metabolic and unknown mechanisms. Metabolites identified in urine were generally active. Of the total dose 13% was found in feces. It was not clear whether this was due to a lack of absorption, to biliary excretion or

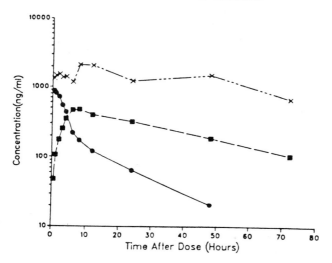

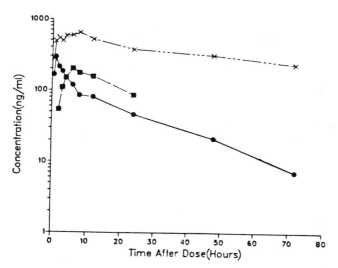

FIGURE 5 Mean blood concentration-time data for ^{14}C (x), isotretinoin
(○), and 4-oxoisotretinoin (■) in four healthy volunteers (upper)
and in two patients with biliary T-tube drainage following 80 mg oral
dose. (With permission from Ref. 47.)

to secretion back into the gastrointestinal tract. However, previous
studies had indicated that cibenzoline was completely absorbed, thus
supporting a biliary excretion or gastrointestinal secretion mechanisms.

The importance of the results from metabolism and mass balance
studies cannot be overemphasized for the development process. In
addition, with the advent of new technologies and regulations, the
investigator should begin to consider stable isotope mass-balance and
metabolism studies for the future.

5. Effect of Food

Food can increase or decrease the absorption of drugs (50). This
study is pivotal to the successful development of a controlled- or
sustained-release oral dosage form and can be pivotal to the development of conventional oral dosage forms as well. Therefore, it should
be treated as a comparative bioequivalence study. There are two
approaches to resolve this problem. One approach is to test the
hypothesis using a 12-subject, two-way crossover pilot study in
which the subjects receive the dose during a complete fast or immediately following a high-fat meal. If there is no food effect, all bets
are off. However, if there is a food effect, a second complete four-
way crossover in 12–24 subjects must be conducted to compare bioavailability with food, 1 hr after food, and 1 hr before food to a
complete fast. This study is needed to establish the specific package
insert statement for dosage administration in relation to food ingestion.
The second approach is to do the complete study in 12–24 subjects
from the outset. The physiochemical characteristics of the drug generally makes this decision easier. The single objective of this study
is to determine if food influences drug pharmacokinetics.

Examples of conventional dosage form food effect studies are
contained in References 51–53. These examples were chosen to show
the wide differences in drug pharmacokinetics that can be attributed
to concomitant administration with food. In the first case (51), food
was shown to decrease the absorption of [14C]captopril. Food reduced
both the 14C and the captopril AUC to about two-thirds of its value
in the gasting state. Lack of absorption was confirmed by a threefold increase in the fecal excretion of 14C in the presence of food.

In two other cases (52,53), the relative bioavailability of two
retinoids, isotretinoin and etretinate, were increased in the presence
of food. Isotretinoin AUC values were increased twofold in the presence of food. Based on the physiochemical properties of the drug
it was surmised that the increased absorption resulted from increased
solubility of isotretinoin in bile. Etretinate plasma concentrations
were increased three- to fivefold when the dose was administered
with a fat load, such as a high-fat meal or whole milk, compared with
the fasting state or a high-carbohydrate meal.

In contrast, plasma concentrations of the two active metabolites were not altered (Fig. 6). The data indicate that food decreases the first-pass conversion of etretinate to etretin. In addition to this mechanism, an artifactual increased bioavailability may occur owing to redistribution of etretinate into the plasma due to elevated lipoproteins from the fat load; that is, etretinate binds predominatly to lipoproteins. This observation points to the fact that these studies must be critically evaluated to avoid potential misinterpretation.

Examples of food effect studies with sustained-release dosage forms are contained in References 54—57. With sustained-release dosage forms, the critical concern is for dose dumping; for example, when the sustained-release dosage form is administered with a high-fat meal, a significant portion of the dose may be released without control (57). The tenor of this issue was set with theophylline. The drug substance, per se, is not significantly influenced by the presence of food (54). However, certain of the sustained-release dosage forms dose dump whereas others do not (55,56). Therefore, the onus has been put on manufacturers to ascertain not only whether the product dose dumps but, if it does, under what conditions it does so (56).

6. Effect of Age

In many cases, a drug may be administered to patients ranging in age from 20 to >90 years. Under these circumstances, it is necessary to evaluate the pharmacokinetics across the entire age range to see if dose adjustments may be required in the older age groups compared to the 20- 55-year-old adult. Alternatively, neonates and children may require the drug for therapy. The younger age groups are usually included in post-NDA studies. An example of one way to investigate this age group is to minimize sampling from any individual child (58).

In older age groups, inclusion involves empaneling 6--10 subjects in each 10- to 20-year age range, such as 20—30, 31--40, 41—50, 51—60, 61—70, 71—80, and 81—90 years. Data analyses require the establishment of a continuum from 20 to 90 years that shows the influence of age on the pharmacokinetics. Again, rigorous control of dosing and sampling schedules is required to successfully achieve the objective of the study. In this case, some flexibility in the inclusion and exclusion criteria is required to recruit the elderly volunteer. However, the single objective of this study is to identify age-dependent differences in the pharmacokinetics.

An example of this type of intensive study design was performed with cibenzoline (59). The data analysis methods employed in this study are exemplary. These methods are shown in Figure 7 and Table 2. Note that data analysis is not conducted by groups, but rather as a continuum. In contrast, if age dependence is not anticipated, a two-group study, old and young, should suffice to prove this point (60).

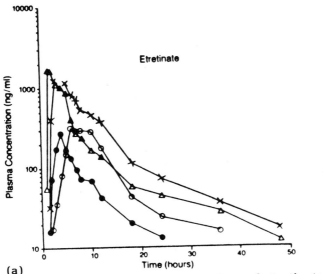

(a)

FIGURE 6 Mean plasma concentrations of etretinate (a), etretin (b), and isoetretin (c) following 100 mg oral doses during a fast (●), high-carbohydrate meal (○), high-fat meal (x), and 16 oz of whole milk (△). (With permission from Ref. 53.)

7. Effects of Gender

In certain cases, a drug may exhibit significantly different pharmacokinetic profiles in males than in females. When evidence surfaces during the development process, the classic pharmacokinetic approach dictates that a specific study be conducted to isolate gender as the only variable. Age- and weight-matched males and females are empaneled to evaluate the influence of gender. A statistical analysis comparing pharmacokinetic and pharmacodynamic parameters between the two genders is required to establish whether dose adjustments are required.

The pharmacokinetics, and therefore the pharmacodynamics, of certain drugs, such as the benzodiazepines, are anticipated to be influenced more by gender than other drugs (61). In some cases this may reflect gender differences but may also reflect the influence of oral contraceptive steroids in those women who use them (62,63). Nevertheless, the influence of gender, both direct and indirect, on pharmacokinetics and pharmacodynamics may be important for certain drugs.

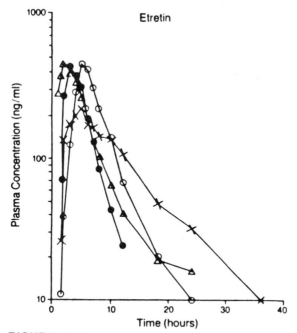

FIGURE 6b

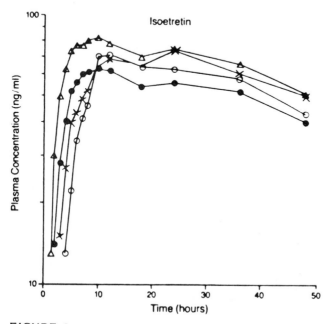

FIGURE 6c

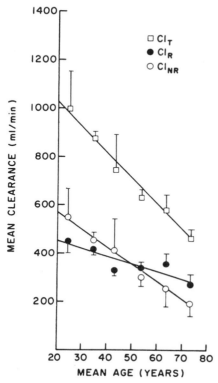

FIGURE 7 Cibenzoline renal, nonrenal, and total clearances as a function of age. Solid lines represent linear regression of clearance on age. (With permission from Ref. 59.)

If the development process allows inclusion of both men and women it may be possible to employ both sexes in all pharmacokinetic studies to avoid the need for a specific study to isolate gender as the only variable. However, this requires that a significant number of subjects be included for adequate comparisons to be made across studies.

8. Multiple-Dose Studies Using the Package Insert Doses and Regimens

Restrictive inclusion studies in patients who will receive the drug for benefit or, if the characteristics of the drug permit, healthy volunteers should be conducted at each dose level and according to the package insert regimens. Restrictive patient inclusion is required to minimize

TABLE 2 Demographic and Pharmacokinetic Data for the Six Age Groups

	Subjects 1–6 (20–29 years)	Subjects 7–12 (30–39 years)	Subjects 13–18 (40–49 years)	Subjects 19–24 (50–59 years)	Subjects 25–30 (60–69 years)	Subjects 31–36 (70–80 years)
Sex	4 M, 2 F	5 M, 1 F	3 M, 3 F	2 M, 4 F	3 M, 3 F	4 M, 2 F
Age (years)	24 ± 2	35 ± 4	43 ± 3	54 ± 3	65 ± 3	74 ± 4
Weight (kg)	69 ± 9	64 ± 12	73 ± 11	66 ± 13	70 ± 6	73 ± 17
Cl_{cr} (ml/min)	89 ± 17	78 ± 9	71 ± 14	64 ± 11	75 ± 13	58 ± 5
C_{max} (ng/ml)	465 ± 144	413 ± 46	578 ± 215	593 ± 81	704 ± 238	626 ± 121
t_{max} (hr)	1.6 ± 0.6	1.4 ± 0.4	1.5 ± 0.3	1.4 ± 0.4	1.8 ± 0.5	1.8 ± 0.5
$t_{\frac{1}{2}}$ $(hr^{-1})^a$	7.0	10.5	8.7	9.1	9.9	10.5
Cl_T (ml/min)	999 ± 371	876 ± 65	740 ± 363	636 ± 57	607 ± 117	465 ± 78
Cl_R (ml/min)	451 ± 123	421 ± 59	327 ± 72	337 57	354 ± 96	208 ± 102
Cl_{NR} (ml/min)	548 ± 294	454 ± 81	412 ± 310	299 ± 84	225 ± 112	197 ± 134
V_d (liters)	588 ± 219	515 ± 38	435 ± 213	374 ± 34	340 ± 92	274 ± 46
X_u (mg)	75 ± 13	77 ± 12	79 ± 20	85 ± 17	99 ± 17	94 ± 39

^{a}Harmonic mean.

the effect of concomitant medications, whereas healthy volunteers avoid this restriction. Extensive sampling after the first dose and again during a dosing interval at steady state identifies any time-dependent changes and or dose-dependent differences. Within-subject statistical comparisons identify time-dependent changes, whereas across-regimen and across-dose level comparisons are used to identify multiple-dose, dose-dependent differences. The singular objective of this study design is to identify any multiple-dose differences or changes in the pharmacokinetic profile.

Several examples using classic pharmacokinetic methods to evaluate single- to multiple-dose data are presented in References 64–68. In certain cases, volunteer patients with the intended disease were studied (64, 67). In other cases (65, 66, 68) healthy volunteers were studied. Regardless of the volunteer status, rigorous protocols were applied to assure that dosing and sampling were adequate to achieve the study objective. In some cases (64,66) noncompartmental methods were used, whereas, for others, (65,67,68) simple to complex curve-fitting procedures were applied.

In the most complex situation (68), severe psoriatic patients received a 6-month course of etretinate therapy followed by a 6-month to 1-year washout period. This study was conducted to understand the apparent change in half-life from approximately 7 hr following the first dose to approximately 120 days following 6 months of dosing. Data were evaluated by curve fitting all the blood concentration-time data with a polyexponential equation. Lengthening of half-life resulted from accumulation of blood concentrations into a measurable range rather than from time-dependent changes (67).

9. Effect of Disease States

Congestive heart failure, hepatic failure, and renal failure are the three most commonly considered disease states for testing. Depending on the pharmacokinetic characteristics of the drug, one or more of these disease states may alter its pharmacokinetics.

a. *Renal Failure* If early phase I data indicate that renal clearance is a primary mode of elimination of active parent or active metabolite, then a renal failure study should be conducted. If renal failure is to be tested, at least four study groups should be studied: (1) creatinine clearance > 60 ml/min (healthy), (2) creatinine clearance 31–60 ml/min (mild renal failure), (3) creatinine clearance 15–30 ml/min (moderate renal failure), and (4) creatinine clearance < 15 ml/min (severe renal failure). When drug pharmacokinetics is considered in relationship to creatinine clearance values, the data should be considered as a continuum to establish how creatinine clearance dictates dose admustment. The inclusion and exclusion criteria for this study may require some leeway to assure adequate patient entry. However, if secondary end-organ failure is implicated, these patients *must* be excluded so that only one variable is tested. To evaluate the effect of Cl_{cr} less than 15 ml/min and the hemodialyzability of the drug, a separate hemodialysis study must be conducted in this subpopulation. An example for each of these studies is presented in References 69 and 70. It must be noted that renal failure does not generally alter the pharmacokinetics of a drug unless it is cleared predominantly by the kidney. Hemodialysis clear-only a significant fraction of those drugs that are filtered by the kidney and have small volumes of distribution. When renal failure alters the pharmacokinetics of a drug that is cleared predominantly by nonrenal mechanisms, secondary disease should be considered.

b. *Hepatic Failure* This is probably the most problematic disease state study for two reasons: (1) difficulty in establishing the appropriate hepatic disease(s) that should be of interest and (2) the criteria used for entry. For example, should one consider hepatitis, cirrhosis, or cholestasis? If one is to consider cirrhosis, should it be active or in remission? If one is to consider cirrhosis, should it be biopsy proven? Also, is the disease of interest primary or secondary in nature? Examples of the difficulties encountered are presented in References 71–73. For these reasons, it may be worthwhile to use pharmacokinetic models to simulate the possible influence of these disease processes on the hparmacokinetics of the drug of interest.

c. *Congestive Heart Failure* For drugs that undergo extensive first-pass clearance, congestive heart failure (CHF) may significantly influence this process. If the process is saturable, the influence becomes even greater. The importance of this disease process on the pharmacokinetics of most drugs is irrelevant unless reduced cardiac output influences the drug of interest.

d. *Recommendations* For each disease state, a compromise must be reached by which a sufficient number of patients can be entered, yet the primary objective of the study is retained. One may need to allow concomitant medications that do not alter the pharmacokinetics of the drug of interest. Secondary disease processes that may alter the drug pharmacokinetics should be excluded. Every effort must be made to isolate a single variable for study.

Specific markers that can be used to quantitate the disease process should be determined (creatinine clearance and cardiac index) or administered (including indocyanine green and antipyrine) so that the extent of the disease can be determined. The ultimate goal of

these studies is to determine if dose adjustments may be required
in certain disease states due to pharmacokinetic differences.

Drugs may be developed for both parenteral and oral use. In
these cases, stable isotope methodology can be applied to simultaneously
evaluate intravenous and oral doses in the same healthy or disease
state volunteers (74,75). The efficiency of these study designs and
the increased amount of obtainable information have been documented.
The results of the study in renal failure patients are presented in
Figure 8, and the results of the study in CHF patients are presented
in Figure 9 to exemplify the type of information that one can obtain
from this approach.

10. Pharmacokinetic Drug-Drug Interactions

Drug-drug interactions may be pharmacokinetic, pharmacodynamic,
or both. We are interested in all three but set out to investigate those
that involve a primary pharmacokinetic mechanism. In general, these
types of interactions involve (1) drug displacement from binding
sites, (2) competition for or induction of metabolic reactions, and/or
(3) competition for clearance processes, such as active tubular
secretion. The pharmacokinetic characteristics of the NCE can usually
be used to identify particular interactions of interest. In addition,
studies are routinely conducted because of the widespread use of the
potentially interacting drug, such as warfarin, cimetidine, and
digoxin.

In these studies, healthy volunteers or patients at steady state
on the other medication can be used depending on medical ethics
and risk-benefit ratio (9). The objective of the study can be to
determine what the NCE does to the other drug, the other drug does
to the NCE, or both. The pharmacokinetic and pharmacodynamic
characteristics of the respective compounds dictate which objective
is tested. In certain cases, in vitro protein binding studies or simulation studies can be used in lieu of costly clinical studies.

Classic pharmacokinetic approaches to drug-drug interactions
are exemplified by several publications (76−78). The most common
approach is to measure the single-dose pharmacokinetics of a drug
substance alone and in the presence of the other drug at steady state
in a crossover design. This can be done with conventional assay
methods (76,77) or by using stable isotope methodology (78).

A simple or complex evaluation of the profile will determine the
lack or existence of a pharmacokinetic interaction. This study design
does not address the potential for a pharmacological interaction,
although it can be incorporated into the protocol (79). The relationships between pharmacokinetics and pharmacodynamics are addressed
in the next section.

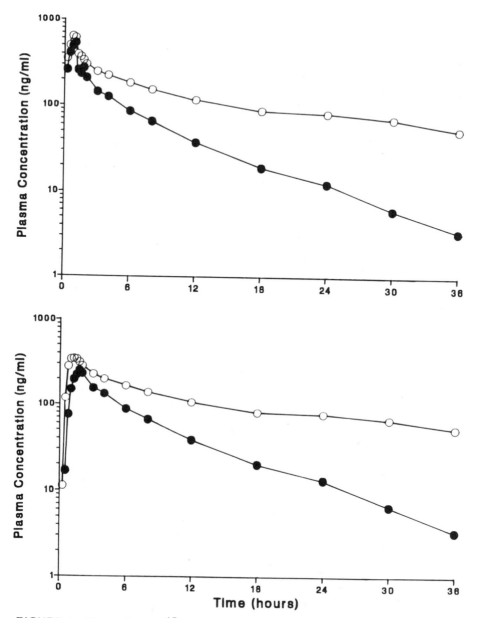

FIGURE 8 Mean plasma $^{15}N_2$-cibenzoline concentration after an 80 mg intravenous dose (top panel) and mean plasma $^{14}N_2$-cibenzoline concentrations after a simultaneous 80 mg oral dose (bottom panel) to a healthy subject (●) and patients with renal failure (○). (With permission from Ref. 74.)

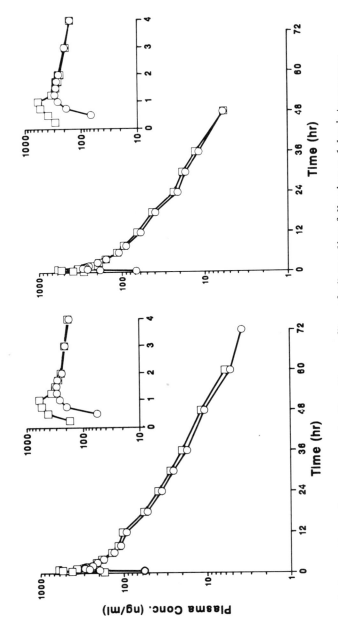

FIGURE 9 Mean plasma concentration-time profiles of cibenzoline following a 1-hr intravenous infusion of 80 mg $^{15}N_2$-cibenzoline (□) administered simultaneously with an 80 mg oral capsule dose of cibenzoline (○) to six patients with congestive heart failure (left) and five healthy subjects (right). The insets represent plasma cibenzoline concentrations during the first 4 hr after administration. (With permission from Ref. 75.)

11. Pharmacokinetics and Pharmacodynamics

Simultaneous pharmacokinetic and pharmacodynamic modeling can serve to streamline the drug development process. To apply this technique, studies must be conducted in the patient population to establish the concentration-effect relationship, to establish single- to multiple-dose correlates, and, when applicable, to establish route-dependent correlates. However, this data analysis method is currently in its infancy and will need to improve to achieve the goal (18,19,80-82). To date, most studies have been conducted with single doses. In the future, intravenous and oral data (83) as well as multiple-dose data (84) will be needed (85). With these data in hand, the intent of the phase III development process can be reduced without compromising the quality of the end product. To achieve this goal, quantifiable pharmacodynamic end points will be needed for both desired and undesired effects. The importance of this study category will continue to grow as our ability to quantitate pharmacological effects in patients expands.

12. Final Bioavailability and Bioequivalence Study

The only *required* study for the clinical biopharmaceutics section of an NDA for a peroral NCE is the final bioequivalence study. The objective of this study is twofold: (1) the relative bioavailability of the proposed market-image formulation is compared to that of the dosage form used in the pivotal clinical trials, and (2) the final market-image formulation is compared to the most readily available oral preparation. The reference is an oral solution when feasible or a suspension when a solution is not possible. In some cases, the oral dosage forms are compared to an intravenous form to determine absolute bioavailability. This study is generally conducted in 18-24 healthy volunteers and is a single-dose design for conventional oral dosage forms. The protocol is rigorous with respect to inclusion and exclusion criteria, times for meal ingestion, dosing times, and sampling schedules. The sampling times are based on prior information about the drug and its dosage form. The protocol should be designed in such a way as to highlight differences between the various treatments.

If a nonconventional dosage form, such as a controlled or sustained-release oral dosage form or a transdermal patch or intranasal dosage form, is compared to an existing dosage form, this is usually conducted as a steady-state study. Relevant parameters are compared during a common dosing interval.

Whether compared following single doses or at steady state, the rate and extent of absorption are statistically compared to determine if there are significant differences among the dosage forms. In all cases, the extent of absorption is the most critical parameters. The rate of absorption is critical only when adverse effects and/or efficacy

is associated with peak plasma concentrations, for example efficacy
for hypnotics, orthostatic hypotension for antihypertensives, or
sedation for anticonvulsants and anxiolytics.

Many of these studies are never published since the results are
often archival in nature. However, certain of the study design concepts
have been published when the results were interesting (86,87) or
the methodology used was unique (88—90). The use of stable isotopes
has reduced the number of subjects required to achieve statistical
power and has therefore optimized the study design.

13. Summary

It should be noted that although there are a multitude of study objectives during the classic pharmacokinetic drug development process,
there are also common underlying factors: (1) prospective, well-
defined study objectives; (2) well-controlled study protocol; (3)
adequate sampling to achieve the objective; and (4) sufficient numbers
to derive a conclusion, whether or not it is statistically based.

Most of these studies begin during phase II and continue through
the completion of phase III. The more extensive and time-consuming
studies are conducted once the firm is confident that it has a high
probability of a successful NDA filing.

C. Results from Classic Analyses

The end product of this collage of studies, each designed with a
specific objective, is a broad generalized understanding of the pharmacokinetics and biopharmaceutics of the NCE. Each study is designed
to answer a specific question and thereby place yet another piece
into the pharmacokinetic puzzle. At each step along the way, the
investigator gains more insight into the NCE and how better to design
the next study. In the later stages, pharmacokinetic understanding
may be great enough to use simulation techniques to avoid, or at
least minimize, human exposure in certain studies. For example,
aging generally reflects end-organ failure and therefore if renal
failure results in increased $t_{\frac{1}{2}}$ and decreased clearance, one can anticipate the same results as patients move beyond 65 years of age.

The result of classic pharmacokinetic analysis is a well-rounded
pharmacokinetic understanding of the NCE in the individual. The
composite across all these individuals should generate useful information
pertaining to intersubject and/or interpatient pharmacokinetic variability. The larger and more diverse the composite data base, the
more comfortable one will be about understanding the population
pharmacokinetics. Upon completion of the classic pharmacokinetic
development process, the responsible investigator should be the most

knowledgeable about the NCE and what the human body does to the drug. The investigator should be able to file a comprehensive acceptable biopharmaceutics volume to the NDA.

III. POPULATION METHODS

The principal characteristic that separates population-based pharmacokinetic methods from classic methods is point of view. Classic methods focus on individual response, but population-based methods focus on central tendency in response across a patient population and the variability in response between individuals. This difference in point of view requires a dramatically different approach to modeling and parameter estimation. A variety of approaches have been proposed in recent years and have been reviewed elsewhere (91). This discussion focuses on one of these approaches: only the nonlinear mixed effect model has been studied in detail and warrants consideration at the present time for use in the drug development process.

Classic compartmental pharmacokinetic models invariably assume error or unexplained deviation from expected response is simply added to predicted response. Simple least-squares nonlinear regression methods suffice with such an error structure. Population-based models assume a more complex error structure and are generally expressed as mixed effect models, indicating that complex interactions and effects are responsible for an observed response. Such models require that extended least-squares regression methods be applied in the estimation of parameters (12,13). A brief discussion of these mixed effect models, their use in population pharmacokinetic analysis, and a discussion of their utility in drug development follows.

A. Basic Concepts

Expression of a population pharmacokinetic model in a form that lends itself to extended least-square analysis allows explicit estimation of components of variance as well as estimation of central tendencies. It is the explicit estimation of inter- and intraindividual variability and the exploration of factors that account for this variability that form the heart of a population pharmacokinetic analysis (12,13,92,93).

Formal expression of the population-based model is accomplished through application of basic principles of analysis of variance. In fact, the similarities between traditional ANOVA or, more accurately, analysis of covariance and nonlinear mixed effect modeling underscores the importance of variance in population modeling.

Just as with simple linear or nonlinear regression models, mixed effect nonlinear regression models estimate a central tendency for parameters that predict average response. The principal difference between simple nonlinear regression and mixed effect regression is the level of complexity allowed in the subsequent expression of variability. Simple nonlinear regression allows a single component of random error about the predicted response. This error is added to the predicted response to account for deviations from prediction and may or may not arise from a distribution of constant variance. Mixed effect nonlinear regression, on the other hand, allows a more complex expression of variance based on principles firmly established for traditional ANOVA (93).

In one of its most basic forms, the population model must recognize two levels or sources of deviation from a predicted response. Assuming that the central tendency in a population model represents the response of an average individual, any particular individual response will be different for the simple reason that that particular individual is not average. Herein lies the source of interindividual variability. In a classic pharmacokinetic study it is this variability that is estimated when individual parameter estimates are averaged and the variance obtained by following a study of a panel of subjects. The second level or source of variability arises from deviations from predicted response after allowing for interindividual variability. After adjusting the predicted response differences between individuals, one must accept that there will remain residual variability for each individual about the adjusted expected response. This residual error is the same as that estimated in simple nonlinear regression except that it does not have to assume an additive relationship to the individual predicted response.

Although interindividual variation and residual or intraindividual error arise from similar sources in classic and populaiton pharmacokinetic models, the methods used to estimate these two components of variability differ dramatically between simple nonlinear and mixed effect nonlinear regression approaches. For simple nonlinear regression, intraindividual error is estimated after a structural model is fit to the data of single individuals. It is obtained as a function of the squared deviations between observed and predicted response. Interindividual variability is then obtained, as already described, by determining the variance of individual pharmacokinetic parameters after fitting the simple nonlinear regression model separately to each individual data set. Estimation of these variance components using mixed effect models, on the other hand, is accomplished at the same time that parameters of the pharmacokinetic model are estimated. Both central tendency, through the structural model, and variability, through the components of variance model, are determined by explicit, simultaneous estimation of their respective parameters.

A proposed advantage to parameter estimation using mixed effect regression models is that the individual need not be characterized as completely as when using simple regression methods in order to obtain useful information about population central tendency and variability in response. This result implies that fewer samples need be taken from each individual because the individual is no longer of central interest. Drug concentrations are pooled to characterize a central tendency for the population rather than the individual. That individual response is usually different from population mean response is preserved through characterization of interindividual variance. Individual contributions to the characterization of this variance are adequately defined with fewer samples than are required for characterization of individual central tendency. Thus, although mixed effect modeling with data obtained by limited sampling of each individual does not allow detailed characterization of each individual response, it does allow characterization of population central tendency in response and the magnitude of variability between individuals about this central tendency.

1. The Pharmacokinetic Model

As with simple nonlinear regression, virtually any pharmacokinetic model can be evaluated using mixed effect regression and population-based analysis (94–96). In advancing a particular model for consideration, one is constrained by the same sorts of considerations that apply to models fitted using classic methods. The model should be as parsimonious as possible and yet at the same time adequately account for the data. The data should cover the entire range of a dosing interval or some similar unit of time. Samples obtained just prior to dose during an oral steady-state study provide no useful information about the rate of absorption. Conversely, samples obtained only during an active absorption phase provide little useful information about clearance. In order to characterize mean drug absorption, distribution, and elimination for the population one must adequately sample all portions of the population plasma concentration-time profile influenced by these processes.

A pharmacokinetic restriction that applies in mixed effect modeling is the requirement that the same distributional and clearance processes apply to all individuals under study. In traditional pharmacokinetic modeling in which the individual response is modeled, data may suggest that different compartmental depictions apply for different individuals. This situation is particularly apt to occur when individuals receive different amounts of drug and receive it by different routes. Slow absorption of a drug may mask a distributional phase that is apparent on intravenous administration. Elimination profiles obtained following administration of a small dose may appear linear, and elimination profiles obtained following administration of larger doses that produce higher plasma concentrations may appear distinctly nonlinear.

When using mixed effect models, a single underlying structural or pharmacokinetic model is developed that characterizes behavior of the drug in the population as a whole. Thus, although slow absorption may confer an apparent one-compartment nature on a two-compartment drug, one may model the two-compartmental aspects of distribution providing information is available regarding the initial distribution phase. This additional information may come from other individuals who have received intravenous doses or rapidly absorbed oral doses that allow characterization of initial distribution. Nonlinear elimination may similarly be modeled for all individuals under study if information is available over a sufficiently large concentration range. Individuals receiving small doses of drug and exhibiting low concentrations would supply information about the terminal elimination rate when plasma concentration is much less than that required for the half-maximal elimination rate and elimination appears linear. Still other individuals, with higher plasma concentrations, would supply information about the maximum rate of elimination. Note that before the maximum rate of elimination can be adequately characterized, concentrations from this latter group of individuals must be high enough to saturate the physiologic process responsible for a nonlinear plasma concentration profile.

The important point to be made of both these examples is that information obtained from individuals is not used to develop individual models but is instead used to develop the overall model that applies to the population in general. Although slow absorption following oral administration prevents characterization of multicompartmental distribution, one need not rely on a less appropriate model if information is available from other individuals that allows such characterization. Similarly, apparent linear elimination of a drug in individuals with relatively low plasma concentrations does not prevent the use of this data in modeling a nonlinear process, providing information is available regarding the elimination rate at higher concentrations. Generally, the ability to use all available information regrading a particular process, whether pharmacokinetic or not, is desirable. However, by integrating all information through a single model, one runs the risk of missing a possible dichotomy. An underlying assumption in population pharmacokinetic modeling using mixed effect methods is that plasma concentration profiles are generated by processes consistent with a single model. To generalize a single model for the population, particularly when only a few plasma concentrations are available from each individual, is to risk missing the presence of subpopulations that have fundamental pharmacokinetic differences.

Any development of a population model should take into consideration the potential for this type of error. At the same time one should recognize the potential benefits of population-based mixed effect modeling, specifically, the opportunity to take advantage of any reliable plasma concentration data available in characterizing the underlying pharmacokinetic profile of a drug.

For the purpose of example we apply the concepts just discussed to the development of a population pharmacokinetic model. Structural or pharmacokinetic aspects of the model are addressed first. Development and discussion of the statistical or variance model are addressed second. Although estimation of parameters occurs simultaneously, it is convenient to isolate and address separately these two aspects of a population model.

A basic one-compartment open model with first-order absorption and elimination is used as the structural or pharmacokinetic model in this development. The model is parameterized to allow determination of the population central tendency in clearance and volume of distribution. Interindividual variation in clearance and distribution volume is assumed, at lteast in part, to be accounted for through interindividual variability in concomitant variables for which individual values are available. We assume that volume of distribution for the hypothetical compound is proportional to body weight. Additionally, we assume that elimination is principally by urinary excretion and that, for this reason, we wish to determine if a relationship exists between drug clearance and serum creatinine clearance. Individual clearance and volume of distribution are ultimately expressed through Equations (1) and (2), respectively:

$$\ln \hat{C}L_j = \ln CL + \Theta_{CR} \ln CL_j^{CR} \tag{1}$$

$$\ln \hat{V}D_j = \ln VD + \Theta_{Wt} \ln Wt_j \tag{2}$$

where $\hat{C}L_j$ and $\hat{V}D_j$ represent model predicted clearance and volume of distribution for the jth individual, respectively; CL and VD represent population central tendencies for the same respective parameters; and CL_j^{CR} and Wt_j represent creatinine clearance and body weight for the jth individual. Creatinine clearance may be estimated using Equation (3) or may be obtained directly from urinary creatinine excretion and plasma creatinine concentration data.

$$CL_j^{CR} = \frac{(116 - 0)age_j}{CR_j} \tag{3}$$

Estimates of individual creatinine clearance could be normalized for population central tendency so that the average individual $\ln CL^{CR}$ equals zero and estimates of population central tendency for drug clearance need no correction for renal function. A similar argument may be made for the normalization of body weight. Scaling of population clearance and distribution volume to individual pharmacokinetic expressions is accomplished through the concomitant variables CL_j^{CR} and Wt_j and their respective scaling parameters Θ_{CR} and Θ_{Wt}. Note that Equations (1) and (2) are, in reality, linear regression equations with $\ln \hat{CL}_j$ and $\ln \hat{VD}_j$ as dependent variables, $\ln CL$ and $\ln VD$ as intercepts, $\ln CL_j^{CR}$ and $\ln Wt_j$ as independent variables, and Θ_{CR} and Θ_{Wt} as slopes relating the independent comcomitant variables (creatinine clearance and body weight) to the dependent variables (drug clearance and distribution volume).

Hypotheses regarding the very existence of a regression relationship between a concomitant variable and a pharmaockinetic parameter may be tested through the scaling Θ values as well. When the appropriate Θ is constrained to zero, the corresponding normalized concomitant variable becomes zero, and thus the contribution of the variable to the expression of individual clearance or distribution volume, as defined by Equations (1) and (2), becomes zero. Such an expression of the population model is tantamount to stating that the particular concomitant variable provides no significant information about interindividual variability in the kinetic parameter of interest. By fitting the model twice, once with one or more scaling Θ values constrained to hypothesized values (usually zero) to obtain a fit to a reduced model, and a second time with the same Θ values unconstrained, to obtain a fit to a full model, one is able to determine the statistical significance of any improvement in fit for the fully parameterized model over the reduced model.

2. Variance Model

a. *Interindividual Variability* Unexplained or residual interindividual variability in clearance and volume of distribution are, in this example, modeled as log normally distributed about the predicted values:

$$\ln CL_j = \ln \hat{CL}_j + \eta_j^{CL} \tag{4}$$

$$\ln VD_j = \ln \hat{VD}_j + \eta_j^{VD} \tag{5}$$

where η_j^{CL} and η_j^{VD} are independent random variables with mean zero and variances ω_{CL}^2 and ω_{VD}^2, respectively, and CL_j and VD_j represent the actual clearance and volume of distribution for the jth individual.

$\hat{C}L_j$ and $\hat{V}D_j$ are defined by Equations (1) and (2). Interindividual variability, expressed in this form, is approximately proportional to individual central tendency, and ω_j approximates an interindividual coefficient of variation for the associated parameters (94).

For example, unexplained interindividual variability in absorption rate is modeled as logarithmically normally distributed about its central tendency but interindividual variability in F, the bioavailability parameter, is modeled as normally distributed:

$$\ln \, ka_j = \ln \, \hat{k}a_j + \eta_j^{ka} \tag{6}$$

$$F_j = \hat{F}_j + \eta_j^F \tag{7}$$

where η_j^{ka} and η_j^F are, as earlier, independent random variables with mean zero and variance ω_{ka}^2 and ω_F^2, respectively. Although we have chosen to model interindividual variability in absorption rate as logarithmically normally distributed, we have modeled interindividual variability in bioavailability as normally distributed. The choice of variance structure is a principal asset of mixed effect modeling. Complex error or variance matrices may be postulated that mirror the complex multidimensional nature of pharmacokinetic response with a target population. In addition, two or more components of variance may be assumed to covary and to do so independently of other variance components. For instance, the volume of distribution may be assumed to be correlated with clearance but at the same time both these processes may vary between individuals in complete independence of rate or extent of absorption.

b. *Intraindividual Variability* The final step in developing this population model is that of characterizing intraindividual variability. This component of variance is commonly thought of as a statistical or residual error and quantifies, in this case, deviations of plasma concentration from the overall model predicted response:

$$\ln \, Cp_{ij} = \ln \, \hat{C}p_{ij} + \hat{C}p_{ij}^{\theta\,err} \, \varepsilon_{ij} \tag{8}$$

where Cp_{ij} is the observed ith drug concentration in the jth individual, $\hat{C}p_{ij}$ is the true ith drug concentration in the jth individual, and ε_{ij} are unexplained, independent residual errors, with mean zero and variance σ^2. Intraindividual residual error, defined by Equation (8), accounts for all sources of deviation between modeled and observed plasma concentration. Some sources of intraindividual error include drug concentration measurement, model specification, protocol

deviation, and sample time documentation. These last two sources
can be of particular concern in mixed effect modeling of large phase
III studies in which the collection of plasma samples for drug assay
occurs secondary to the collection of data regarding efficacy.

The parameter θ_{err} in Equation (8) acts in much the same way as
the scaling θ values associated with concomitant variables. Restricting
θ_{err} to zero implies that intraindividual error about $\ln Cp_{ij}$ is homo-
scedastic. Restricting θ_{err} to unity implies that errors are directly
proportional to the natural logarithm of Cp_{ij}. If θ_{err} is left unconstrained, intraindividual error can assume virtually any increasing
or decreasing monotonic dependency on Cp_{ij}.

This characterization of a population pharmacokinetic model
exhibits some of the key components of such a model. Just as with
traditional compartmental pharmacokinetic models, complexity is limited
only by good scientific judgment. The investigator must be aware,
perhaps more so than ever before, of the limitations of regression
analysis and modeling in general. Physiological as well as statistical
considerations must be continuously evaluated during the modeling
process to assure the development of a meaningful, relatistic model
of drug behavior in the population studied.

B. Problems Addressed by Population Analysis

Initial concepts of where population pharmacokinetic analysis fit into
the drug development process have evolved over the few short years
that these methods have been under development and evaluation.
Initial attitudes seemed to suggest that population pharmacokinetics
would provide an approach to diverse and incomplete data sets that
would not yield to traditional analysis. Any data that were fragmentary
or "soft" could be analyzed using population methods because complete plasma concentration-time profiles were not required of each
individual in the data base. Although it was not the intent of those
that developed the concept and methodology to portray population
pharmacokinetic methods as the answer to bad data, many initial
investigators believed that such was the case. With the exposure
that comes with use, the method's limitations, as well as its assets,
are being realized. Some analyses that have met with success are
summarized here.

1. Effects of Physiological Variables

A number of clinical population pharmacokinetic applications have
explored the effects of weight on pharmacokinetic variables. This is
a natural starting point for an investigation of physiological effects
on the pharmacokinetic behavior of a drug. A positive relationship

between weight or body size and volume of distribution has been observed for digoxin (13), gentamicin in young children and neonates (97), procainamide (98), mexiletine (99), and lidocaine (100). Clearance has been shown to depend on weight or body size for gentamicin (97), lidocaine (100), warfarin (101), and mexiletine (102) in these same studies. Studies have demonstrated a positive relationship between phenytoin V_{max} and weight (94,103,104).

2. Effects of Disease States

The effects of disease states are commonly explored indirectly through clinical chemical indices. Plasma creatinine concentration, creatinine clearance, and plasma urea concentration are used as indices of renal function and disease. Plasma alkaline phosphatase activity, plasma bilirubin concentration, and serum glutamic oxaloacetic transferase (SGOT) activity are used as indices of hepatic function and disease. Somewhat subjective criteria, such as the New York Heart Association (NYHA) functional classification scheme, and more objective criteria, such as left ventricular ejection fraction and cardiac output, are used as indices of congestive heart failure severity.

A correlation has been demonstrated between the severity of congestive heart failure as assessed by NYHA functional class and both lidocaine clearance and volume of distribution (100). Imazodan clearance in congestive heart failure patients has been found to be positively correlated with severity of disease as assessed by cardiac output (105). The later study also demonstrated an inverse relationship between clearance and either SGOT or serum bilirubin concentration. This would imply a relationship between imazodan clearance and hepatic function. Assessment of hepatic function through SGOT or bilirubin is difficult in congestive heart failure patients because elevations in these indices may reflect only imparied end-organ perfusion, a characteristic symptom of CHF.

3. Drug-Drug Interactions

Population pharmacokinetic methods have been applied to the analysis of a drug-drug interaction between alprazolam and imipramine (106). Results indicated a 10% decrease in imipramine clearance in the presence of alprazolam. The results obtained in this study compared favorably with those obtained by classic pharmacokinetic methods.

4. Pharmacogenetics

One of the more interesting results of a population pharmacokinetic study comes from an analysis of phenytoin data obtained from Japanese as well as European patients (104). Results of this study indicate a significantly lower K_m for patients of Japanese origin. This shift in K_m when considered in light of an observed reduction in K_m for younger patients points to a patient population in which phenytoin dosage adjustment may be difficult.

5. Pooling of Data

The complete generality of a population pharmacokinetic model allows incorporation of any reliable concentration-time data if accurate information is available regarding dosing history and relevant concomitant variables. Many questions remain regarding the properties of variance and correlation when data are pooled from many different studies. The success of this approach to fragmentary data remains to be determined.

C. Developing a Clinical Pharmacokinetic Program for an NDA

Ideally, population pharmacokinetic methodology would provide information from patients under study in the early phase of drug development that could be used to direct the clinical pharmacokinetic program during later stages of development (107). For instance, qualitative or semiquantitative observations of heaptic status changes and the effect of these changes on drug clearance may provide the impetus for a formal pharmacokinetic study in hepatic failure. Similarly, evidence of a significant drug-drug interaction may be observed using population pharmacokinetic methods early in patient trials. This evidence, in turn, could guide protocol development for a formal pharmacokinetic study of the suspected interaction.

Unfortunately, this ideal situation has not yet been realized. Many questions remain regarding the validity of various population pharmacokinetic methods. Proper validation of population-based methods will require a broad base of user experience. However, the relatively sophisticated statistical background required for the successful application of population-based methods limits the number of investigators using the methods and the number of analyses that are performed. At the present time, data entry and data-base management are tedious and time-consuming tasks. These tactical aspects of a population-based study must be refined before such a study can provide pharmacokinetic information early enough during the development of a drug to prove useful in guiding later development.

Finally, there is a fundamental concern about whether population-based analyses can address questions with sufficient statistical power to provide answers. The number of potentially confounding variables, such as age, weight, renal function, hepatic function, severity of primary illness, concurrent illnesses, and concomitant medications, combined with poor documentation of drug-related variables, such as dosage, time since last dose, missed doses, relationship of dose to food, position, activity, sample handling, and assay variability, may combine to render the results of all but the most meticulous of population pharmacokinetic data bases useless. Only extensive application and time-tested experience with this new approach to pharmacokinetics will provide answers to the utility of these methods.

IV. THE FUTURE: AN INTEGRATED APPROACH?

So now we know the current status, the pros and cons, for both classic and population pharmacokinetics. What will the future hold? How and where can population pharmacokientics impact on the drug development process? What must happen for population pharmacokinetic methods to assure a position of credibility in the development process? It should be clear that population methods will never replace classic methods in the drug development process. There is, no doubt, some question about whether population methods have any place in drug development, however. Proponents say that it should be integrated throughout. Opponents say it has no place. So where are we?

A. Classic Foundation

Classic pharmacokinetic methods are essential to development of a new drug entity in the pharmaceutical industry. The application of classic methods generates data that become an integral part of a new drug application. This information is generally accepted as reliable, useful, and predictive because the methods used to generate it are time tested and well understood. Classic methods form the foundation for all pharmacokinetic data interpretation. In contrast, population methods are relatively new, are not time tested, and are far from well understood.

Pharmacokinetic studies, regardless of design and analysis methods, are designed to determine the characteristics of a drug in the patients who will receive it for benefit. With classic methods, this is accomplished through intensive study of a relatively small number of individuals and subsequent extrapolation to the target population. Studies are generally well controlled and provide specific answers to specific questions regarding distinct aspects of drug ADME. In this, classic methods excel: reliable information is obtained through intensive study in a relatively small number of individuals. Regardless of this intensity, these methods are often applied to the study of drug ADME in healthy volunteers rather than in individuals intended to receive the drug. Questions regarding the

extrapolation of information obtained in healthy volunteers to the
target population can, and have, been raised. It is in part this
questioning that has led to consideration of poulation-based methods
to obtain information regarding drug ADME directly in the patient
poulation. A select few studies need to be conducted in the patient
population to assure the data from healthy subjects can be extrapolated to the patients for whom the drug is intended. If not, then
the data should be generated in the patients of interest. However,
as we noted elsewhere (9), most often the data obtained in healthy
volunteers can be extrapolated to the patients who will receive
the drug for benefit.

B. Population Pharmacokinetics in Large
   Patient Groups

Population concepts and methods deviate from those that support
classic pharmacokinetics. Population methods do not use intensive
sampling in an individual to define the pharmacokinetic profile but
rather a few samples from a larger number of patient volunteers to
determine the central tendency. Because of the shift in perspective
away from the individual that results from analysis of a population
central tendency, intensive characterization of the individual is not
critical to the method. This result allows investigation that is compatible
with ethical considerations regarding pharmacokinetic studies in a
patient population. Additionally, relaxation of restrictions concerning
the number of samples required from each individual allows cost-
effective sampling of a greater number of individuals. This in turn
permits the generation of a broad base of pharmacokinetic information
in the target population at costs equivalent to those required to conduct formal, intensive, classic pharmacokinetic studies in a relatively
small number of volunteers. However, this advantage has been
perceived by some critics as a major flaw in the current approach to
population pharmacokinetic analysis. Many are concerned that reduced
restrictions on sampling will result in a loss of control over study
conditions and sample documention.

Similarly, population methods are often held apart from classic
methods because they are not well understood, time proven, or readily
accepted. The advantages of population methods need to be elucidated
for them to assume a position alongside classic methods. Currently,
the cost in time and resources is too high to be competitive in the
development process. Prospective studies must be designed in such
a way as to assure *quality* data. The future of population pharmacokinetics depends on the implementation of prospective protocol designs
in which the quality of the data is equivalent to that obtained from
classic studies.

The fervor with which the proponents of population kinetics have attempted to infiltrate the classic development process has created a schism; in fact, it has created opponents with cause. Population kinetics has been confused with NONMEM (13) and the pharmacokinetic screen that was proposed by Temple (108). Proponents have applied the method without first testing it to understand it. Time proven means exactly that. One cannot "validate" a method by simply testing it on a few unknown data sets or on simulated data sets with one type of known error structure.

C. Result: An Improved NDA

Population pharmacokinetic methods cannot be expected to replace traditional or classic pharmacokinetic methods in the NDA process. Although the actual utility of population-based pharmacokinetic models in the pharmaceutical industry is still under evaluation, their actual role will probably be one of supporting or one of establishing the significance of observations made during the development of a pharmacokinetic profile using classic methods.

The time of the population input will be critical to its utility. At present, the likelihood that population results can be obtained in a timely enough manner to guide the classic study designs is not great. On the other hand, the use of population studies to extend the observations made during classic studies could be a major contribution to the NDA process expanded data bases during phase III and through phase IV epidemiological studies.

This is where population methods can, in fact, supplement the classic methods to improve the current package, to expand the patient pharmacokinetic data base, and to understand and evaluate ADRs. However, to achieve this goal, population pharmacokineticists will need to generate data comparable to those that are currently available from classic methods.

V. SUMMARY

We have detailed the background of both classic and population pharmacokinetics. Classic methods are well accepted and are time proven. In contrast, population methods are like the new kid on the block. Population kineticists have something to prove before the method is generally accepted or its place is generally established.

The classic pharmacokinetic process was outlined in detail. The NDA package can be achieved without population kinetics if a few classic studies in patients are conducted to assure that data in healthy volunteers can be extrapolated to the patient population(s) of interest. Specifically, multiple-dose studies should be conducted in the patients who will receive the drug for benefit.

Prospective study designs that allow comparison of classic and population results will need to be implemented for a variety of drugs. Unbiased interpretation of these results will be needed to determine if one would come to the same conclusions with both methods. If the results from population methods are consistent with those from time-proven classic methods, we will then begin to integrate population methods into the classic development process so that both methods can be used to improve the quality of the product, the NDA.

REFERENCES

1. P. G. Welling. Graphic methods in pharmacokinetics: The basics. J. Clin. Pharmacol. 26: 510–514, 1986.
2. K. Yamaoka, T. Nakagawa, and T. Uno. Statistical moments in pharmacokinetics. J. Pharmacokinet. Biopharm. 6: 547–558, 1978.
3. J. G. Wagner. Linear pharmacokinetic equations allowing direct calculation of many needed pharmacokinetic parameters from the coefficients and exponents of polyexponential equations which have been fitted to data. J. Pharmacokinet. Biopharm. 4: 443–467, 1976.
4. G. Segre. Pharmacokinetics—compartmental representation. Pharmacol. Ther. 17: 111–127, 1982.
5. J. J. DiStefano, III, and E. M. Landaw. Multiexponential multi-compartmental and noncompartmental modeling. I. Methodological limitations and physiologic interpretations. Am. J. Physiol. 246: R651–R654, 1984.
6. E. M. Landaw and J. J. DiStefano, III. Multiexponential, multi-compartmental and noncompartmental modeling. II. Data analyses and statistical considerations. Am. J. Physiol. 246: R665–R667, 1984.
7. M. Gibaldi and D. Perrier. Pharmacokinetics, 2nd ed. Marcel Dekker, New York, 1982.
8. J. J. DiStefano, III. Noncompartmental vs. compartmental analysis: Some bases for choice. Am. J. Physiol. 243: R1–R6, 1982.
9. R. K. Brazzell and W. A. Colburn. Controversy I: Patients or healthy volunteers for pharmacokinetic studies. J. Clin. Pharmacol. 26: 242–247, 1986.
10. T. Teorell. Kinetics of distribution of substances administered to the body. I. The extravascular modes of administration. Arch. Int. Pharmacodyn. 57: 205–225, 1937.

11. T. Teorell. Kinetics of distribution of substances administered to the body. II. The intravascular modes of administration. Arch. Int. Pharmacodyn. 57: 226–240, 1937.
12. L. B. Sheiner, B. Rosenberg, and K. L. Melmon. Modeling of individual pharmacokinetics for computer-aided drug dosage. Comput. Biomed. Res. 5: 441–459, 1972.
13. L. B. Sheiner, B. Rosenberg, and V. V. Marathe. Estimation of population characteristics of pharmacokinetic parameters from routine clinical data. J. Pharmacokinet. Biopharm. 5: 445–479, 1977.
14. W. A. Colburn. A pharmacokinetic model to differentiate pre-absorptive, gut epithelial and hepatic first-pass metabolism. J. Pharmacokinet. Biopharm. 7: 407–415, 1979.
15. W. A. Colburn. First-pass clearance of lidocaine in healthy volunteers and epileptic patients: Influence of effective liver volume. J. Pharm. Sci. 70: 969–971, 1981.
16. W. A. Colburn. First-pass, formation-rate-limiting metabolism. J. Pharm. Sci. 72: 711–713, 1983.
17. L. B. Sheiner, D. R. Stanski, S. Vozeh, R. D. Miller, and J. Ham. Simultaneous modeling of pharmacokinetics and pharmacodynamics: Applications to de-tubocurarine. Clin. Pharmacol. Ther. 25: 358–371, 1979.
18. W. A. Colburn. Simultaneous pharmacokinetic and pharmacodynamic modeling. J. Pharmacokinet. Biopharm. 9: 367–388, 1981.
19. N. H. G. Holford and L. B. Sheiner. Kinetics of pharmacologic response. Pharmacol. Ther. 16: 143–166, 1982.
20. E. Fuseau and L. B. Sheiner. Simultaneous modeling of pharmacokinetics and pharmacodynamics with a nonparametric pharmacodynamic model. Clin. Pharmacol. Ther. 35: 733–741, 1984.
21. J. D. Unadkat, F. Bartha, and L. B. Sheiner. Simultaneous modeling of pharmacokinetics and pharmacodynamics with nonparametric kinetic and dynamic models. Clin. Pharmacol. Ther. 40: 86–93, 1986.
22. D. J. Tucker. Linear systems analysis in pharmacokinetics. J. Pharmacokinet. Biopharm. 6: 265–282, 1978.
23. J. F. Cocchetto, D. M. Cocchetto, T. D. Bjornsson, and T. Belgan. Initial slope technique for estimation of the apparent volume of distribution during constant-rate intravenous infusion. J. Pharm. Sci. 73: 58–62, 1984.
24. V. K. Piotrovskii. Model-independent definition of the initial volume of distribution of drugs in the body. Int. J. Clin. Pharmacol. Ther. Toxicol. 24: 403–407, 1986.
25. R. K. Brazzell and S. A. Kaplan. Factors affecting the accuracy of estimated mean absorption times and mean dissolution times. J. Pharm Sci. 72: 713–715, 1983.

26. I. H. Patel, L. Bornemann, and W. A. Colburn. Evaluation of drug absorption by nonlinear regression, statistical moments, and Loo-Riegelman methods. J. Pharm. Sci. 74: 359–360, 1985.

27. K.-C. Khoo, M. Gibaldi, and R. K. Brazzell. Comparison of statistical moments parameters to C_{max} and T_{max} for detecting differences in in vivo dissolution rates. J. Phar. Sci. 74: 1340–1342, 1985.

28. J. C. K. Loo, and S. Riegelman. New method for calculating the intrinsic absorption rate of drugs. J. Pharm. Sci. 57: 918–928, 1968.

29. J. G. Wagner and E. Nelson. Percent absorbed time plots derived from blood level and/or urinary excretion data. J. Pharm. Sci. 52: 610–611, 1963.

30. J. G. Wagner. Application of the Wagner-Nelson absorption method to the two-compartment open model. J. Pharmacokinet. Biopharm. 2: 469–486, 1974.

31. M. Nicklasson, K. Ellstrom, R. Sjoquist, and J. Sjovall. Linear systems analysis and moment analysis in the evaluation of bacampicillin bioavailability from microcasule suspensions. J. Pharmacokinet. Biopharm. 12: 467–478, 1984.

32. W. R. Gillespie and P. Veng-Pedersen. Gastrointestinal bio-availability: Determination of in vivo release profile of solid oral dosage forms by deconvolution. Biopharm. Drug Dispos. 6: 351–355, 1985.

33. J. H. Proost. Application of a numerical deconvolution technique in the assessment of bioavailability. J. Pharm. Sci. 74: 1135–1136, 1985.

34. B. Blackwell. For the first time in man. Clin. Pharmacol. Ther. 13: 812–823, 1973.

35. L. Weissman. Multiple-dose phase I trials—normal volunteers or patients? One viewpoint. J. Clin. Pharmacol. 21: 385–387, 1981.

36. T. Chang, R. M. Young, J. R. Goulet, and G. J. Yakatan. Pharmacokinetics of oral pramiracetam in normal volunteers. J. Clin. Pharmacol. 25: 291–295, 1985.

37. W. A. Colburn, R. Lucek, R. Dixon, and M. Parsonnet. Pharmacokinetics of single ascending oral doses of the antiallergenic agent 2 methoxy-11-oxo-11H-lyrido,[2,1-B]quinazoline-8-carboxylic acid in man. Drugs Exp. Clin. Res. 7: 609–617, 1981.

38. L. D. Bornemann, H. E. Spiegel, Z. E. Dziewanowska, S. E. Krown, and W. A. Colburn. Intravenous and intravascular pharmacokinetics of recombinant leukocyte A interferon. Eur. J. Clin. Pharmacol. 28: 469–471, 1985.

39. R. K. Brazzell, W. A. Colburn, K. Aogaichi, A. J. Szuna, J. C. Somburg, N. Carliner, J. Hegur, J. Morganroth, R. A. Winkle, and P. Block. Pharmacokinetics of oral cibenzoline in arrhythmia patients. Clin. Pharmacokinet. 10: 178–186, 1985.

40. R. J. Whitley, B. C. Tucker, A. W. Kinkel, N. H. Barton, R. F. Pass, J. D. Whelchel, C. G. Cobbs, A. G. Diethelm, and R. A. Buchanan. Pharmacology, tolerance and antiviral activity of vidarabine monophosphate in humans. Antimicrob. Agents Chemother. 18: 709–715, 1980.

41. P. K. Noonan and L. Z. Benet. The bioavailability of oral nitroglycerin. J. Pharm. Sci. 75: 241–243, 1986.

42. J. J. Ferry, A. M. Horvath, I. Bekersky, E. C. Heath, C. F. Ryan, and W. A. Colburn. Relative and absolute bioavailability of prednisone and prednisolone after separate oral and intravenous doses. J. Clin. Pharmacol. (Submitted).

43. W. A. Colburn, A. R. DiSanto, S. S. Stubbs, R. E. Monovich, and K. A. DeSante. Pharmacokinetic interpretation of plasma cortisol and cortisone concentrations following a single oral administration of cortisone acetate ot human subjects. J. Clin. Pharmacol. 20: 428–436, 1980.

44. K.-C. Khoo, A. J. Szuna, W. A. Colburn, K. Aogaichi, J. Morganroth, and R. K. Brazzell. Single-dose pharmacokinetics and dose proportionality of oral cibenzoline. J. Clin. Pharmacol. 24: 283–288, 1984.

45. W. A. Colburn and D. M. Gibson. Isotretinoin kinetics after 80 to 320 mg oral doses. Clin. Pharmacol. Ther. 37: 411–414, 1985.

46. L. D. Bornemann, B. H. Min, T. Crews, M. M. Rees, H. P. Blumenthal, W. A. Colburn, and I. H. Patel. Dose-dependent pharmacokinetics of midazolam. Eur. J. Clin. Pharmacol. 29: 91–95, 1985.

47. W. A. Colburn, F. M. Vane, C. J. L. Buggé, Dean E. Carter, R. Bressler, and C. W. Ehmann. Pharmacokinetics of ^{14}C-isotretinoin in healthy volunteers and volunters with biliary T-tube drainage. Drug Metab. Dispos. 13: 327–332, 1985.

48. R. W. Lucek, J. Dickerson, D. E. Carter, C. J. L. Buggé, T. Crews, F. M. Vane, W. Cunningham, and W. A. Colburn. Pharmacokinetics of ^{14}C-etretinate in healthy volunteers. Biopharm. Drug. Dispos. (In press).

49. J. W. Massarella, A. C. Loh, T. H. Williams, A. J. Szuna, D. Sandor, R. Bressler, and F-J Leinweber. The disposition and metabolic fate of ^{14}C-cibenzoline in man. Drug Metab. Dispos. 14: 59–64, 1986.

50. P. G. Welling. Interactions affecting drug absorption. Clin. Pharmacokinet. 9: 404–434, 1984.

51. S. M. Singvi, D. N. McKinstry, J. M. Shaw, D. A. Willard, and B. H. Migdalof. Effect of food on the bioavailability of captopril in healthy subjects. J. Clin. Pharmacol. 22: 135–140, 1982.
52. W. A. Colburn, D. M. Gibson, R. E. Wiens, and J. J. Hanigan. Food increases the bioavailability of isotretinoin. J. Clin. Pharmacol. 23: 534–539, 1983.
53. W. A. Colburn, D. M. Gibson, L. C. Rodriguez, C. J. L. Bugge, and H. P. Blumenthal. Effect of meals on the kinetics of etretinate. J. Clin. Pharmacol. 25: 583–589, 1985.
54. N. Leeds, P. Gal, A. A. Purohit, and J. B. Walter. Effect of food on the bioavailability and pattern of release of sustained-release theophylline tablet. J. Clin. Pharmacol. 22: 196–200, 1982.
55. A. Karim, T. Burns, L. Wearley, J. Streicher, and M. Palmer. Food induced changes in theophylline absorption from controlled-release formulations. Part I. Substantial increased and decreased absorption with Uniphyl Tablets and Theo-Dur Sprinkles. Clin. Pharmaol. Ther. 38: 77–82, 1985.
56. A. Karim, T. Burns, D. Janky, and A. Hurwitz. Food induced changes in theophylline absorption from controlled-release formulations. Part II. Importance of meal composition and dosing time relative to meal intake in assuring changes in absorption. Clin. Pharmacol. Ther. 38: 642–647, 1985.
57. FDA Drug Bull. Theo-24 absorption with meals. 14(1): April 1984.
58. W. A. Colburn and D. M. Gibson. Composite pharmacokinetic profiling. J. Pharm. Sci. 73: 1667–1669, 1984.
59. R. K. Brazzell, M. M. C. Rees, K.-C. Khoo, A. J. Szuna, D. Sandor. and J. Hanigan. Age and cibenzoline disposition. Clin. Pharmacol. Ther. 36: 613–619, 1984.
60. A. Selen, A. W. Kinkel, A. C. Darke, D. S. Green, and P. G. Welling. Comparative single dose and steady-state pharmacokinetics of bevantolol in young and elderly subjects. Eur. J. Clin. Pharmacol. 30: 699–704, 1986.
61. R. B. Smith, M. Divoll, W. R. Gillespie, and D. J. Greenblatt. Effect of subject age and gender on the pharmacokinetics of oral triazolam and temazepam. J. Clin. Psychopharm. 3: 172–176, 1983.
62. D. R. Abernethy, D. J. Greenblatt, H. R. Ochs, D. Weyers, M. Divoll, J. S. Harmatz, and R. I. Shader. Lorazepam and oxazepam kinetics in women on low-dose oral contraceptives. Clin. Pharmacol. Ther. 33: 629–632, 1983.
63. D. R. Abernethy, D. J. Greenblatt, and R. I. Shader. Imipramine disposition in users of oral contraceptive steroids. Clin. Pharmacol. Ther. 35: 792–797, 1984.

64. R. K. Brazzell, F. M. Vane, C. W. Ehmann, and W. A. Colburn. Pharmacokinetics of isotretinoin during repetitive dosing to patients. Eur. J. Clin. Pharmacol. 24: 695–702, 1983.
65. W. A. Colburn and M. Gibaldi. Use of MULTDOS for pharmacokinetic analysis of ethosuximide data during repetive administration of single or divided daily doses. J. Pharm. Sci. 67: 574–575, 1978.
66. R. J. Wills and W. A. Colburn. Multiple-dose pharmacokinetics of diazepam following once-daily administration of a controlled-release capsule. Ther. Drug Monit. 5: 423–426, 1983.
67. J. Massarella, F. Vane, C. Buggé, L. Rodriguez, W. J. Cunningham, T. Franz, and W. A. Colburn. Etretinate kinetics during chronic dosing in severe psoriasis. Clin. Pharmacol. Ther. 37: 439–446, 1985.
68. W. A. Colburn, A. R. DiSanto, and M. Gibaldi. Pharmacokinetics of erythromycin on repetitive dosing. J. Clin. Pharmacol. 17: 592–600, 1977.
69. R. E. Polk, D. A. Sica, T. M. Kerkering, B. J. Kline, P. M. Patterson, and J. W. Baggett. Cefmenoxime pharmacokinetics in patients with renal insufficiency. Antimicrob. Agents Chemother. 26: 322–327, 1984.
70. A. D. Blair, B. M. Maxwell, S. C. Forland, L. Jacob, and R. E. Cutler. Cefonicid kinetics in subjects with normal and impaired renal function. Clin. Pharmacol. Ther. 35: 798–803, 1984.
71. C. M. MacLeod, E. A. Bartley, J. A. Payne, E. Hudes, K. Vernan, and R. G. Devlin. Effect of cirrhosis on kinetics of aztreonam. Antimicrob. Agents Chemother. 26: 493–497, 1984.
72. A. A. Holazo, S. S. Chen, G. McMahon, J. R. Ryan, J. J. Konikoff, and R. K. Brazzell. The influence of liver dysfunction on the pharmacokinetics of carprofen. J. Clin. Pharmacol. 25: 109–114, 1985.
73. R. H. Bergstrand, T. Wang, D. M. Roden, G. R. Avant, W. W. Sutton, L. A. Siddoway, H. Wolfenden, R. L. Woosley, G. R. Wilkinson, and A. J. J. Wood. Encainide disposition inpatients with chronic cirrhosis. Clin. Pharmacol. Ther. 40: 148–154, 1986.
74. G. R. Aranoff, M. L. Mayer, M. Barbalas, K. Aogaichi, R. S. Sloan, R. K. Brazzell, J. B. Walters, and J. W. Massarella. Bioavailability and elimination kinetics of cibenzoline in healthy volunteers and patients with renal failure. Clin. Pharmacol. Ther. (In Press).
75. J. W. Massarella, T. Silvestri, F. DeGrazia, B. Miwa, and D. Keefe. Effect of congestive heart failure on the pharmacokinetics of cibenzoline. J. Clin. Pharmacol. 27: 187–192, 1987.

76. J. P. Phillips, E. J. Antal, and R. B. Smith. A pharmacokinetic drug interaction between erythromycin and triazolam. J. Clin. Psychopharmacol. 6: 297–299, 1986.

77. R. A. Prince, D. S. Wing, M. M. Weinberger, L. S. Hendels, and S. Riegelman. Effect of erythromycin on theophylline kinetics. J. Allergy Clin. Immunol. 68: 427–431, 1981.

78. M. Eichelbaum. Pharmacokinetic drug interactions. J. Clin. Pharmacol. 26: 469–473, 1986.

79. P. D. Kroboth. Design and analyses of drug interaction studies. In Pharmacokinetics and Pharmacodynamics—Research Design and Analysis. Edited by R. B. Smith, P. D. Kroboth, and R. P. Juhl. Harvey Whitney Books, Cincinnati, Ohio, 1986.

80. N. H. G. Holford and L. B. Sheiner. Kinetics of pharmacologic response. Pharmacol. Ther. 16: 143–166, 1982.

81. W. A. Colburn and R. K. Brazzell. Pharmacokinetics as an aid to understanding drug effects. In Advances in Pain Research and Therapy. Vol. 8. Edited by K. M. Foly and C. E. Inturrisi. Raven Press, New York, 1986.

82. R. B. Smith, P. D. Kroboth, and R. P. Juhl (eds.). Pharmacokinetics and Pharmacodynamics—Research Design and Analysis. Harvey Whitney Books, Cincinnati, Ohio, 1986.

83. W. A. Colburn, R. K. Brazzell, and A. A. Holazo. Verapamil pharmacodynamics after intravenous and oral dosing: Theoretic consideration. J. Clin. Pharmacol. 26: 71–73, 1986.

84. A. A. Holazo, R. K. Brazzell, and W. A. Colburn. Pharmacokinetic and pharmacodynamic modeling of cibenzoline plasma concentrations and antiarrhythmic effect. J. Clin. Pharmacol. 26: 336–345, 1986.

85. W. A. Colburn. Pharmacokinetics/pharmacodynamic modeling: Study design considerations. In Pharmacokinetics and Pharmacodynamics—Research Design and Analysis. Edited by R. B. Smith, P. D. Kroboth, and R. P. Juhl. Harvey Whitney Books, Cincinnati, Ohio, 1986.

86. A. A. Holazo, W. A. Colburn, J. H. Gustafson, R. L. Young, and M. Parsonnet. Pharmacokinetics of bumetanide following intravenous, intramuscular and oral administrations to normal subjects. J. Pharm. Sci. 73: 1108–1113, 1984.

87. T. Ishizaki, Y. Horai, T. Sasaki, K. Chiba, A. Ohnishi, T. Suganuma, G. Tsujimoto, H. Eckizen, and T. Okaniwa. Bioavailability and pharmacokinetics of theophylline following plain uncoated and sustained-release dosage forms in relation to smoking habit subjects. Eur. J. Clin. Pharmacol. 24: 361–369, 1983.

88. H. d'A. Heck, S. E. Butrill, N. W. Flynn, R. L. Dyer, M. Anbar, T. Cairns, S. Dighé, and B. E. Cabana. Bioavailability of imipranine tablets relative to a stable isotope-labeled internal standard: Increasing the power of bioavailability tests. J. Pharmacokinet. Biopharm. 7: 233−248, 1979.

89. U. Meresaar, M.-I. Nilsson, J. Holmstrand, and E. Anggard. Single-dose pharmacokinetics and bioavailability of methadone in man studied with a stable isotope method. Eur. J. Clin. Pharmacol. 20: 473−478, 1981.

90. A. Kannikoski, M. Marvola, P. Ottoila, and S. Nykanen. Assessment of bioavailability of two experimental sustained release capsules of varapamil hydrochloride using the stable isotope technique. Acta Pharm. Fenn. 94: 23−29, 1985.

91. J. L. Steimer, A. Mallet, J. L. Golmard, and J. F. Boisvieux. Alternative approaches to estimation of population pharmacokinetic parameters; comparison with the nonlinear mixed effect model. Drug Metab. Rev. 15: 265−292, 1984.

92. L. B. Sheiner and S. L. Beal. Analysis of nonexperimental pharmacokinetic data. In Drug Absorption and Disposition: Statistical Considerations. Edited by K. Albert. American Pharmaceutical Association, Washington, D.C., 1980.

93. S. L. Beal and L. B. Sheiner. Estimating population kinetics. CRC Crit. Rev. Biomed. Eng. 8: 195−222, 1982.

94. L. B. Sheiner and S. L. Beal. Evaluation of methods for estimating population pharmacokinetic parameters. I. Michaelis-Menton model routine clinical data. J. Pharmacokinet. Biopharm. 8: 553−571, 1980.

95. L. B. Sheiner and S. L. Beal. Evaluation of methods for estimating population pharmacokinetic parameters. II. Biexponential model; experimental pharmacokinetic data. J. Pharmacokinet. Biopharm. 9: 635−651, 1981.

96. L. B. Sheiner and S. L. Beal. Evaluation of methods for estimating population pharmacokinetic parameters. III. Monoexponential model; routine pharmacokinetic data. J. Pharmacokinet. Biopharm. 11: 303−319, 1983.

97. A. W. Kelman, A. H. Thomson, B. Whiting, S. M. Bryson, and D. A. Steedman. Estimation of gentamicin clearance and volume of distribution in neonates and young children. Br. J. Clin. Pharmacol. 18: 685−692, 1984.

98. T. H. Grasela and L. B. Sheiner. Population pharmacokinetics of procainamide from routine clinical data. Clin. Pharmacokinet. 9: 545−554, 1984.

99. S. Vozeh, G. Katz, V. Steiner, and F. Follath. Population pharmacokinetic parameters in patients treated with oral mexiletine. Eur. J. Clin. Pharmacol. 23: 445−451, 1982.

100. S. Vozeh, M. Berger, M. Wenk, R. Ritz, and F. Follath. Rapid prediction of individual dosage requirements for lignocaine. Clin. Pharmacokinet. 9: 354–363, 1984.

101. D. R. Mungall, T. M. Ludden, J. Marshall, D. W. Hawkins, and R. T. Talbert. Population pharmacokinetics of racemic warfarin in adult patients. J. Pharmacokinet. Biopharm. 13: 213–227, 1985.

102. S. Vozeh, M. Wenk, and F. Follath. Experience with NONMEN: Analysis of serum concentration data in patients treated with mexilitine and lodocaine. Drug Metab. Reve. 15: 305–315, 1984.

103. S. Vozeh, K. T. Muir, L. B. Sheiner, and F. Follath. Predicting individual phenytoin dosage. J. Pharmacokinet. Biopharm. 9: 131–146, 1981.

104. T. H. Grasela, L. B. Sheiner, B. Rambeck, H. E. Boenick, and A. Dunlop. Steady-state pharmacokinetics of phenytoin from routinely collected patient data. Clin. Pharmacokinet. 8: 355–364, 1983.

105. S. C. Olson. A population pharmacokinetic profile of imazodan in congestive heart failure patients. Pharmaceutical Res. (submitted).

106. L. Ereshefsky, A. R. Richards, R. L. Evans, B. Wells, and T. H. Grasela. Detection of drug-drug interactions using population pharmacokinetic analysis. Pharmaceutical Res. (submitted).

107. L. B. Sheiner and L. Z. Benet. Premarketeing observational studies of population pharmacokinetics of new drugs. Clin. Pharmacol. Ther. 38: 481–487, 1985.

108. R. Temple. Discussion paper on the testing of drugs in the elderly. (memorandum). U.S. Department of Health and Human Services, Food and Drug Administration Washington, D.C., September 30, 1983.

10

Drug Metabolism Factors in Drug Discovery and Design

K. SANDY PANG and XIN XU *University of Toronto, Toronto, Ontario, Canada*

I. INTRODUCTION

The duration of therapeutic agents in the body is dictated by events
for absorption and disposition underlying drug distribution and
elimination. Appreciation for the relative importance of metabolic and
excretory factors in drug removal requires consideration of the
following aspects.

>   The maximum metabolic clearance may be as high as cardiac output
>   when a substrate in circulation is almost completely removed
>   in a drug-metabolizing tissue, such as the lung, which receives
>   the entire cardiac output (1), whereas for renal drug ex-
>   cretion, the highest renal clearance is renal blood flow, or
>   25% of total cardiac output.
>   The metabolic activities of the intestine, liver, and lung may
>   significantly reduce the proportion of an orally administered
>   drug reaching the systemic circulation, known as the first-
>   pass effect (2).
>   Biotransformation acts as both a deactivation and an activation
>   pathway, leading to termination of drug action and/or
>   production of pharmacologically potent or toxic metabolites.

Metabolic pathways have been categorized as phase I and phase
II reactions. Phase I reactions entail oxidation, reduction, and
hydrolysis, and phase II reactions are conjugation pathways, such
as sulfoconjugation, glucuronidation, glutathione and amino acid
conjugations, methylation, acetylation, glucosidation, and hydration
(opening of epoxide in diol formation), and require the presence of
cofactors. Specific enzymes for such reactions are, in general, most
abundant in the liver, but almost all other organs and tissue, namely
the kidney (3), intestine (4), lung (5), adrenals (6), and skin (7),
are found to posses metabolic activities.

Biotransformation of xenobiotics usually renders metabolites of
high polarity for renal excretion, leading to inactivation of drug and
short duration of action. However, the notion of biotransformation
as synonymous with detoxication is no longer valid. Recent advances
in drug metabolism and isolation of drug metabolites have firmly
established the identities of drug metabolites as pharmacologically
active and toxic species (8,9). In fact, this principle is well recognized in the prodrug approach to drug design, and the realization
has evoked the necessity for a detailed description of the formation,
distribution, and elimination of drug metabolite in the body.

Metabolite existence, by definition, depends on the presence
of a drug and a subsequent biotransformation process. Consequently,

factors that influence drug disposition also exert influences on metabolite disposition, in addition to factors that influence metabolite behavior. A classic example is that the apparent $t_{1/2}$ for the metabolite may parallel that for drug but is shorter after intravenous administration of the metabolite. This is due to a slower formation rate constant of the metabolite (the formation rate constant of metabolite is embodied in the total elimination rate constant for drug) relative to its faster elimination rate constant, resulting in a "flip-flop" model. Theoretical treatments of metabolite kinetics based on simple compartmental approaches are therefore more complex than those for drug kinetics, as mass balance relationships necessarily evoke consideration of both drug and metabolite(s). For this reason, descriptions of metabolite data have been relatively numbered (10–32) and are rarely extended to include secondary and tertiary metabolites.

A recent and important observation on metabolite formation is that metabolites, when formed in situ in an eliminating organ, may undergo immediate elimination (metabolism or excretion) before leaving the organ (15), furnishing less metabolite than formed to the systemic circulation. The phenomenon of this "sequential first-pass effect of a formed metabolite" is inherent in the genesis of the nascently formed metabolite in situ in the organ, is analogous to the first-pass effect of drugs, and must be considered in an accurate description of metabolite behavior. In compartmental modeling, the fate of a generated (derived from drug entry and followed by uptake and biotransformation within an eliminating organ) and a preformed (entering an eliminating organ via the circulation as the metabolite) metabolite is frequently taken to be identical, as described by venous equilibration. In this sense, the fraction available for a metabolite derived from drug may be approximated by that found for its preformed counterpart (18,20,24,27).

There is, however, an increasing body of evidence showing disparity in fate between a generated versus preformed metabolite within a major metabolite formation organ, such as the liver. If such concerns hold, preformed metabolite behavior does not necessarily predict handling of generated metabolites. By the same token, prediction of drug behavior following prodrug administration will not be attainable from drug administration. This chapter reviews the causes for discrepancies and brings attention to the phenomenon and the consequences. Because many of the observations arise from studies on the liver, emphasis is placed on the description of events for the liver and its encompassing microcirculatory patterns and heterogeneities. Similar observations may be perceived for other eliminating organs, but these may be modulated by unique features of circulation patterns or anatomy within these eliminating organs.

II. THE LIVER

The liver is the most important drug-metabolizing organ, as it usually
contains the most abundant enzyme systems that mediate a variety
of diverse metabolic reactions. The structure of the liver is unique
and must be considered when defining the manner in which this
organ exerts its influence on the metabolic disposition of substrates.
It is composed of parallel sinusoids of similar lengths lined by endothelial cells with fenestrated cellular processes, a free accessible
space of Disse (a functional extracellular space) beyond this, and
plates of hepatocytes adjacent to the space of Disse (Fig. 1). The
first potentially substantial barrier to the passage of materials into
the liver is the liver cell membrane, a lipid domain that may retard
the entry of some polar compounds but facilitates the entry of other
substrates into cells with carrier systems (32–35). These membrane-
limited transport mechanisms contrast with those underlying the
movement of lipophilic substrates, which experience flow-limited
transport, that is, free passage into and out of hepatocytes as rapidly
as presented, the organ perfusion rate being the limiting factor.

Materials passing through this membrane gain access to the
metabolic machinery in the liver cell. When a substrate is removed
by hepatocytes lining the length of the sinusoid, a concentration
profile is created in space during steady state, declining from inlet
(mixed supply of hepatic arterial blood and portal vein, 25 and 75%
of total liver blood flow, respectively) to outlet (terminal hepatic
venule) (36–38). This concentration profile of substrate in space
(with its corresponding input-output concentration difference) must
be accounted for by the underlying hepatic microcirculatory structure
and physiological and biochemical processes. The phenomenon holds,
for example, for the flow of oxygen, being highest at the entrance
of the dual supply of the hepatic artery and portal vein, or zone 1,
and dwindling to lower levels at the exit of the liver, or zone 3 of
the liver acinus (39). An overlapping zone 2 region exists, where
the cells are prone to recruitment to become zone 1 or 3 cells, con-
tingent upon oxygen tension and flow (39,40). Morphologically, the
sinusoids (41), cell types, and their occurrence (42) also differ
among different zones of the liver. Zone 1 cells are known to be
more equipped to support normal biliary excretion (43) and gluconeogenesis (44), and zone 3 cells favor glycolysis (45).

Metabolic zonation for the metabolism of drugs (46–62) is also
a well-known phenomenon in the periportal, midzonal, and pericentral

---

FIGURE 1 Transmission electron micrograph of liver in periportal region.
Numerous microvilli (M) project into the spaces of Disse (D), the narrow
space between the hepatocytes (H), and endothelial cells (E) lining the
sinusoid. Bile ducts (B) are evident in the micrograph (magnification ×
8750); section was stained with lead citrate.

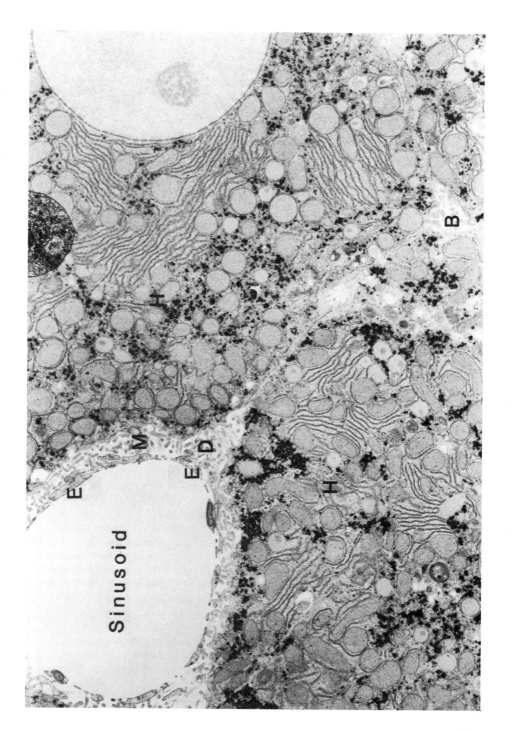

389

regions of the liver, and the regions are analogous to zones 1, 2, and 3 in the description of flow of oxygen along the acinus. Within the intact organ, a drug (an already existing chemical entity) enters the liver at a high concentration and is removed during traversal as a result of uptake by the liver. Uptake occurs as a distributed-in-space phenomenon, directed by flow along the sinusoids, and described according to its position along the sinusoidal flow path. Drug uptake is governed by time-related events, including drug transport into and out of hepatocytes, drug binding to red cell, plasma, and tissue proteins, and metabolism by enzymes or excretion into bile, which occurs as a function of unbound intracellular substrate concentration. The rates at which these elimination processes occur, however, are dependent upon the amounts of eliminatory activity for metabolism and excretion within hepatocytes located at discrete regions of the liver. As a consequence of drug uptake into cells and irreversible loss due to elimination, drug concentration in liver decreases from inlet to outlet, and the outlet concentration becomes the outflow concentration (36, 63).

Metabolite formation is also a distributed-in-space phenomenon (32). A metabolite formed in situ hepatocytes will behave differently from a corresponding already formed or preformed metabolite introduced as an input into the system (53,54,62). Differences are expected because of differing points of entry of the metabolite into the liver (at each site of formation and at the origin of the sinusoid). Metabolite formation is highly dependent upon drug uptake and biotransformation and, therefore, parameters associated with drug uptake and biotransformation. For the preformed metabolite, its access to hepatocytes is dependent only on cell permeability and space distribution and is independent of drug uptake and metabolic transformation of the drug. When the metabolite is further metabolized or excreted into bile, the sojourns of the generated metabolite, defined in the space and time domain of the system, are dependent on drug uptake as well as on the enzymatic processes for metabolite elimination (32,53). Metabolite formation ordinarily precedes metabolite elimination, either by metabolic or excretory processes, in a highly ordered reaction sequence. Without metabolite formation from its precursor, further metabolite elimination does not proceed. A preformed metabolite, which already exits in the system as metabolite, is potentially acted on immediately by succeeding enzyme systems, but only following uptake of the preformed metabolite. However, events underlying the elimination of metabolite generated from a precursor and preformed metabolite are interrelated because of involvement of the same enzyme system(s) for metabolite metabolism. Whether a transport barrier for drug or metabolite exists further augments the difference between preformed and generated metabolite metabolism (64–66).

III. FACTORS AFFECTING DRUG METABOLISM AND METABOLITE FORMATION AND ELIMINATION IN LIVER

From the preceding description, it is clear that factors affecting drug uptake, biotransformation, metabolite formation, and efflux of the compounds are highly dependent on physical, biochemical, physiological and kinetic factors. In order to delineate the roles of each component, simple metabolic schemes are used for removal of a drug solely to a single (primary) metabolite that may be further metabolized and/or excreted (scheme 1) or to two or more (primary) metabolites via competitive pathways (scheme 2). Within an intact organ, modulation of uptake characteristics due to drug binding to tissue and/or plasma proteins or inherent features of a lipid membrane in facilitating or delimiting substrate transport is considered. The uniqueness of the hepatic vasculature and microcirculation in conjunction with the distribution of enzymatic metabolic activities is viewed in terms of inlet substrate concentration. For the traversal of a substrate from inlet to outlet of the liver, recruitment of hepatocyte metabolic and excretory activities occurs along the sinusoidal flow path. Metabolite formation results only when both substrate and enzyme are present. In the absence of substrate, enzymatic activity, albeit present, may not be recruited. The ensuing sections describe in more detail how the distribution of enzymatic activities and the K_m, the Michaelis-Menten constant, of the enzymic systems, influence substrate recruitment of hepatocyte activities.

A. Kinetic Phenomenon in Metabolite Formation and Elimination

Because metabolite formation must necessarily precede metabolite elimination, such events as drug uptake followed by biotransformation affect further metabolism and excretion of the immediately formed metabolite, compared with that of the preformed metabolite, which enters as input to the organ and is independent of drug characteristics. As an illustration of the kinetic phenomenon in shceme 1, [^{14}C]phenacetin, at tracer concentrations, is metabolized primarily to [^{14}C]acetaminophen and [^{14}C]acetaminophen sulfate conjugate in rat isolated hepatocyte experiments (67). In the absence of a physical barrier for the transport of acetaminophen into cells, preformed acetaminophen (labeled with tritium in these studies) readily enters hepatocytes and becomes sulfated. For the lipophilic precursor, phenacetin, such barriers also appear to be absent such that both drug and metabolite gain ready access into cells. Since hepatocytes represent cells from

zones, 1, 2, and 3, the system is an apparent "homogeneous" pool
of enzymatic activities from all zones. In this apparently well-mixed
system, [^{14}C]acetaminophen generated from [^{14}C]phenacetin forms
proportionally less labeled sulfate than preformed [^{3}H]acetaminophen
under first-order conditions (Fig. 2).

The kinetic succession of drug biotransformation to the primary
and then secondary metabolites may fully explain the phenomenon.
This phenomenon is easily demonstrated by a simulated comparison
of the extents of sequential metabolism of the generated primary metabolite and the metabolism of a preformed metabolite in a well-mixed
compartment, as in isolated hepatocytes (68). In the simulation, a
drug (D) is solely converted to a primary (MI) then secondary (MII)
metabolite. Different enzymatic activities (drug intrinsic clearances

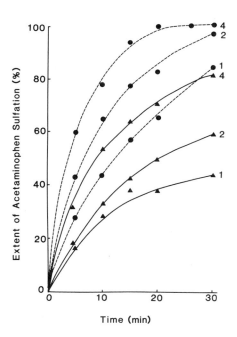

FIGURE 2 A comparison of the extents of sulfation of acetaminophen
at low concentrations of preformed [^{3}H]acetaminophen (● and – – – –),
and [^{14}C]acetaminophen (▲ and ———) generated from low concentrations of [^{14}C]phenacetin in isolated rat hepatocytes. The numbers
adjacent to each curve represent the volume of hepatocyte cell
suspension employed in the incubation mixture (5 ml). (Data were
obtained from Ref. 67.)

are 0.4, 0.1, and 0.025 ml/sec) are used for drug disappearance in metabolite formation, but the activity in metabolizing both preformed and generated metabolite is identical (0.05 ml/sec). The simulation of the time course of drug and primary (generated), and secondary metabolites reveals a decay of drug, a rise and fall of the primary metabolite, and accumulation of the secondary metabolite. When formation of primary metabolite is rapid (high formation intrinsic clearance), metabolite concentrations rise and fall rapidly, as does the accumulation of the secondary metabolite. The converse is also true. When formation of the primary metabolite is slow (poor intrinsic clearance of formation), the primary metabolite displays a less steep rise and prolonged fall, with a longer peak time shifted to the right; less rapid accumulation of the secondary metabolite occurs (Fig. 3). In contrast, preformed metabolite decay is independent of parameters describing drug disappearance but occurs because of its underlying removal mechanisms, which are identical to those operating for the generated metabolite.

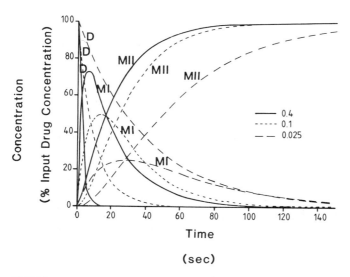

FIGURE 3 Drug disappearance and metabolite formation from a sequential pathway of drug (D) to its primary (MI) and secondary (MII) metabolites in a evenly distributed system, such as the isolated rat hepatocytes. Simulation was performed by the computer program MLAB using various formation intrinsic clearances for MI (0.4, 0.1, and 0.025 ml/sec). The elimination intrinsic clearance of MI to form MII was 0.05 ml/sec. (Data were obtained from Ref. 68.)

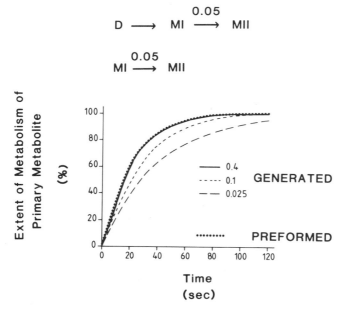

FIGURE 4 A comparison of the extents of metabolism of generated versus preformed metabolites (transformed data of Fig. 3). (Data were obtained from Ref. 68.)

Transformation of these data further shows that the greatest extent of metabolism exists for the preformed (primary) metabolite owing to its pre-existence, allowing this metabolite maximal exposure to the enzymatic machinery. The extent of sequential metabolism of a generated metabolite, however, is maximal when associated with the precursor having the highest intrinsic clearance for formation of the metabolite (0.4 ml/sec) and is lesser with precursors with smaller formation intrinsic clearances (Fig 4). Rapid formation of the metabolite furnishes metabolite for avid metabolism, and less of a "lag" is observed when its extent of sequential metabolism is compared to that found for the preformed metabolite. When formation of the metabolite is extremely rapid, the extents of metabolism of preformed and generated primary metabolites become identical; whereas if formation of the metabolite is slow, sequential metabolism lags behind that for preformed metabolite. This kinetic phenomenon is augmented in the intact liver, when hepatocytes are aligned adjacent to the sinusoidal flow paths, such that metabolites formed downstream are unable to utilize enzymatic activities within hepatocytes upstream, even with an even distribution of formation and metabolism enzymes for metabolite. The presence of heterogeneities in drug-metabolizing activities further modulates the expected kinetic differences. This last aspect is covered in the ensuing sections.

B. Enzymic Distributions in Intact Liver

Metabolic zonation of enzyme system(s) within the liver lobule has been well studied within the past few years. Direct and indirect techniques have shown an enriched presence of the cytochrome P-450, epoxide hydrolase, glutathione-S-transferases, and UDP-glucuronosyltransferases in the perivenous region (zone 3) and sulfotransferases in the periportal region of the liver (32–62,69,70).

In considering relative enzymic distributions, the liver is viewed simplistically as a series of parallel units of length L, each denoting a single sinusoid lined by sheets of hepatocytes, one cell thick on either side. Enzymatic activity within a cell located at any point x, or $V_{max,x,cell}$, may be summed for all hepatocytes at point x, such that a distribution of the overall $V_{max,x}$ results. Analogously, the distribution pattern of another enzyme system (for either durg removal or metabolism of metabolite) may be similarly constructed (Fig. 5). Despite that $V_{max,x}$ varies along L, K_m for the metabolic pathway is considered constant for the same system. The relative distribution patterns for enzyme systems may be described by the median (or center) of enzymic distribution, or the plane that divides total enzymatic activity (total V_{max} or $\int_0^L V_{max,x} \, dx$) into halves. The median or the "median distance" serves to interrelate the distance between inlet of the liver and the bulk of the enzyme. For example, by examining the "median distances," system I is of anterior distribution to system II, since its median (or center) of distribution precedes that for system II (Fig. 5). System I may represent enzyme activity for metabolite metabolism with system II supporting metabolite formation (scheme 1), or system I and system II are competing metabolic pathways (scheme 2). Adopting this approach one may proceed to examine the effects of zonation of enzymes ($V_{max,x}$) and their respective K_m values on drug disappearance and metabolite formation and metabolism.

1. Sequential Metabolic Pathways (Scheme 1)

a. Uneven Distribution of Enzymes The precursor-metabolite pair, phenacetin-acetaminophen (Sec. III.A) serves as an example of sequential pathways. The kinetic phenomenon of metabolite formation preceding the metabolism of metabolite is expected to result in a lag in the metabolism of the generated metabolite compared with that found for a preformed metabolite (Fig. 4). The same kinetic phenomenon

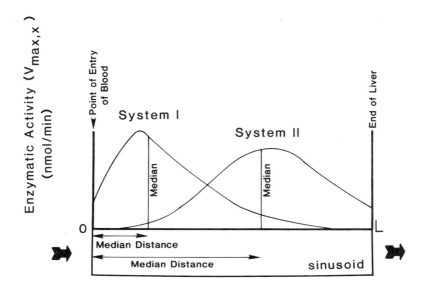

FIGURE 5 Schematic presentation of the liver. Effectively, the liver is viewed as a unit that consists of bulk flow (bold arrows) through sinusoids of identical length L. When all enzymatic actitivies at any point x along L are assumed, a distribution for $V_{max,x}$ results. Heterogeneous enzymic distribution of systems I and II are shown in liver tissues. Enzymic distributions may be described with respect to the "median" or plane that divides total enzymatic activity ($\int_0^L V_{max,x}$ dx) into halves.

will manifest itself in an intact organ, where finite transit times for drug and metabolites exist. Attendant heterogeneities in the intact organ, with a pericentral distribution of the cytochrome(s) P-450 system and a periportal enrichment of sulfotransferases, should augment differences in sequential metabolism between generated and preformed acetaminophen for the same drug-metabolite pair (Fig. 5; system I applies to metabolite metabolism and system II applies to metabolite formation). Since the cytochrome P-450 system that effects 0-deethylation of [14]phenacetin is preferentially localized pericentrally, formation of [14C] acetaminophen, mostly by downstream hepatocytes, precludes [14C]acetaminophen sulfation by upstream hepatocytes in once-through rat liver perfusion studies. However, preformed [3H]acetaminophen recruits sulfation activities from all hepatocytes and is removed

TABLE 1   Extent of Sulfation of Acetaminophen as a Generated and Preformed Metabolite in the Once-through Perfused Rat Liver Preparation[a]

Study	[^{3}H]acetaminophen (preformed)	[^{14}C]acetaminophen (generated)
1	0.62	0.46
2	0.77	0.64
3	0.78	0.72
4	0.56	0.55
5	0.61	0.44
6	0.69	0.67
7	0.69	0.58
8	0.64	0.56
Mean ± SD	0.67 ± 0.8	0.58 ± 0.1

[a]First-order case: Extent of sulfation

$$= \frac{\text{rate of formation of AS}}{\text{rate of formation or presentation of acetaminophen}}$$

AS is acetaminophen sulfate.
Source: Data from Reference 71.

predominantly by periportal hepatocytes, which possess the most abundant sulfation activity (Table 1) (71). With a procedure known as retrograde perfusion of the liver preparation, in which substrates enter the liver through the hepatic vein and exit through the portal vein, the localization patterns of enzymes with respect to substrate recruitment are effectively reversed (53). In this case, the cytochrome P-450's are now upstream and the sulfotransferases downstream. Metabolite generated upstream is then exposed to downstream hepatocytes for sulfation, and sulfation of acetaminophen generated from phenacetin occurs to similar extents as does preformed acetaminophen (reverse bold arrows in Fig. 5). The difference, previously demonstrated during normal flow (Table 1), now disappears (Table 2).

TABLE 2 Extent of Sulfation of Acetaminophen (Preformed [^{3}H]-Acetaminophen or [^{14}C]Acetaminophen Generated from [^{14}C]Phenacetin) During Normal N and Retrograde R Flows in the Once-through Perfused Rat Liver Preparation[a]

Study	[^{3}H]acetaminophen (preformed)	[^{14}C]acetaminophen (generated)
1 N	0.65	0.51
R	0.65	0.62
2 R	0.73	0.73
N	0.69	0.52
3 N	0.76	0.50
R	0.72	0.70
N	0.73	0.45
4 N	0.78	0.67
R	0.77	0.76
N	0.77	0.58
5 N	0.77	0.72
R	0.78	0.79
N	0.80	0.70
6 N	0.70	0.65
R	0.76	0.74
N	0.72	0.60

[a]First-order cases: Extent of sulfation

$$= \frac{\text{rate of formation of AS}}{\text{rate of formation or presentation of acetaminophen}}$$

Source: Data from Reference 53.

    b. Enzymatic Constants in Total Drug Disappearance, Metabolite Formation, and Metabolism of Metabolite Simulations (Sec. III.A) also reveal that a high sequential first-pass metabolism of the metabolite occurs with high drug intrinsic clearance in the previous example of a sequential pathway, in which a drug forms a primary and a secondary metabolite. When a drug is eliminated by pathways other than metabolite formation, metabolite formation intrinsic clearance is a fraction

TABLE 3 Extent of Sulfation of Acetaminophen as a Generated Metabolite from Phenacetin (E = 0.91) and Acetanilide (E = 0.45) in the Once-through Perfused Rat Liver Preparation[a]

Study	Precursor of acetaminophen		
	(I) Acetanilide	(II) Phenacetin	(III)[b] Acetanilide
1	0.37	0.51	0.43
2	0.30	0.44	0.25
3	0.28	0.32	0.22
4	0.23	0.37	0.26
5	0.35	0.53	0.39

[a]First-order case: Extent of sulfation

$$= \frac{\text{rate of efflux of AS}}{\text{rate of efflux of A + AS}}$$

[b]I, II, and III are the three steady-state perfusion periods within the same rat liver preparation.
Source: Data from Reference 54.

of (total) drug intrinsic clearance. The manner in which metabolite formation intrinsic clearance affects metabolite formation and sequential metabolism of the generated metabolite is further investigated in a computer simulation (unpublished data). This simulation was carried out with either even or heterogeneous distribution of formation and metabolism enzymes in the intact liver by (1) keeping drug intrinsic clearance (10–100% of total drug intrinsic clearance), and (2) repeating the procedure with varying drug intrinsic clearances. Accordingly, high intrinsic clearances for metabolite formation lead to high formation rates of the metabolite. At a constant total drug intrinsic clearance, metabolite formation clearance, either as 10 or 100% of total drug intrinsic yields identical extents of sequential metabolism of the metabolite. The result is not unexpected, since prevailing first-order conditions ensure that metabolite formed intrecellularly is processed proportionally. The lack effect of metabolite formation intrinsic clearance on its extent of sequential metabolism is shown in a series of acetaminophen precursors (N-propyl-, isopropyl-, N-butyl-, and isobutyl-acetanilide) (Fig. 6).

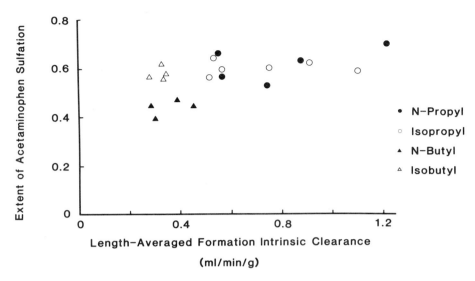

FIGURE 6 Lack of dependence of sequential first-pass sulfation of acetaminophen on the formation intrinsic clearance of acetaminophen from various precursors in the once-through perfused rat liver preparation. In these studies, input precursor concentrations (1–500 μM) were increased and metabolite formation at each steady state was quantified. The length-averaged V_{max} and K_m were estimated by fitting rates of formation of acetaminophen at steady-state and the logarithmic concentration according to the Michaelis-Menten equation by the computer program BMDP. The length-averaged intrinsic clearance for the formation of acetaminophen (length-averaged $\bar{V}_{max}/K_m$) was plotted against the extent of acetaminophen sulfation when input precursor concentration was low ($\simeq$ 1 μM) to ensure first-order conditions. (Data were obtained from Ref. 55.)

In contrast, the total drug intrinsic clearance, which influences intrahepatic drug concentrations, is an important parameter that affects the extent of sequential metabolism of metabolite. The influence is shown in the examples of acetanilide and phenacetin in acetaminophen formation in the once-through perfused rat liver. Acetanilide is of an extraction ratio of 0.4 to 0.5, and that for phenacetin is around 0.9 in the once-through perfused rat liver preparation (54). The extents of sulfation of acetaminophen, generated from these precursors, are found to be correlated to the total intrinsic clearance (or extraction ratios) of the precursors (Table 3).

Pang has explained these observations by linking time-related events that influence the duration of a generated metabolite in liver: drug uptake, drug-metabolizing activity, transport of the formed metabolite to its site(s) of removal, and the enzymatic activities in the formation and metabolism of metabolite. These time-related events are dependent on the localization of enzymes for drug disappearance, as determined by the "median distance" from inlet to the center of distribution for the enzymes, their K_m and V_{max} values, the relative distribution patterns of the formation and metabolizing enzymes for metabolite, and enzymatic constants K_m and V_{max} for metabolism of metabolite. Since a drug has a finite transit time in the liver (found by volume of distribution of drug/blood flow), the faster a drug reaches the enzymes for formations of metabolite and the more rapid the formation of metabolite due to high enzymatic activity, the greater is the likelihood that formed metabolite will reach its sites of metabolism for sequential metabolism. The converse is also true (68).

Pang and Stillwell (72) further examined the effect of total drug intrinsic clearance, and total metabolite intrinsic clearance, and various enzyme distributions on the extent of sequential metabolism of the generated (primary metabolite) versus preformed metabolite for a drug forming solely a primary and a secondary metabolite. In a simulation, they confirmed that drug intrinsic clearance and metabolite intrinsic clearance affect the extent of sequential metabolism of the formed metabolite (Table 4). They showed that different enzymic distribution patterns for metabolite formation and metabolism accordingly influence the extents of sequential metabolism. When the intrinsic clearances (V_{max}/K_m) for drug disappearance and metabolism of metabolite are high, enzymic distribution patterns become unimportant. The slightest overlap of the enzymic distributions ensures avid formation and metabolism of the metabolite. When the formation intrinsic clearance and metabolite intrinsic clearance are low, enzymic distribution patterns, however, are of paramount importance in the extent of sequential metabolism of the metabolite (Table 4). An overlap of enzyme activities, or a distribution of formation enzymes preceding sequential metabolism enzymes, allows the occurrence of sequential metabolism of metabolite. When formation enzymes are distributed posterior to metabolism enzymes for the metabolite, the extent of sequential metabolism is diminished (72).

These aspects should be seriously considered in drug development. First, recognition of organs of biotransformation and enzymic distribution patterns for formation and metabolism of metabolite and their activities (K_m and V_{max}) allow some predictions of the extent of sequential metabolism. Second, prodrug administration evokes the principles of sequential metabolism (for drug) in biotransformation organs. For eliminating organs that effect prodrug conversion solely to drug as well as sequential metabolism of drug, a facile conversion

TABLE 4 Simulation of the Extent of Sequential Metabolism of Generated Metabolite: Roles of Length-Averaged Drug and Metabolite Intrinsic Clearances[a]

Length-averaged intrinsic clearance[b] Drug	Metabolite	Extents of sequential metabolism according to models A to E $E_{ss}(mi)$ A	B	C	D	E	E_{ss}	$E_{ss}(pmi)$
1	50	0.844	0.976	0.988	0.998	1.00	0.632	1.00
1	10	0.641	0.875	0.935	0.967	0.996	0.632	1.00
1	4	0.452	0.697	0.816	0.892	0.957	0.632	0.982
1	2	0.301	0.499	0.632	0.732	0.815	0.632	0.865
1	1	0.179	0.311	0.418	0.506	0.578	0.632	0.632
1	0.5	0.099	0.176	0.245	0.305	0.353	0.632	0.394
1	0.25	0.052	0.094	0.133	0.168	0.197	0.632	0.221
0.1	5	0.417	0.687	0.808	0.889	0.968	0.0952	0.993
0.1	1	0.142	0.269	0.373	0.467	0.558	0.0952	0.632
0.1	0.4	0.064	0.123	0.179	0.231	0.283	0.0952	0.330
0.1	0.2	0.033	0.065	0.095	0.125	0.154	0.0952	0.181
0.1	0.1	0.017	0.033	0.049	0.065	0.080	0.0952	0.095
0.1	0.05	0.009	0.017	0.025	0.033	0.041	0.0925	0.049
0.1	0.025	0.004	0.008	0.013	0.017	0.021	0.0952	0.025

[a]First-order case when drug forms one primary and secondary metabolite and both drug and metabolites do not experience permeability barriers. The amount of enzyme (intrinsic clearacne) in systems I (formation of metabolite) and II (metabolism of metabolite) are constant among models. Enzymic distributions for models are as follows: model A, system I, zero initial value at inlet, increasing with linear slope to high value at outlet; system II, high initial value at inlet, decreasing linearly to zero at outlet; model B, system I, same as model A; system II, evenly distributed; model C, systems I and II, evenly distributed; model D, system I, evenly distributed; system II, zero initial value at inlet, increasing with linear slope to high value at outlet; model E, system I, high initial value at inlet, decreasing with linear slope to zero at outlet; system II, zero initial value at inlet, increasing with linear slope to high value at outlet. $E_{ss}(mi)$, E_{ss}, and $E_{ss}(pmi)$ are the apparent steady-state hepatic extraction ratios for the generated metabolite, drug, and preformed metabolite, respectively.
[b]Multiples of flow.
Source: Data from Reference 72.

of prodrug to drug furnishes rapid release of drug and also avid sequential metabolism; the converse also holds true (Fig. 3). In this sense, a drug that is formed rapidly from a prodrug may exhibit a rapid onset but a short duration of action, whereas the same drug originating from another prodrug associated with a slower conversion clearance may show a slow onset but a prolonged duration of action (Fig. 3).

c. *Enzyme Induction and Inhibition* Enzyme induction in vivo in drug removal is evidenced by increased drug clearance. However, metabolite concentrations in the systemic circulation are a net result of formation and removal. If formation of the metabolite is induced but its removal pathways remain unchanged, metabolite concentrations increase. If both formation and metabolism pathways are induced, metabolite levels alone do not reflect the extent of induction of each process (73). Metabolite formation is also modulated when induction of other competing pathways occurs, wherein drug is channeled away from metabolite formation, thereby reducing metabolite concentrations (73). This aspect is covered in more detail under Sec. III.B.2.c.

2. Competing Metabolic Pathways (Scheme 2)

a. *Uneven Distribution of Enzymes* The consequences of enzymic distributions in the liver on competitive metabolic pathways are ex-exemplified by sulfation and glucuronidation of phenolic substrates. These concepts may be applied to any two competing drug-metabolizing systems. In these examples, sulfation poses as a high-affinity, low-capacity system, whereas glucuronidation is a low-affinity, high-capacity pathway. When considering conjugation of these substrates, the distribution of conjugating activities, as well as the K_m and V_{max}, must be regarded in conjunction with inlet substrate concentration and recruitment of enzymatic activities by substrate presented by flow.

Much evidence exists on the periportal abundance of sulfation activity and a more posterior (even or pericentrally enriched) gluc-uronidation system (56–62). The distribution (V_{max} at any point x, $V_{max,x}$) and the K_m for these two systems greatly modify metabolite formation at varying inlet substrate concentrations. Intuitively, the anterior sulfation system (Fig. 5, system I) is highly efficient. A low substrate concentration entering the liver at the inlet undergoes avid sulfation, leaving little residual substrate to reach the distal region for recruitment of glucuronidation activity (Fig. 5, system II). As inlet substrate concentration increases (>K_m for sulfation and <K_m for glucuronidation), saturation of the sulfation system allows substrate to reach downstream hepatocytes, where glucuronidation occurs. As inlet substrate concentration increases beyond the K_m for sulfation and glucuronidation, little intrahepatic concentration gradient is present and both enzyme systems are "fully" recruited for maximal activities (74).

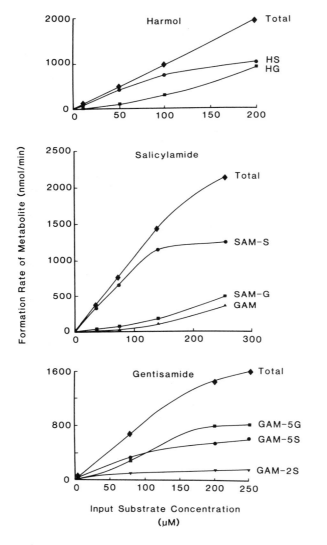

FIGURE 7 Rates of formation of metabolites from harmol, salicylamide, and gentisamide at varying input substrate concentrations in the once-through perfused rat liver preparations at constant flow rate (10 ml/min). Rates of formation are taken as the efflux of metabolite in bile and perfusate at steady-state. Harmol forms harmol sulfate (HS) and harmol glucuronide (HG); salicylamide (SAM) forms its sulfate (SAM-S) and glucuronide (SAM-G) conjugates and gentisamide (GAM, conjugated and unconjugated). When total rates of formation of metabolites are presented against input substrate concentration, a linear relationship may be found at <200, <150, and <120 μM for harmol. salicylamide, and gentisamide, respectively. (Data were obtained from Refs. 75, 62, and 61, respectively.)

Several examples are provided here to illustrate the concept of substrate recruitment of zonal hepatocyte activities. In addition to the periportal and perivenous distributions of sulfation and glucuronidation activities, respectively, in liver, the distribution of hydroxylation activity toward salicylamide (SAM) in the formation of gentisamide (GAM) is also posterior to sulfation activities (62). Three phenolic substrates are used at present as examples: harmol, which forms sulfate and glucuronide conjugates (75); gentisamide, which forms two monosulfates (GAM-2S and GAM-5S) and a monoglucuronide conjugate (GAM-5S) (61); salicylamide, which forms the sulfate (SAM-S) and glucuronide (SAM-G) as well as the hydroxylated metabolite GAM in once-through rat liver perfusion studies (62). The lack of recruitment of posterior activites (glucuronidation and hydroxylation) at low inlet concentrations of harmol, SAM, and GAM is shown by the predominance of the sulfate conjugates (harmol sulfate, HS, SAM-S, GAM-5S, and GAM-2S) (Fig. 7); glucuronidation and hydroxylation rates are low. At increasing substrate input, however, saturation of sulfation is approached whereby disproportionate increases in glucuronidation and hydroxylation rates result (Fig. 7). When substrate is spared by inhibiting the sulfation pathway with specific inhibitors, such as 2,6-dichloro-4-nitrophenol (57), glucuronidation reveals itself as an effective conjugation pathway, displaying high activity and simple Michaelis-Menten behavior (Fig. 8).

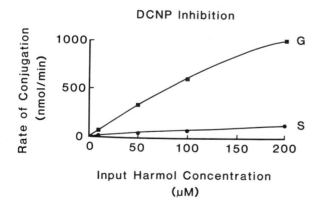

FIGURE 8 Conjugation rates of harmol at varying input concentrations in the once-through perfused rat liver preparation in the presence of a specific inhibitor of sulfation, DCNP (2,6-dichloro-4-nitrophenol, 40 µM). Suppression of sulfation and high glucuronidation rates were seen compared with Figure 7, where the inhibitor of sulfation was absent. (Data were obtained from Ref. 57.)

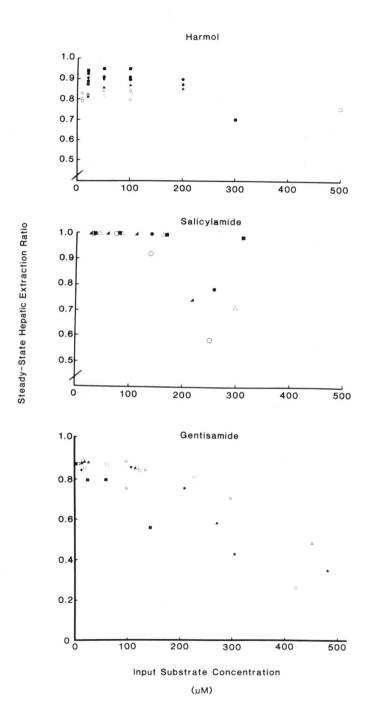

Harmol

Salicylamide

Gentisamide

Steady–State Hepatic Extraction Ratio

Input Substrate Concentration

(µM)

Upon examination of substrate recruitment of conjugation activities by the liver, drug removal (denoted by total rate of metabolism and the steady-state hepatic extraction ratio E_{ss}) has remained apparently constant whereas the formation of metabolites has not (Figs. 7 and 9). This behavior is a consequence of a gradual saturation of an anterior pathway, allowing metabolic recruitment of the posteriorly positioned metabolic pathways, which act as "backup" systems. Within this concentration range, first-order drug disappearance does not mandate first-order metabolite formation. Rather, the apparent first-order behavior of drug may elicit the formation of different proportions of metabolites. This condition was also found in vivo in humans following single and chronic dosing of acetaminophen, when both cases furnished the same $t_{1/2}$ and area under the concentration-time curve (AUC) but different proportions of sulfate and glucuronide conjugates; the ratio of sulfate to glucuronide decreased for chronic dosing and correlated with a decrease in sulfation. The case was presumed to be depletion of body stores of sulfate, a precursor of the cosubstrate in sulfation (76).

The differential recruitment of activity from hepatocytes with different drug input rates bears important implications in drug design. Different oral dosage forms are associated with varying absorption rate constants. This results in varying rates of substrate input into the portal circulation. A rapidly absorbed dosage form may lead to rapid saturation of the first (anterior) enzyme, allowing residual substrate to be recruited by downstream hepatocytes (posterior enzyme) in facile formation of the second (primary) metabolite. A slowly absorbed dosage form renders low-input concentrations to the liver, avoids saturation of the anterior pathway, and conduces to the formation of the first (primary) metabolite and little of the second (primary) metabolite. One may even consider that sustained-release dosage forms provide a burst effect followed by trickling of drug into the circulation. This condition is akin to a combination of rapidly and slowly absorbed dosage forms, respectively, resulting in the formation of different metabolites. If pharmacological and toxicological activities are associated with metabolite formation, for example posterior pathway, unexpected higher proportions of this

---

FIGURE 9 The steady-state hepatic extraction ratios of harmol, salicylamide, and gentisamide at varying input substrate concentrations in the once-through perfused rat liver at constant flow rate (10 ml/min per liver). Note the constant extraction ratios of harmol, salicylamide, and gentisamide at input concentrations <200, 150, and 120 μM, respectively. Data from each preparation are represented by the same symbol. (Data were obtained from Refs. 75, 62, and 61.)

metabolite may result from rapid absorption (release) of the dosage form. Moreover, overall parent drug removal during the first-pass effect by the liver may be constant. This condition does not stipulate that formation of metabolites also obeys apparent first-order kinetics, however. This explanation is a consequence of staggered enzyme systems in liver on drug removal.

   b. *Enzymatic Parameters* The extent of modulation of metabolite formation by another parallel and competing metabolic pathway is in accord with the effectiveness of the parallel pathway. The relative distributions of the two enzymes with respect to substrate entry and the relative magnitudes of the enzymatic parameters, K_m in particular, are important. A recent simulation study (74) assigned the same amount of enzymes (total V_{max}), systems I and II, in different regions of the liver (shown in Fig. 10) and compared the extent of modulation of system II by system I. When system II has the same even distribution as system I (model A), or is exclusively placed in the second half of the liver with system I in the first half (model B), a reduction of metabolites is seen emanating from system II (compared with model C). This is especially true for model B because of the anterior distribution of system I with its lower K_m and allows initial removal of substrate by system I, thereby reducing the substrate available to system II. When system I competes simultaneously with system II for substrate removal (model A), the lower K_m of system I effectively reduces the substrate available for system II. No modulation of system

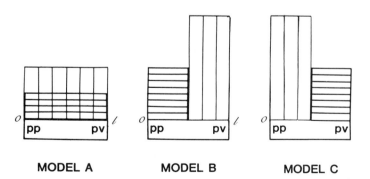

MODEL A   **MODEL B**   **MODEL C**

FIGURE 10 Schematics of enzymic distribution for system I (horizontal lines) and system II (vertical lines) activities in liver toward a substrate for models A, B, and C. Symbols pp and pv denote the periportal and perivenous regions of the liver, respectively. See text for details.

II by system I, however, is seen for model C, in which the distribution of system II is exclusively before that for system I. Similar statements describe the modulating effects of system II on the formation of metabolites from system I. No effect, however, is anticipated for model B, whereas the highest effect should be seen for model C, in which system II is exclusively before system I. An intermediate effect is expected for model A, in which system II is present simultaneously with system I (Fig. 11).

System II becomes an effective competing pathway of system I when its K_m (Fig. 12) is lower or when the V_{max} is higher than those for system I (Fig. 13). The effectiveness also varies with inlet substrate concentration. Conversely, when system I, the anterior-coincidential pathway, is easily saturated, its modulation on a posterior-coincidental pathway (system II) diminishes with increasing concentration (Fig. 11). This is due to failure of the anterior pathway to create a large intrahepatic concentration gradient for the posterior pathway, allowing substrate to reach downstream for recruitment of activity of the posterior pathway.

  c. *Enzyme Induction and Inhibition* Induction effects within an intact organ must be interpreted with caution, inasmuch as there are heterogeneities in drug-metabolizing activities among competitive pathways. An equal induction of both anterior and posterior pathways may lead to an increased formation rate of metabolite from the anterior, not posterior, pathway because of almost complete substrate recruitment by upstream hepatocytes, sparing little substrate for downstream hepatocytes. In fact, a reduction in the formation of metabolite from the posterior pathway is observed, albeit the pathway is induced (73,74). Inductive effects on the posterior pathway will only be appreciated at high enough inlet substrate concentrations when the anterior pathway becomes saturated.

Inhibition of drug metabolism pathways is subject to similar considerations. An inhibited posterior pathway has little influence on an anterior pathway, whereas inhibition of an anterior pathway may bring about increased formation of metabolites from the posterior pathway (57), although the latter is unaffected by the inhibitor (Fig. 8). Again, the reasoning draws upon the availability of substrate for enzyme recruitment.

3. Competitive and Sequential Pathways

An illustration of mixed competitive and sequential biotransformation patterns of drug and metabolites may be found in the previous example of salicylamide and gentisamide in rat liver perfusion studies (61,62). Formation of GAM-2S and GAM-5S from preformed GAM is found to predominate at low GAM concentrations because of the low K_m anterior

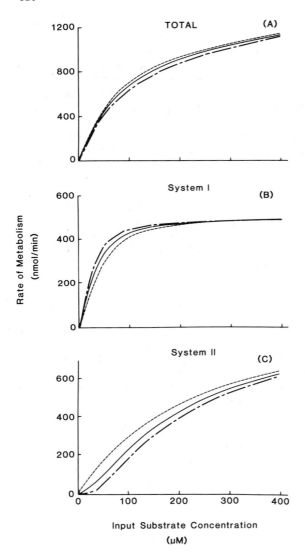

FIGURE 11 Rates of metabolite formation with input substrate concentration for models A, B, and C. Total rate of formation of metabolites (A), and metabolite formation rates from systems I (B) and II (C) at steady state are shown for models A (———), B (— - —), and C (- - - - -).

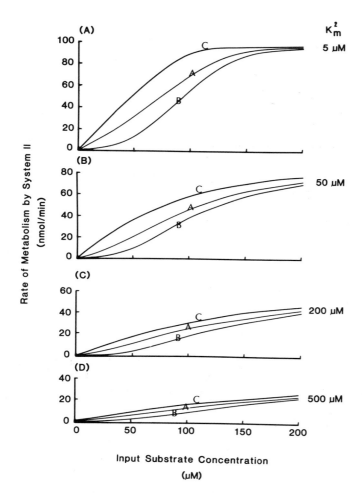

FIGURE 12 Effect of K_m of system II as a competing pathway for system I. K_m for system II (K_m^2) was varied from 5 to 500 μM. Other enzymatic parameters used for simulations were length-averaged $\bar{V}_{max}$ for system II, 1000 nmol/min per liver; K_m and length-averaged $\bar{V}_{max}$ for system I, 10 μM and 500 nmol/min per g liver. (Simulations were taken from Ref. 74.)

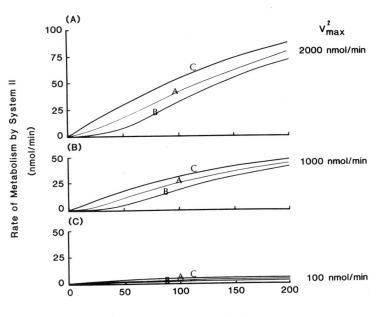

FIGURE 13   Effect of length-averaged $\overline{V}_{max}$ of system II as a competing pathway for system I. The length-averaged $\overline{V}_{max}$ for system II ($\overline{V}^2_{max}$) was varied from 100 to 2000 nmol/min). Other enzymatic parameters used for simulations were K_m for system II, 200 μM; K_m and length-averaged $\overline{V}_{max}$ for system I, 10 μM and 500 nmol/min. (Simulations were taken from Ref. 74.)

sulfation pathways; increasing input GAM concentrations result in more than proportional increases in rates of glucuronidation (Fig. 14) (61). Analogously, sulfation of SAM is a readily saturable anterior pathway; at increasing SAM concentrations, increased metabolite formation by the posterior pathways is seen for glucuronidation and hydroxylation (Fig. 7). Upon examination of the GAM metabolites arising from SAM and GAM administration, however, distinctly different proportions of metabolites are found. GAM-5G is the only metabolite formed from GAM after SAM adminstration (Fig. 15). At comparable input rates of preformed GAM into the rat liver preparation, however, GAM-2S and GAM-5S are the predominant metabolites formed (Fig. 14).

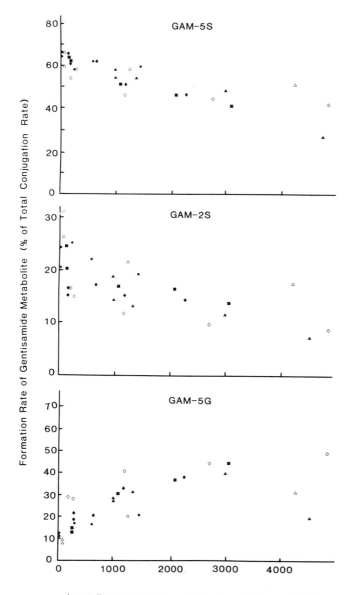

FIGURE 14 Formation of gentisamide metabolites at varying input rates (concentrations of preformed gentisamide × flow rate at 10 ml/min) in the once-through perfused rat liver preparation. GAM-5S and GAM-2S were the predominant metabolites formed, especially at low input concentrations of preformed GAM; GAM-5G was only a minor metabolite at low input concentrations, but more GAM-5G was formed at increasing GAM input concentrations to the once-through rat liver. (Data were obtained from Ref. 61.)

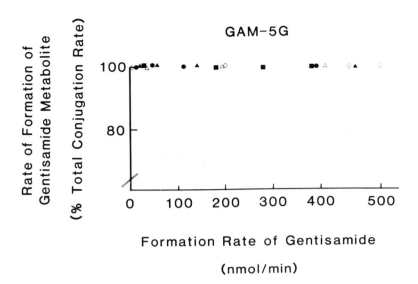

FIGURE 15 Formation of gentisamide metabolites from gentisamide, generated from varying input concentrations of salicylamide into the once-through perfused rat liver preparation. The plot was performed by plotting formation rate of gentisamide metabolite(s) versus formation rate of gentisamide from salicylamide. Only gentisamide-5-glucuronide (GAM-5G) was formed. (Data were taken from Ref. 62.)

The astounding dissimilarity in gentisamide metabolism, generated (Fig. 15) or preformed (Fig. 14), evident in the once-through liver preparation is due to heterogeneous enrichment of enzymes for metabolite formation and metabolism along the sinusoidal flow path. When SAM enters the liver, GAM formed by downstream hepatocytes is in close proximity to the glucuronidation enzymes preferentially localized in downstream hepatocytes. GAM is thereby conduced mainly to form GAM-5G. Preformed GAM entering the liver, however, initially recruits sulfation activity in upstream hepatocytes to form predominantly GAM-2S and GAM-5S. Such removal of substrate by upstream activities results in reduced formation of GAM-5G by downstream hepatocytes.

The in vivo administration of SAM gives rise to a complex situtation, comprised of both forms of GAM (preformed and generated). Consider the liver as the only organ involved in GAM formation and GAM metabolism. During traversal of SAM through the liver, GAM and GAM-5G are the only hydroxylated products formed that re-enter the circulation. Upon reaching the liver, now as a preformed metabolite, GAM forms GAM-2S and GAM-5S predominantly and GAM-5G marginally

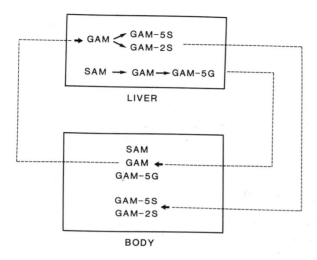

FIGURE 16 Schematic of the body in its formation of gentisamide (GAM) metabolites resulting from salicylamide (SAM) administration. GAM formation from SAM in liver results only in GAM-5G formation, whereas GAM, on re-entering the body and liver as preformed metabolite, forms primarily GAM-5S and GAM-2S.

(Fig. 16). A mixture of the metabolites GAM-2S, GAM-5S, and GAM-5G is anticipated in the circulation, with the sulfates arising from preformed GAM and the glucuronide conjugate arising from SAM entering the liver. In fact, all three metabolites are found in urine of intact rats after administration of SAM (unpublished results). If GAM-5G were a potent toxic metabolite, formed only with SAM and minimally with preformed GAM to the liver, toxicity would manifest itself only after SAM administration. The identity of the toxicant will not be readily revealed, nor will GAM metabolites be implicated as causal to the manifestation of toxicity. Failure to recognize enzymic distribution patterns in metabolite formation and metabolism may therefore lead to erroneous interpretations.

C. Drug and Metabolite Transport Across Lipoidal Membranes

The rate of influx of substrates into sites of elimination is another important factor in consideration of overall substrate uptake. The general mode of transport of a drug into cells is via transport through

biologic membranes that are lipoidal in nature. Mechanisms for such
transport by the membrane entail passive diffusion, carrier-mediated
and active processes (33), pore diffusion, and phagocytosis. Passive
diffusion usually serves as the prevailing mechanism. Compounds
whose structures resemble endogenous substances likely share the
carrier-mediated or active transport systems of their endogenous
counterparts. These mechanisms, associated with membrane transport,
may sometimes pose as rate-controlling factors, when the flux across
the membrane is slower than the delivery of substrate by flow. The
delivery of substrate can thus be differentiated as a membrane- or
perfusion-controlled process.

Perfusion limitation exists when the rate of drug permeation into
an organ or tissue is faster than the rate of delivery by the organ
perfusion rate. A diffusion limitation to intracellular transport, however, implies that the rate of permeation through a membrane is
slower than the organ or tissue perfusion rate. Diffusion rate-limited
transport usually pertains to compounds that are of high polarity or
exist in the charged or ionized forms rather than to lipophilic and
un-ionized drugs, which penetrate lipoidal membranes readily. Other
membrane-controlled processes, namely carrier-mediated systems or
active transport, also facilitate the passage of drugs or substrates
into the intracellular milieu and operate against an electrochemical
gradient (1). It has been shown that for such compounds as bile
acids (77) and organic anions, such as bilirubin, indocyanine green,
and bromosulfophthalein (78), and ouabain (79), morphine and nalor-
phin (80), such carrier systems exist in liver to facilitate their transport into hepatocytes. Similarly, a carrier system has been found to
transport glutathione out of liver cells (81).

Less attention has been given to passive diffusion as a possible
rate-controlling step in drug elimination. The manner in which the
presence of a diffusional barrier influences vascular and intracellular
events has been illustrated only recently (64—66). The probability
of metabolites encountering membrane barriers for diffusion is even
greater than for drug since drug biotransformation usually furnishes
metabolites of higher polarity than the parent compound in order to
facilitate excretion. This is readily demonstrated by drug conjugates,
such as sulfates and glucuronides, which are transferred polar
functional groups. Other examples may be found in prodrug-drug
pairs or precursors and their metabolites, as found in enalapril and
enalaprilat (82).

1. Drug Elimination and Diffusion Barriers

The manner in which a diffusional barrier affects drug removal has
been described by Gillette and Pang (83), who revealed that the diffusional clearance CL^d of a drug must be considered in the overall
removal rate or clearance. In considering a venous equilibration of

drug in effluent blood and in organ, the steady-state rate equations that describe the rate of change of drug in organ blood and organ tissue are

$$\text{Blood: } 0 = QC_{A_{ss}} - QC_{V_{ss}} + f_T C_{T_{ss}} CL^d - f_B C_{B_{ss}} CL^d \tag{1}$$

$$\text{Tissue: } 0 = f_B C_{B_{ss}} CL^d - f_T C_{T_{ss}} (CL_{int} + CL^d) \tag{2}$$

where C_{ss} is the steady-state concentration in either arterial (subscript A), venous (subscript V), organ blood (subscript B), or tissue (subscript T); Q is organ blood flow rate, and f is the unbound fraction in either organ blood (subscript B) or tissue (subscript T). CL_{int} is the intrinsic clearance and is $V_{max}/(K_m + [S])$, where V_{max} is the maximum velocity, K_m the Michaelis-Menten constant of the enzyme system and [S] the substrate concentration in liver. When diffusion is via a carrier-mediated system as well as by passive diffusion, the term CL^d may be further resolved into the two respective components:

$$CL^d = \frac{V_{max}^c}{K_m^c + [S]} + CL^{pd} \tag{3}$$

where V_{max}^c and K_m^c are the Michaelis-Menten parameters associated with the carrier system that is saturable, and CL^{pd} is the clearance associated with the passive diffusion component.

On solving Equation (2), the steady-state unbound tissue concentration may be found.

$$f_T C_{T_{ss}} = \frac{f_B C_{B_{ss}} CL^d}{CL_{int} + CL^d} \tag{4}$$

On substitution of Equation (4) into Equation (1), the rate of drug loss at steady state becomes

$$Q(C_{A_{ss}} - C_{V_{ss}}) = \frac{f_B C_{B_{ss}} CL^d CL_{int}}{CL_{int} + CL^d} \tag{5}$$

and the steady-state hepatic extraction ratio E_{ss} and clearance CL_{ss} become (83)

$$
E_{ss} = \frac{C_{A_{ss}} - C_{V_{ss}}}{C_{A_{ss}}} = \frac{f_B CL_{int} CL^d}{CL_{int}(Q + f_B CL^d) + QCL^d}
\tag{6}
$$

$$
CL_{ss} = \frac{Q f_B CL_{int} CL^d}{CL_{int}(Q + f_B CL^d) + QCL^d}
\tag{7}
$$

illustrating that when CL^d is comparable or less than organ flow rate Q, the barrier effect should be considered in the overall clearance or removal rate by that organ. The unbound tissue concentration $f_T C_{T_{ss}}$ is not equal to the unbound concentration in organ blood that leaves the organ ($f_B C_{B_{ss}}$). When perfusion limitation prevails ($CL^d \gg Q$), the equations are simplified to

$$
E_{ss} = \frac{f_B CL_{int}}{Q + f_B CL_{int}}
\tag{8}
$$

$$
CL_{ss} = \frac{Q f_B CL_{int}}{Q + f_B CL_{int}}
\tag{9}
$$

and the unbound tissue concentration equals the effluent blood concentration.

While incorporating the effect of ideal tubular flow behavior in liver, Sato et al. (65) considered the effect of a diffusional barrier on the behavior of steady-state extraction ratio of drug (E_{ss}). With equal enzymatic activity present among hepatocytes that show identical permeability to the substrate along the sinusoidal flow path, the steady-state hepatic extraction ratio of a drug is dependent on the diffusional clearance and the intrinsic clearance, which are identical along any point x of the sinusoidal flow path of length L:

$$
E_{ss} = 1 - e^{- f_B CL^d CL_{int} / Q(CL^d + CL_{int})}
\tag{10}
$$

When diffusional clearance greatly exceeds intrinsic clearance at point x, the relationship simplifies to

$$
E_{ss} = 1 - e^{- f_B CL_{int} / Q}
\tag{11}
$$

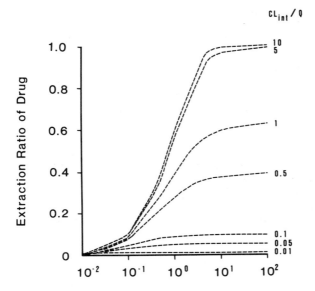

Flow Normalized Diffusional Clearance

(CL^d/Q)

FIGURE 17 Effect of a diffusional barrier on the extraction ratio of drug. Simulation was based on a homogeneous system of enzymes and barrier for drug. When drug diffusional clearance is low ($CL^d/Q <$ 10^{-2}; Q is flow rate to organ), diffusion becomes the rate-limiting factor for the extraction of a highly cleared compound (intrinsic clearance $CL_{int}/Q = 10$). A diffusional barrier ($CLd/Q < 10^{-2}$) has little effect on the rate of removal of poorly cleared compounds ($CL_{int}/Q < 0.1$) of low intrinsic clearances.

The effect of a diffusional barrier on drug extraction is depicted in Figure 17. As can be seen, for a drug with a small intrinsic clearance ($CL_{int}/Q = 0.01$), CL^d has little effect on E_{ss}. In this case, overall drug removal is dictated by the poor inherent ability within cells (or the intrinsic clearance), not by the arrival of substrate through membrane permeation. In contrast, the extraction of ordinarily high intrinsic clearance compounds ($CL_{int}/Q = 10$) may be reduced dramatically by membrane permeation. This phenomenon may be readily explained by considering that the rate-controlling step in elimination is not the enzymatic or excretory capacity but permeation through the membrane. As stated earlier, the rate of permeation can be limited by either membrane permeation or organ perfusion rate.

With uneven distribution of metabolizing activities for drug removal, a lack or presence of a diffusion barrier of drug is anticipated to affect overall rates of uptake. Sato et al. (65) further examined the presence of a common drug diffusion barrier into hepatocytes that contain varying enzymatic activities at different regions of the liver. The effect of a barrier, retarding transport of drug on overall drug removal(E_{ss}) is least for the efen enzyme case and greatest for skewed enzyme distributions (enzyme exclusively in one-half of liver). When an abundance of enzymes is present at a discrete site in liver, poor substrate entry due to a barrier may pose as the rate-limiting step in elimination because substrate is precluded from coming into contact with enzyme sites. In other cases when enzymes are scanty or absent, enzymatic activity, not substrate entry, becomes rate controlling in elimination. Drug extraction in the presence of a barrier is less than that in the absence of a barrier.

2. Metabolite Formation and Elimination and Diffusional Barriers

Membrane barrier effects on metabolite formation and elimination have also been explored by de Lannoy and Pang (64,66). In a comparison of two compounds ordinarily with a high (0.9) versus a low (0.1) extraction ratio, widely different intrahepatic concentrations are predicted during steady-state substrate delivery to the liver. In the comparison, enzymatic activities, binding to tissue and plasma, and diffusional barriers for drug and metabolite are considered identical at any point x along the liver. The liver may be modeled as a three-compartment model (Fig. 18), with blood, liver, and bile as the compartments. Enzymatic activities, binding to tissue and plasma, and diffusional barriers for drug and metabolite are considered identical at any point x along the liver. Accordingly, the mass balance relationships for the change of drug concentrations in blood and tissue with respect to their position x in liver are, for drug in blood,

$$\frac{dC_x}{dx} = - \frac{f_B C_x CL^d CL_{int}}{LQ(CL^d + CL_{int})} \tag{12}$$

and for drug in tissue,

$$\frac{dC_{T,x}}{dx} = 0 = \frac{1}{L\,Q}(f_B C_x CL^d - f_T C_{T,x} CL^d - f_T C_{T,x} CL_{int}) \tag{13}$$

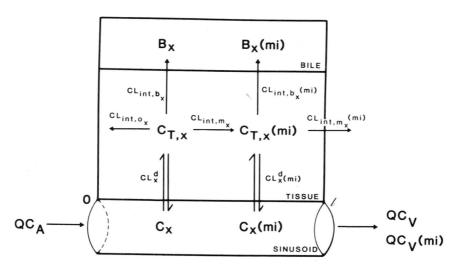

FIGURE 18 A three-compartment model for the liver; the blood or sinusoid, the tissue, and bile compartments. Events are enlarged at any point x along the length of the sinusoid of length L. Drug and metabolite concentrations at point x, C_x and $C_x(mi)$, enter the liver tissue with diffusional clearances CL_x^d and $CL_x^d(mi)$, respectively, to result in tissue concentrations of drug and metabolite $C_{T,x}$ and $C_{T,x}(mi)$. Conversion of drug to metabolite occurs with metabolic intrinsic clearance $CL_{int,mx}$; the total drug intrinsic clearance at point x is represented by a sum of all eliminatory pathways $CL_{int,mx} + CL_x^b + CL_{int,ox}$. Metabolite elimination may occur by either biliary excretion [intrinsic clearance = $CL_{int,bx}(mi)$] or metabolism [intrinsic clearance = $CL_{int,mx}(mi)$; total intrinsic clearance for metabolite $CL_{int,x}(mi) = CL_{int,bx}(mi) + CL_{int,mx}(mi)$]. B_x and $B_x(mi)$ represent the rates of biliary excretion of drug and metabolite, respectively, at point x. QC_A, AC_V, and $QC_V(mi)$ represented input rate of drug and output rates of drug and metabolite, respectively. See text for further details.

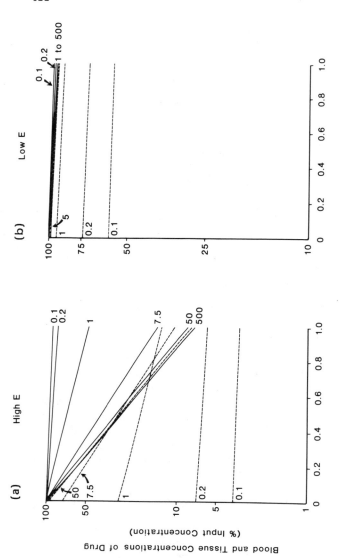

FIGURE 19 The effect of diffusional clearance CL^d on the spatial distributions of a high intrinsic clearance (a) versus a low intrinsic clearance (b) compound. Blood (———) and tissue (– – –) concentrations along the sinusoidal flow path were simulated at different diffusional clearances for a highly (a) and poorly cleared (b) drug (extraction ratios are 0.9 and 0.1, respectively, when free passage of drug occurs). The numbers adjacent to the graphs represent diffusional clearance normalized to flow rate to the organ. (Simulated data were taken from Ref. 66.).

where C_x and $C_{T,x}$ are the concentrations of drug in blood and tissue at point x, respectively, f_B and f_T, denote the unbound fractions of drug to blood and tissue components, respectively; and CL^d and CL_{int} denote the drug diffusional and intrinsic clearances, respectively.

Assuming a lack of binding of drug to tissue and blood components (f_B and $f_T = 1$), the spatial tissue and blood concentrations are compared with the preceding mass balance relationships [Eqs. (12) and (13)]. Tissue concentrations parallel blood concentrations regardless of the diffusional clearance and the intrinsic clearance for evenly distributed enzymes and diffusional clearances (Fig. 19). When the diffusional clearance is small relative to hepatic blood flow, concentrations in blood greatly exceed those in tissue as a result of poor penetration through the membrane. With increasing diffusional clearance, differences in blood and tissue concentrations diminish until the blood equals tissue concentrations (at high ratios of CL^d to Q).

There is a distinct difference between the spatial concentration patterns in liver for a highly cleared (Fig. 19a) versus a poorly cleared compound (Fig. 19b). Despite the high CL_{int} for drug, liver concentrations decrease only slightly from x = 0 to x = L at low CL^d ($CL^d/Q = 0.2$) when drug elimination is rate limited by diffusion. At increasing CL^d, however, the rate-limiting process for elimination changes from drug diffusion to organ perfusion rate (since the intrinsic clearance of drug is high and $\gg$ Q). This is evidenced by the increasing slope for drug concentration profiles with CL^d. In contrast, the slopes for the concentration profiles of poorly cleared drug along the flow path have not varied among all values of diffusional clearances (Fig. 19b). The lack of change in slope of the concentration profiles indicates that the rate-limiting condition for the distribution and elimination of this poorly cleared compound remains the intrinsic clearance ($CL_{int} < CL^d$ and Q).

In the next example, a highly extracted drug ($E_{ss} = 0.9$ when no diffusional barrier is present) is metabolized to a metabolite that is poorly extracted [preformed metabolite extraction ratio $E_{ss}(pmi) = 0.1$ when diffusional barrier is absent for metabolite]. The equations describing the generated metabolite in blood and tissue following input of drug to liver are (66), for generated metabolite in blood,

$$\frac{dC_x(mi)}{dx} = -\frac{CL^d(mi)}{L\,Q} \times$$

$$\left\{ \frac{f_B(mi)C_x(mi)CL_{int}(mi) - [f_B C_x CL^d CL_{int,m}/(CL^d + CL_{int})]}{[CL^d(mi) + CL_{int}(mi)]} \right\}$$

$$(14)$$

and for generated metabolite in tissue,

$$\frac{dC_{T,x}(mi)}{dx} = 0 = \frac{1}{L\,Q}\,\{f_B(mi)C_x(mi)CL^d(mi) + f_T C_{T,x}CL_{int,m}$$

$$- f_T(mi)C_{T,x}(mi)[CL^d(mi) + CL_{int}(mi)]\,\} \qquad (15)$$

where $C_x(mi)$ and $C_{T,x}(mi)$ are the concentrations of generated metabolite in blood and tissue at any point x, respectively; $f_B(mi)$ and $f_T(mi)$ correspond to the unbound fractions of metabolite in blood and tissue; $CL_{int,m}$ is the formation intrinsic clearance of metabolite; and $CL^d(mi)$ and $CL_{int}(mi)$ denote the the diffusional and elimination clearance for metabolite, respectively.

Assuming a lack of binding of drug and metabolite to tissue and blood components, the spatial tissue and blood metabolite concentrations are compared with the preceding mass balance relationships [Eqs. (12) and (15)]. In contrast to that for preformed metabolite, which is independent of barrier effect on drug [Fig. 19b; Eqs. (12) and (13) for drug also apply to this preformed entity], generated metabolite distribution and elimination become highly dependent on drug diffusional clearance CL_d, the total intrinsic clearance for metabolite formation $CL_{int,m}$, and total drug disappearance CL_{int}, in addition to parameters that govern (preformed) metabolite disposition [intrinsic and diffusion clearance for metabolite, $CL_{int}(mi)$ and $CL^d(mi)$].

In examining the intrahepatic concentrations, metabolite concentrations generated in blood and tissue (Fig. 20) differ dramatically from those of preformed metabolite (Fig. 19b): with free passage of drug ($CL^d \gg Q$) but not of metabolite [$CL^d(mi) < Q$], intrahepatic concentrations of the generated metabolite exceed blood metabolite concentrations at any point x; tissue metabolite concentrations are high at the inlet and gradually decrease toward the outlet, whereas blood concentrations increase with distance along the flow path. As $CL^d(mi)$ increases ($\gg Q$), tissue metabolite concentrations accrue with distance along L, as do blood concentrations. The difference in metabolite concentrations in tissue and blood diminishes progressively and eventually disappears at high $CL^d(mi)$ (Fig. 20a).

When a diffusional barrier for drug is present ($CL^d/Q = 0.2$), drug concentrations in tissue remain low and parallel those in blood. Although the general patterns seen at high CL^d are also seen at low CL^d (similar metabolite tissue and blood concentration profiles with x), the magnitudes of the concentrations differ (Fig. 20). At low CL^d, low drug tissue concentrations result in reduced formation and low tissue concentrations of the generated metabolite.

Since the overall rate of drug and metabolite removal is equal to the unbound tissue concentration and their respective intrinsic

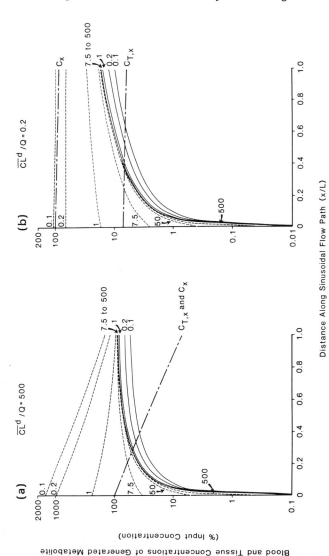

Distance Along Sinusoidal Flow Path (x/L)

FIGURE 20 Spatial distributions of the generated metabolite concentrations along the sinusoidal flow path when its precursor exhibits high (a) or low (b) diffusional clearances. Blood (———) and tissue (— – —) concentrations of generated metabolite along the sinusoidal flow path were simulated for a poorly extracted metabolite (preformed metabolite extraction ratio = 0.1 with free passage of metabolite across membrane) at its various diffusional clearances. When free passage across hepatocyte membrane occurs ($CL_d/Q = 500$), drug exhibits a high extraction ratio (0.9). The formation intrinsic clearance of metabolite is 97% of the total drug intrinsic hepatic clearance. The numbers appearing next to the graphs represent the diffusional clearance of metabolite, CL^d(mi) normalized to Q. C_x and $C_{T,x}$ (— – —) represent both blood and tissue concentrations for drug at point $\bar{x}$.

clearances, tissue concentrations for drug (same equation for preformed metabolite) and generated metabolite are obtained by rearrangement of Equations (13) and (15): for drug,

$$
C_{T,x} = \frac{f_B C_x CL^d}{f_T(CL^d + CL_{int})} \tag{16}
$$

and for generated metabolite.

$$
\begin{aligned}
&C_{T,x}(mi) \\
&= \frac{f_B(mi)C_x(mi)CL^d(mi) + [f_B C_x CL^d CL_{int,m}/(CL^d + CL_{int})]}{f_T(mi)[CL^d(mi) + CL_{int}(mi)]}
\end{aligned} \tag{17}
$$

The changes of elimination rates of drug v_x and metabolite $v_x(mi)$
and the formation rates of metabolite $v_{m,x}$ at any point x become

$$
\frac{dv_x}{dx} = - \frac{f_T C_{T,x} CL_{int}}{L} = - \frac{f_B C_x CL_{int} CL^d}{L(CL^d + CL_{int})} \tag{18}
$$

$$
\begin{aligned}
\frac{dv_x(mi)}{dx} &= - \frac{f_T(mi)C_{T,x}CL_{int}(mi)}{L} \\
&= - \frac{CL_{int}(mi)}{L} \times
\end{aligned}
$$

$$
\left\{ \frac{f_B(mi)C_x(mi)CL^d(mi) + [f_B C_x CL_{int,m}CL^d/(CL^d + CL_{int})]}{[CL^d(mi) + CL_{int}(mi)]} \right\} \tag{19}
$$

$$
\frac{dv_{m,x}}{dx} = \frac{f_T C_{T,x} CL_{int,m}}{L} = \frac{f_B C_x CL_{int,m} CL^d}{L(CL^d + CL_{int})} \tag{20}
$$

The overall removal, expressed as E_{ss}(pmi), for the preformed metabolite may be expressed as

$$E_{ss}(\text{pmi}) = \frac{QC_A(\text{pmi})_{ss} - \bar{v}(\text{pmi})}{QC_A(\text{pmi})_{ss}} \qquad (21)$$

where $\bar{v}$(pmi), the length-averaged rate of removal of preformed metabolite, may be ascertained by integration of Equation (18) (equation same as drug), and the observed steady-state hepatic extraction ratio of the generated metabolite E_{ss}(mi) is

$$E_{ss}(\text{mi}) = \frac{\bar{v}_m - \bar{v}(\text{mi})}{\bar{v}_m} \qquad (22)$$

where $\bar{v}_m$ and $\bar{v}$(mi), the length-averaged rate of formation and removal of primary metabolite, respectively, are obtained by integration of Equations (19) and (20).

A barrier effect has differential implications for the generated and preformed metabolites. For a generated metabolite, a barrier leads to intracellular accumulation of the generated metabolite by preventing efflux after its formation. The accumulated generated metabolite is prone to further elimination by either excretion or metabolism. The hepatocyte membrane, however, poses as a transport barrier and retards entry, thereby preventing removal of the preformed species. As expected, widely different extents of metabolite removal are seen between generated and preformed metabolites, despite the similarity in mechanism.

The steady-state extraction ratios of a preformed metabolite versus a generated metabolite may be pictorially represented (Fig. 21). Variations in hepatic extraction of a preformed metabolite with diffusional clearances of metabolite follow the same trend for drug, another preformed entity (Fig. 17). The apparent hepatic ratio of the generated metabolite E_{ss}(mi), however, shows an inverse relationship with CL^d(mi) and is largely influenced by CL_{int}(mi); CL_{int} and CL^d both exert their effects, albeit to a lesser degress (Fig. 21b and c). Given the same CL_{int}(mi), decreases in CL^d(mi) retard preformed metabolite entry and result in a reduction of the hepatic extraction ratio of the preformed metabolite E_{ss}(pmi) (Fig. 21a). Additionally, a general statement may be made on metabolite extraction and diffusional barrier for the metabolite. In absence of a barrier (CL^d(mi)/Q is large), E_{ss}(pmi) is greater than E_{ss}(mi), a phenomenon explained in Section III.A. With a diffusional barrier, E_{ss}(mi) exceeds E_{ss}(pmi).

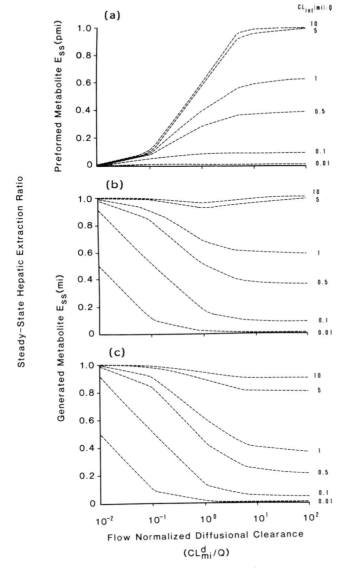

Steady-State Hepatic Extraction Ratio

D. Drug and Metabolite Binding to Blood and Tissue Components

1. Drug and Metabolite Binding to Albumin and Red Blood Cells

It is generally considered that the unbound species traverses lipid membranes and is eliminated. Recent findings have alluded to the fact that drugs bound to albumin are removed at higher clearances than predicted by the unbound fraction (84,85) and have led to the concept of an albumin receptor on the sinusoidal membrane of hepatocytes that couples with albumin and facilitates dissociation of the albumin-drug complex to furnish unbound drug for entry and removal. This concept, however, is highly controversial and has been disputed in some studies (86,87).

Binding of drug and metabolite to blood and/or tissue proteins has been found to inhibit drug removal and metabolite formation and elimination. Intuitively, one expects to observe an inhibitory effect of binding (blood and tissue) on the rate of elimination, although different degrees of influence are expected for highly versus poorly extracted compounds (88−92). Binding of drugs to plasma proteins is perceived to be rapid compared with dissociation of the drug-

---

FIGURE 21 Simulation of the effect of diffusional barrier of metabolite $CL^d(mi)$ and intrinsic clearance of metabolite $CL_{int}(mi)$ on the observed extraction ratio of a preformed $E_{ss}(pmi)$ (a) and generated metabolite $E_{ss}(mi)$ (b) and (c). All enzymic and diffusional clearances are evenly distributed at any point x along L. Drug intrinsic clearance and diffusional clearance were varied: the intrinsic clearance normalized to flow CL_{int}/Q were 10, 5, 1, 0.5, 0.1, 0.01, of which 50% conduces to metabolite formation; drug diffusional clearance normalized to flow were 10^2, 10^1, 10^0, 10^{-1} and 10^{-2}. The steady-state hepatic extraction ratio of preformed metabolite $E_{ss}(pmi)$ increases with $CL^d(mi)$, especially for highly cleared metabolites $[CL_{int}(mi)/Q \gg 1]$. In contrast, $E_{ss}(mi)$ decreases with increasing $CL^d(mi)$ and displays similar trends (b) and (c) and is altered minimally with CL_{int} and CL^d. Qualitatively similar trends are seen for $CL_{int}/Q = 10$ and at $CL^d/Q = 100$ or 10 (b). For other combinations of CL_{int}/Q and CL^d/Q, trends as in c ($CL_{int}/Q = 0.01$ and $CL^d/Q = 10^{-2}$) are seen. $Cl_{int,m}$, when varied from 10 to 100% of CL_{int}, failed to alter the shapes of the graphs (b and c) (data not shown). The numbers adjacent to each graph represent $CL_{int}(mi)/Q$.

protein complex; that is, the on-rate constant k_{on} greatly exceeds the off-rate constant k_{off}. For bound drug, dissociation of this species ($t_{1/2}$ estimated as $0.693/k_{off}$) may exceed the transit time of drug across the organ and delimit elimination (92). The manner in which the dissociation of the bound albumin-drug complex delimits elimination has been demonstrated (93–95).

Drug binding to red cells may be viewed in a manner analogous to that of drug binding to albumin (96). Drug may bind either to red cell proteins on the membrane or to hemoglobin. The on rate is considered rapid. It has been found for some drugs, such as acetazolamide, that equilibrium for binding to red cells, more specifically hemoglobin, is achieved relatively slowly, however, presumably due to slow penetration of drug across the red cell membrane (97).

2. Drug and Metabolite Binding to Tissue Proteins

The effect of tissue binding and partitioning on drug removal was initially shown by Rowland et al. (98). Tissue binding effectively increases the volume of distribution V of drug in the system and, in turn, increases $t_{1/2}$ since $t_{1/2} = 0.693\ V/CL$. By expressing the relative tissue to emergent blood concentrations as the drug partitioning ratio K_p, they found that drugs with a high K_p in liver exhibit a biphasic drug disappearance curve (initial phase, distribution; terminal phase, and elimination) in a recirculating liver perfusion system. With compounds of low K_p and the same hepatic intrinsic clearance, a monophasic curve results, denoting only elimination. Rubin and Tozer (99) further examined the effect of the k_{on} and k_{off} for tissue binding on the rate of drug metabolism according to Michaelis-Menten kinetics. By keeping the ratio of k_{on} to k_{off} as 99:1, a higher K_p has the tendency to increase metabolic clearance with tissue binding, which maintains low unbound concentrations in liver, thereby reducing the tendency for saturation of metabolism.

Differential effects are seen for steady-state conditions with constant drug input to the organ, however. Although the steady-state tissue drug (also for preformed metabolite) and generated metabolite concentrations at point x are dependent on tissue binding [Eqs. (16) and (17)], the rates of drug elimination and metabolite formation and elimination are not [Eqs. (18) through (20)]. Rather, the removal rates are dependent on the unbound concentrations in blood, that is, the unbound fractions in blood for drug and metabolite f_B and $f_B(mi)$.

E. Organ Blood Flow

Blood flow Q affects the transit time $\bar{t}$ of a drug within an eliminating organ in the inverse relationship (99)

$$\bar{t} = \frac{V}{Q} \tag{23}$$

where V is the volume of distribution of drug. A prolonged transit of drug through the liver promotes contact between drug and enzymes, enhancing drug loss, whereas a shortened transit of drug results in reduced removal. The importance of blood flow on drug removal, however, is also dependent on whether a drug is highly or poorly cleared (89,90). Since the overall rate of drug loss is dependent on the presence or absence of diffusional barriers, the enzyme system (K_m and V_{max}) and cofactors, unbound intracellular drug concentration, and organ blood flow, any of these factors may become rate limiting.

1. Drug Elimination and Blood Flow Rate

In an absence of a barrier, free passage of drug occurs, as outlined previously (Sec. III.C.1). For highly cleared drugs, the enzymic system is highly efficient and greatly exceeds blood flow rate. Removal of unbound drug is rapid and affects the equilibrium between bound and unbound drug. Dissociation of the drug-protein complex occurs in an attempt to re-establish equilibrium. Effectively, both unbound and bound drug are removed across the organ. For these highly cleared compounds, with the extraction ratio approaching unity and clearance approaching blood flow, organ blood flow becomes the rate-limiting step in removal. For poorly extracted compounds, the rate-controlling step is not organ blood flow in delivering drug to the organ but the limited capacity of the enzyme system. To be readily eliminated, drug should be in its unbound form. For this reason, blood flow has a greater influence on the clearance of highly rather than poorly extracted compounds. With a higher than normal flow, reduced drug extraction is seen, whereas a reduced flow promotes drug elimination (89,90). These qualitative changes with flow have been shown for highly extracted compounds, such as lidocaine (101,102) and propranolol (102).

2. Metabolite Formation and Elimination and Blood Flow Rate

a. *Sequential Pathways (Scheme 1)* The manner in which organ blood flow affects metabolite removal subsequent to formation has not been well studied. Changes in blood flow rate may affect formation and/or elimination of the metabolite, depending on whether the drug or the metabolite is highly cleared. An increase in flow generally increases metabolite concentrations for those formed and eliminated with high intrinsic clearances (unpublished simulations according to the "well-stirred" and "parallel tube" models of hepatic drug clearances, Ref. 103). When lidocaine is delivered to the once-through perfused rat liver, increased concentrations of MEGX (monoethyl-glycine xylidide), the N-deethylated metabolite of lidocaine (drug and metabolite are highly cleared), are found with increasing flow rates (Fig. 22a) (102,103). When the formation and elimination clearances of metabolite are low or when a drug is removed by competing pathways other than formation of the metabolite in question, however, a succinct relationship may not be readily found between flow and the outflow metabolite concentration (unpublished simulations).

    b. *Competitive Pathways (Scheme 2)* The manner in which blood flow influences the formation of metabolites by competitive pathways is analogous to the relationship between drug disappearance (due to metabolite formation) and flow. Formation of metabolite by an anterior pathway increases with reduced flow, rendering less substrate available for recruitment of downstream hepatocyte activity. With an increase in flow rate, formation of an anterior metabolite is lessened and allows nonmetabolized substrate to reach downstream hepatocytes. This phenomenon has been shown for harmol, which is sulfated (anterior) and glucuronidated (posterior enrichment). On varying

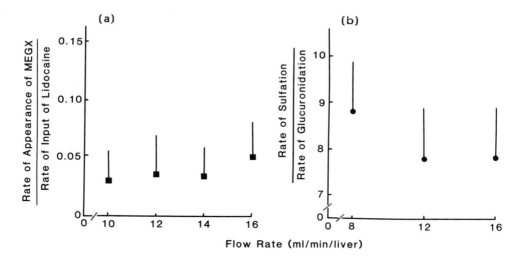

FIGURE 22 Effect of blood flow rate on the efflux of metabolites in a sequential metabolic pathway, as exemplified by MEGX from lidocaine (a) and a competitive pathway, as exemplified by formation of harmol sulfate and glucuronide conjugates (b). The appearance rate of MEGX to input rate of lidocaine (a) and the rate of sulfation to rate of glucuronidation of harmol (b) at steady state were plotted against the flow rates employed in the once-through perfused rat liver preparations. (Data were taken from Refs. 60, 100, and 103).

flow from 12 to 8 and 16 ml/min in the once-through perfused rat liver preparation, the ratio of sulfation to glucuronidation rates at steady-states was shown to increase at decreased flows (Fig. 22b) (60).

F. Cosubstrate Availability

Conjugation pathways require the presence of cofactors or cosubstrates. Limited availability of endogenous cofactors for drug metabolism may produce time-dependent changes in the disposition of drugs. PAPS (3'-phosphoadenosine-5'-phosphosulfate), UDPGA (uridine diphosphoglucuronic acid), GSH (glutathione), acetyl coenzyme A, amino acids (glycine, taurine, and glutamine), S-adenosylmethionine, and UDPG (uridine disphosphoglucose) are cofactors required for conjugation reactions, as outlined in the introduction. The localization of glutathione has been found to be enriched periportally (105), but not much is known about the distribution of other cofactors. These endogenous cofactors exist in varying concentrations (around K_m) in animals and humans (106—108) and are readily depleted (109—112), in which case cosubstrate availability becomes the rate-limiting factor in substrate removal. Levels may be perturbed by ether anesthesia (113), fasting (114—117), ethanol intake (118), the presence of inducers or inhibitors (119), and disease state, such as diabetes (120), that conduce to glucuronide formation.

Although much attention is given to cofactor availability in conjugation reactions, that the supply of nicotinamide and adenine nucleotides may be rate limiting for NADH- and NADPH-dependent mixed-function oxidation has been less emphasized. Biosynthesis of adenine nucleotides from intermediary metabolites is influenced by glycolytic, pentose phosphate pathway, and tricarboxylic acid cycle intermediates. p-Nitroanisole 0-demethylation is shown to be stimulated by low ethanol concentrations (0.2 mM) with fasted rate livers (121) but inhibited at high ethanol concentrations (122). These paradoxical effects have been attributed to the production of NADH from NAD^+ and to ethanol oxdiation (123). At low ethanol concentrations, NADH produced in oxidations of ethanol and acetaldehyde furnished reducing equivalents for mixed-function oxidation, whereas when NADH is produced at high rates it decreases intracellular concentrations of malate, aspartate, and α-ketoglutarate, key intermediates for substrate shuttle mechanisms that transport reducing equivalents between the mitochondrial and cytosolic spaces. Therefore, high concentrations of ethanol produce redox inhibition of mixed-function oxidation in intact cells indirectly by interfering with the transfer of mitochondrial reducing equivalents to the extramitochondrial site of NADPH cytochrome P-450 (122). By contrast, sorbitol stimulated p-nitroanisole

metabolism by producing NADPH via the pentose phosphate shunt
(124).

G. Other Considerations

1. Reversible Metabolism

Interconversion of a drug and its metabolite(s) is readily recognized
when the administration of drug gives rise to metabolite and that of
metabolite produces drug. This relationship between drug and metabolite modulates the disposition of drug and metabolite. The metabolite
acts as a storage compartment for drug and confers compartmental
characteristics to drug (the number of compartments for drug includes
those for metabolite). Drug and metabolite eventually decay in unison
under first-order conditions (125—127). Some examples of reversible
metabolism include oxidation-reduction [prednisone and prednisolone
(127), sulindac and its sulfide (129), and methylprednisone and
methylprednisolone (130)], acetylation and deacetylation [procainamide
and acetylprocainamide (131)], and conjugation-deconjugation reactions.
    Some of these reversible reactions are not readily recognized: a
substrate that is conjugated is prone to deconjugation during its traversal through an eliminating organ, and effectively, formation of a conjugated metabolite is a net result of conjugation-deconjugation. For
example, rates of production of glucuronide and sulfate conjugates
represent a balance of conjugation minus deconjugation rates, as
demonstrated in the formation of 4-methylumbelliferone (4-MU) conjugates in microdissected human liver tissues. Metabolic data for 4-MU
and its conjugates revealed that conjugation-deconjugation activities
overlap among liver tissues: transferase (sulfotransferases and UDP-
glucuronosyltransferases) activities for formation of 4-MU sulfate
and glucuronide are periportal and pericentral, respectively, and
hydrolase activities for deconjugation (arylsulfatase and β-glucuro-
nidases) are evenly distributed (132). The coexistence of conjugation
and deconjugation pathways, however, is demonstrated only when one
of these pathways is stimulated or inhibited, resulting in a change
in the rate of appearance of the conjugate (133). For example, addition
of epinephrine to perfused rat livers reduced the production of p-
nitrophenylglucuronide when epinephrine, reacting with α-adrenergic
receptors and elevating cytosolic free Ca^{2+}, stimulated β-glucuronidase
activities (132). Deconjugation of 4-MU sulfate to 4-MU is followed
by subsequent conjugation to 4-MU glucuronide in the once-through
perfused rat liver (134). Deconjugation rates in vivo (or in intact
liver) for these polar conjugates (4-MU sulfate and glucuronide),
however, drastically underestimate activities of the hydrolases when
a diffusional barrier exists for the polar conjugates and poses as
the rate-controlling step in deconjugation.

2. Enterohepatic Circulation

Enterohepatic circulation of drugs and metabolites, not unlike reversible metabolism, is another mechanism that prolongs the duration of a drug in the body. Biliarily excreted drug and/or metabolite (typically conjugates) enter the intestine for reabsorption. For polar conjugates, reabsorption is facilitated after hydrolysis, effected mostly by bacterial or brush-border enzymes. This enterohepatic cycle presents an effective mechanism of drug storage, either as itself or as metabolites, in the gall bladder or intestine. Re-entry of drug into the body results in accumulation. A close analogy may also be drawn to bladder resorption of drugs (and metabolites); after hydrolysis of metabolites in urine, resorption of drug also leads to drug accumulation. In these cases, the fraction of dose absorbed exceeds 1 when the contribution of enterohepatic circulation is not considered.

The consequence of cholestasis on the accumulation profile of a drug was demonstrated by Harrison and Gibaldi (135). The phenomenon of enterohepatic circulation, with a lag time, has been further elaborated to describe the spurious behavior of concentration versus time profile (136—138). Morphine (137) and phenolphthalein (138), which form the respective glucuronide conjugates, undergo avid enterohepatic circulation. Indomethicin and metabolites (139) and sulindac and metabolites (140), as well as many drug conjugates, partake in the phenomenon. Biliary excretion followed by reabsorption as aglycone leads to drug accumulation (141), and when a narrow therapeutic window exists, the extent of biliary excretion and reabsorption is often found to correlate with toxicity (140). Tse et al. (141) showed that this fraction of biliary excreted drug equivalents that is reabsorbed may be estimated experimentally with knowledge of the areas under the curve of drug, with and without interruption of enterohepatic circulation, and the fraction of dose excreted into bile.

There is a concern about the estimation of drug bioavailability when it is estimated by the relationship AUC^{PO}/AUC^{IV} in the presence of enterohepatic circulation. Assuming that all drug and metabolites excreted into bile are recycled, Pang and Gillette (143) and Shepherd et al. (144,145) revealed that the theoretical relationship holds when the liver is the only organ for drug removal. Intestine drug metabolism conducive to metabolite formation, however, invalidates this estimate (143). However, humans, who possess a gall bladder, release bile at random intervals, more so after stimulation by food intake. This undoubtedly brings about spurious extents of enterohepatic circulation of drugs and metabolites (140). Moreover, when other eliminating organs conduce to either drug removal or metabolite formation (e.g., kidney), different routes of drug administration (intravenous versus po-oral) may result in varying extents of metabolite formation and biliary excretion and, therefore, enterohepatic circulation.

IV. CONCLUDING REMARKS

Compartmental modeling that ignores biochemical, physiological,
anatomical, and circulatory patterns within intact eliminating organs
must be viewed with caution in attempting to describe metabolite
kinetics. A better definition may be arrived at if first-pass sequential
elimination of a generated metabolite is considered. This aspect has
been routinely neglected in compartmental modeling of metabolite
behavior and has yet to be considered in treatments on reversible
metabolism and enterohepatic circulation.

Generated metabolites are categorically different from preformed
metabolites, albeit the same processes for transfer and removal are
present. Additionally, generated metabolites depend on uptake, biotransformation, and competing pathways of drug, not only within
metabolite formation organs but also other eliminating organs (146).
The remarkably different fates between generated and preformed
metabolites and the causative factors and consequences have been
outlined. Knowledge of these biologic factors, when integrated with
kinetics, should pose as a more exacting and powerful tool to our
understanding of the underlying events occurring within eliminating
organs and, ultimately, the body.

EXPLANATION OF SYMBOLS

Terminologies pertaining to drug appear without further classification;
terminologies pertaining to the generated metabolite (mi) and preformed
metabolite (pmi) are further classified.

L = length of the sinusoid, assumed to be identical for all sinusoids
$V_{max,x,cell}$ = maximum velocity (enzymatic activity) for an enzyme
system for cell at any point x along L
$V_{max,x}$ = enzymatic activity for an enzyme system for all hepatocytes
at any point x ($\Sigma\, V_{max,x,cell}$)
$\bar{V}_{max}$ = length-averaged maximum velocity (enzymatic activity) for an
enzyme in liver ($\int_0^L V_{max,x}\, dx/L$)
K_m = Michaelis-Menten constant for an enzymatic reaction, taken to be
identical among cells

For clearance terms, subscript x denotes the concentrations at
point x. When the intrinsic clearance or diffusional clearance is
identical for any point x along L, the intrinsic clearance $CL_{int,x}$ or
diffusional clearance CL_x^d at any point x equals length-averaged
instrinsic clearance $\overline{CL}_{int}$ or $\overline{CL}^d$.

$CL_{int,m,x}$ = hepatic intrinsic clearance of drug in the formation of mi, at point x

$CL_{int,b,x}$ = hepatic biliary intrinsic clearance of drug, at point x

$CL_{int,o,x}$ = hepatic intrinsic clearance of drug of pathways other than biliary excretion and formation of mi, at point x

$CL_{int,x}$ = total hepatic intrinsic clearance for drug elimination, sum of $CL_{int,b,x}$, $CL_{int,m,x}$, and $CL_{int,o,x}$, at point x

$\overline{CL}_{int}$ = length-averaged hepatic intrinsic clearance for drug removal $(\int_0^L CL_{int,x}\, dx/L)$

CL_x^d = diffusional clearance of drug in liver, at point x

$\overline{CL}^d$ = length-averaged diffusional clearance of drug in liver

$CL_{int,m,x}(mi)$ = hepatic metabolic intrinsic clearance of mi, at point x

$CL_{int,b,x}(mi)$ = hepatic biliary intrinsic clearance of mi, at point x

$CL_{int,x}(mi)$ = total hepatic intrinsic clearance for mi elimination; sum of $CL_{int,b,x}(mi)$ and $CL_{int,m,x}(mi)$, at point x

$\overline{CL}_{int}(mi)$ = length-averaged hepatic intrinsic clearance for mi removal $(\int_0^L CL_{int,x}(mi)\, dx/L)$

$CL_x^d(mi)$ = diffusional clearance of mi in liver, at point x

$\overline{CL}^d(mi)$ = length-averaged diffusional clearance for mi in liver

E_{ss} = steady-state hepatic extraction ratio of drug; further qualifications with (mi) and (pmi) denote those for the generated and preformed metabolites, respectively.

C_A, C_V = steady-state input and output concentrations

Q = total hepatic blood flow rate

V = volume of distribution of drug in liver

$\overline{t}$ = mean transit time of drug in liver

B, T = blood and tissue (subscripts)

f = unbound fractions (in blood and tissue)

C = concentration in blood

C_T = concentration in tissue

x = point x (subscript)

mi, pmi = generated and preformed metabolites (subscripts)

v_x = total rate of drug elimination at point x in liver

$v_x(mi)$ = total rate of elimination of generated metabolite (mi) at point x in liver

$v_{m,x}$ = rate of formation of mi from drug at point x in liver

$\overline{v}_m$ = length-averaged rate of formation of mi from drug in liver

$\overline{v}(mi)$ = length-averaged rate of elimination of mi in liver

ACKNOWLEDGMENTS

The authors thank Mary Jean Clements for performance of simulations and Marie V. St-Pierre for electron microscopy. This work was supported by Canadian MRC grants MA-9104, MA-9765, ME-9757, and DG-263 and a grant from US-HHS, GM-38250.

REFERENCES

1. D. A. Wiersma and R. A. Roth. Clearance of 5-hydroxytryptamine by rat lung and liver: The importance of relative perfusion and intrinsic clearance. J. Pharmacol. Exp. Ther. 212: 97–102, 1980.
2. M. Gibaldi, R. N. Boyes, and S. Feldman. Influence of first-pass effect on bioavailability. J. Pharm. Sci. 61: 1338–1340, 1972.
3. K. R. Emslie, M. C. Smail, I. C. Calder, S. J. Hart, and T. D. Tange. Paracetamol and the isolated perfused kideny: Metabolism and functional effects. Xenobiotica 11: 43–50, 1981.
4. J. R. Dawson and J. W. Bridges. Intestinal microsomal drug metabolism. A comparison of rat and guinea-pig enzymes, and of rat crypt and villous tip cell enzymes. Biochem. Pharmacol. 30: 2415–2420, 1981.
5. M. K. Cassidy and J. B. Houston. In vivo capacity and extra-hepatic enzymes to conjugate phenol. Drug Metab. Dispos. 12: 619–624, 1984.
6. H. D. Colby and R. C. Rumbaugh. Adrenal drug metabolism. In Extrahepatic Metabolism of Drugs and Other Foreign Compounds Chap. 5. Edited by T. E. Gram. SP Medical and Scientific, Spectrum Publications, New York, 1980, pp. 239–266.
7. A. Pannather, P. Jenner, B. Testa, and J. C. Etter. The skin as a drug metabolizing-organ. Drug Metab. Rev. 8: 319–343, 1978.
8. D. E. Drayer. Pharmacologically active drug metabolies: Therapeutic and toxic activities, plasma and urine data in man, accumulation in renal failure. Clin. Pharmacokinet. 1: 426–443, 1977.
9. A. J. Atkinson, Jr., and J. M. Strong. Effect of active drug metabolites in plasma level-response correlations. J. Pharmacokinet. Biopharm. 5: 95–109, 1977.
10. A. J. Cummings and B. K. Martin. Excretion and accrual of drug metabolites. Nature 200: 1296–1297, 1963.
11. A. J. Cummings, B. K. Martin and G. S. Park. Kinetic considerations relating to the accrual and elimination of drug metabolites. Br. J. Pharmacol. Chemother. 29: 136–149, 1967.
12. B. K. Martin. Treatment of data from drug urinary data. Nature 214: 247–249, 1967.
13. E. Nelson. Percent absorbed versus time plots from metabolite levels in blood. J. Pharm. Sci. 44: 1075–1076, 1965.
14. M. Rowland and S. Riegelman. Pharmacokinetics of acetylsalicylic acid and salicylic acid after intravenous administration in man. J. Pharm. Sci. 57: 1313–1319, 1968.

15. K. S. Pang and J. R. Gillette. Sequential first-pass elimination of a metabolite derived from a precursor. J. Pharmacokinet. Biopharm. 7: 275–290, 1978.

16. K. S. Pang and J. R. Gillette. Metabolite pharmacokinetics: Methods for simultaneous estimates of elimination rate constants of a drug and metabolite. A commentary. Drug Metab. Dispos. 8: 39–43, 1980.

17. J. R. Gillette. Pharmacokinetic factors governing steady-state concentrations of foreign chemicals and their metabolites. In Environmental Chemicals, Enzyme Function and Human Disease. Ciba Foundation 76. Elsevier/North Holland, Amsterdam, 1980, pp. 191–217.

18. K. S. Pang and K. C. Kwan. A commentary. Methods and assumptions in kinetic estimation of metabolite formation. Drug. Metab. Dispos. 11: 79–84, 1983.

19. K. S. Pang. Metabolite pharmacokinetics: The area under the curve of metabolite and the fractional rate of metabolism of a drug after different routes of administration for renally and hepatically cleared drugs and metabolites. J. Pharmacokinet. Biopharm. 9: 477–487, 1981.

20. J. B. Houston. Drug metabolite kinetics. Pharmacol. Ther. 15: 521–552, 1982.

21. E. A. Lane and R. H. Levy. Metabolite to parent drug concentration ratio as a function of parent drug extraction ratio: Cases of nonportal route of administration. J. Pharmacokinet. Biopharm. 9: 489–496, 1981.

22. K. K. Chan. A simple integrated method for drug and derived metabolite kinetics. An application of statistical moment theory. Drug Metab. Dispos. 10: 474–479, 1982.

23. C. L. Devane and W. J. Jusko. Drug and metabolite concentrations combined in predicting stead-state concentrations from test doses. Biopharm. Drug Dispos. 4: 19–29, 1983.

24. J. B. Houston and G. Taylor. Drug metabolite concentration-time profiles: Influence of route of drug administration. Br. J. Clin. Pharmacol. 17: 385–394, 1984.

25. P. J. M. Klippert and J. Noordhoek. Influence of administration route and blood sampling site on the area under the curve. Assessment of gut wall, liver, and lung metabolism from a physiological model. Drug Metab. Dispos. 11: 62–66, 1983.

26. P. J. M. Klippert and J. Noordhoek. The area under the curve of metabolites for drugs and metabolites cleared by the liver and extrahepatic organs. Its dependence on the route of precursor drug. Drug Metab. Dispos. 13: 97–101, 1985.

27. K. S. Pang. A review of metabolite kinetics. J. Pharmacokinet. Biopharm. 13: 633–662, 1985.

28. E. A. Lane and R. H. Levy. Fractions metabolized in a triangular metabolic system: Cinromide and two metabolites in Rhesus monkey. J. Pharmacokinet. Biopharm. 13: 373–386, 1985.

29. W. F. Bayne and S. S. Hwang. General method for evaluating the fraction of irreversible organ clearance due to conversion of drug to a primary metabolite. J. Pharm. Sci. 74: 722–726, 1985.

30. K. K. Chan, M. Bolger, and K. S. Pang. Statistical moment theory in metabolite kinetics. Anal. Chem. 57: 2145–2151 1985.

31. M. Weiss. Metabolite residence time: Influence of the first-pass effect. Br. J. Clin. Pharmacol. 22: 121–122, 1986.

32. C. A. Goresky, G. G. Bach, and A. J. Schwab. Distributed-in-space product formation in vivo: Its consequences. Submitted.

32. C. A. Goresky. Uptake in the liver: The nature of the process. Int. Rev. Physiol. 21: 65–101, 1980.

33. M. Silverman and C. A. Goresky. A unified kinetic hypothesis of carrier mediated transport and its applications. Biophys. J. 5: 487–509, 1965.

34. C. A. Goresky, W. H. Ziegler, and G. G. Bach. Capillary exchange modeling barrier-limited and flow-limited distribution. Circ. Res. 27: 739–747, 1970.

35. C. A. Goresky and H. L. Goldsmith. Capillary-tissue exchange kinetics: Diffusional interactions between adjacent capillaries. Adv. Exp. Biol. Med. 37B: 733–781, 1973.

36. A. L. Jones, G. T. Hradek, R. H. Renston, K. Y. Wong, G. Karlaganis, and G. Paumgartner. Autoradiographic evidence for hepatic lobular concentration gradient of bile acid derivative. Am. J. Physiol. 238: G233–G237, 1980.

37. J. J. Gumicio, D. L. Miller, M. D. Krauss, and C. C. Zanolli. Transport of fluoroescent compounds into hepatocytes and the resultant zonal labeling of the hepatic acinus in the rat. Gastroenterology 80: 639–664, 1981.

38. D. L. Gumicio, J. J. Gumicio, J. A. P. Wilson, C. Cutter, M. Krauss, R. Caldwell, and E. Chen. Albumin influences sulfobromophthalein transport by hepatocytes of each acinar zone. Am. J. Physiol. 246: G86–G95, 1984.

39. A. M. Rappaport. The structural and functional units in the human liver (liver acinus). Anat. Rec. 130: 673–689, 1958.

40. A. M. Rappaport. Hepatic blood flow: Morphologic aspects and physiologic regulation. Int. Rev. Physiol. 21: 1–63, 1980.

41. J. J. Gumicio and D. L. Miller. Functional implications of liver cell heterogeneity. Gastroenterology 80: 393–403, 1980.

42. A. M. de Leeue and D. L. Knook. The ultrastructure of sinusoidal liver cells in the intact rat at various ages. In Pharmacological, Morphological and Physiological Aspects of Aging. Edited by C. F. A. van Bezooijen. Eurage, Rijswik, 1984, pp. 91–96.

43. J. L. Boyer, E. Elias, and T. J. Layden. The paracellular pathway and bile formation. Yale J. Biol. Med. 52: 61—67, 1979.

44. T. Matsumara, T. Kashiwagi, H. Meren, and R. G. Thurman. Gluconeogenesis predominates in the periportal regions of the liver lobule. Eur. J. Biochem. 144: 409—414, 1982.

45. T. Matsumara and R. G. Thurman. Predominance of glycolysis in pericentral regions of the liver lobule. Eur. J. Biochem. 140: 229—234, 1982.

46. L. W. Wattenberg and J. L. Leong. Histochemical demonstration of reduced pyridine nucleotide dependent polycyclic hydrocarbon metabolizing systems. J. Histochem. Cytochem. 10: 412—420, 1962.

47. J. Baron, J. A. Redding, and F. P. Guengerich. Immunohistochemical localization of cytochromes P-450 in rat liver. Life Sci. 23: 2627—2632, 1978.

48. J. Baron, R. A. Redick and F. P. Guengerich. An immunohistochemical study on the localizations and distributions of phenobarbital- and 3-methylcholanthrene-inducible cytochrome P-450 within the livers of untreated rats. J. Biol. Chem. 256: 5931—5937, 1981.

49. J. A. Redick, J. Baron, and F. P. Guengerich. Immunohistochemical localization of glutathione-S-transferases in livers of untreated rats. J. Biol. Chem. 257: 15200—15203, 1982.

50. D. Ullrich, G. Fisher, N. Katz, and K. W. Bock. Intralobular distribution of UDP-glucuronosyltransferase in livers from untreated, 3-methylcholanthrene- and phenobarbital-treated rats. Chem. Biol. Interact. 48: 181—190, 1984.

51. J. R. deBaun, J. Y. R. Smith, E. C. Miller, and J. A. Miller. Reactivity in vivo of the carcinogen N-hydroxy-2-acetylaminofluorene: Increase by sulfate ion. Science 167: 184—186, 1971.

52. J. H. N. Meerman and G. J. Mulder. Prevention of the hepatotoxic action of N-hydroxy-2-acetylaminofluorene in the rat by inhibition of N-O-sulfation by pentachlorophenol. Life Sci. 28: 2361—2365, 1981.

53. K. S. Pang and J. A. Terrell. Retrograde perfusion to probe the heterogeneous distribution of drug metabolizing activities in rats. J. Pharmacol. Exp. Ther. 216: 339—348, 1981.

54. K. S. Pang, L. Waller, K. K. Chan, and M. G. Horning. Metabolite kinetics: Formation of acetaminophen from deuterated and non-deuterated phenacetin and acetanilide on acetaminophen sulfation kinetics in the perfused rat liver preparation. J. Pharmacol. Exp. Ther. 222: 14—19, 1982.

55. K. S. Pang, W. F. Cherry, and K. K. Chan. Precursor effects on the sequential metabolism of metabolite: p-Alkyl precursors of acetaminophen on acetaminophen sulfation in perfused rat liver. Fed. Proc 46: abstract 30635, 1987.

56. J. G. Conway, F. C. Kauffman, S. Ji, and R. G. Thurman. Rates of sulfation and glucuronidation of 7-hydroxycoumarin in the periportal and pericentral regions of the liver lobule. Mol. Pharmacol. 22: 509—516, 1982.

57. H. Koster, I. Halsema, E. Scholtens, J. H. N. Meerman, K. S. Pang, and G. J. Mulder. Selective inhibition of sulfate conjugation in the rat. Pharmacokinetics and characterization of the inhibitory effect of 2,6-dichloro-4-nitrophenol. Biochem. Pharmacol. 31: 1919—1924, 1982.

58. K. S. Pang, H. Koster, I. C. M., E. Scholtens, R. N. Stillwell, and G. J. Mulder. Normal and retrograde perfusion to probe the zonal distribution of sulfation and glucuronidation activities of harmol in the perfused rat liver preparation. J. Pharmacol. Exp. Ther. 224: 7—653, 1983.

59. J. G. Conway, F. C. Kauffman, T. Tsukada, and R. G. Thurman. Glucuronidation of 7-hydroxycoumarin in periportal and pericentral regions of the liver lobule. Mol. Pharmacol. 25: 487—493, 1984.

60. J. R. Dawson, J. G. Weitering, G. J. Mulder, R. N. Stillwell, and K. S. Pang. Alteration of transit time and direction of flow to probe the heterogeneous distribution of conjugation activities for harmol in the perfused rat liver preparation. J. Pharmacol. Exp. Ther. 234: 691—697, 1985.

61. M. E. Morris, V. Yuen, and K. S. Pang. Metabolism of gentisamide in the perfused rat liver in situ preparation. Fed. Proc. 44: abstract 4944, 1985.

62. X. Xu and K. S. Pang. Gentisamide metabolism in perfused rat liver preparation: As a generated metabolite of salicylamide and as a preformed metabolite. Pharmacologist 28: abstract 157, 1986.

63. R. A. Weisiger, C. M. Mendel, and R. R. Cavalieri. The hepatic sinusoid is not well-stirred: Estimation of the degree of axial mixing by analysis of lobular concentration gradients formed during uptake of thyroxine by the perfused rat liver. J. Pharm. Sci. 75: 233—237, 1986.

64. I. A. M. de Lannoy and K. S. Pang. A commentary. The presence of diffusional barriers on metabolite kinetics. I. Enalaprilat as a generated versus preformed metabolite. Drug Metab. Dispos. 14: 513—520, 1986.

65. H. Sato, Y. Sugiyama, S. Miyauchi, Y. Sawada, T. Iga, and M. Hanano. A simulation study on the effect of a uniform diffusional barrier across hepatocytes on drug metabolism by evenly or unevenly distributed uni-enzyme in the liver. J. Pharm. Sci. 75: 3—8, 1986.

66. I. A. M. de Lannoy and K. S. Pang. Diffusional barriers on drug and metabolite kinetics. Drug Metab. Dispos. 15: 51—58, 1987.

67. K. S. Pang, P. Kong, J. A. Terrell, and R. E. Billings. Metabolism of acetaminophen and phenacetin by isolated rat hepatocytes. A system in which the spatial organization inherent in the liver is disrupted. Drug Metab. Dispos. 13: 42—50, 1985.

68. K. S. Pang. The effect of intracellular distribution of drug metabolizing enzymes on the kinetics of stable metabolite formation and elimination by liver: First-pass effects. Drug Metab. Rev. 14: 61—76, 1983.

69. T. T. Kawabata, F. P. Guengerich, and J. Baron. An immuno-histochemical study on the localization and distribution of epoxide hydrolase within livers of untreated rats. Mol. Pharmacol. 20: 309—314, 1981.

70. J. A. Redick, W. B. Jakoby, and J. Baron. Immunohistochemical localization of glutathione-S-transferase in livers of untreated rats. J. Biol. Chem. 257: 15200—15203, 1982.

71. K. S. Pang and J. R. Gillette. Kinetics of metabolite formation and elimination in the perfused rat liver preparation: Differences between the elimination of preformed acetaminophen and acetaminophen formed from phenacetin. J. Pharmacol. Exp. Ther. 207: 178—194, 1978.

72. K. S. Pang and R. N. Stillwell. An understanding of the role of enzymic localization of the liver on metabolite kinetics: A computer simulation. J. Pharmacokinet. Biopharm. 11: 451—468, 1983.

73. R. H. Levy, E. A. Lane, M. Guyot, A. Brachet-Liermain, B. Cenraud, and P. Loiseau. Analysis of parent drug-metabolite relationship in the presence of an inducer. Application to the carbamazepine-clobazam interaction in normal man. Drug Metab. Dispos. 11: 286—291, 1983.

74. M. E. Morris and K. S. Pang. The competition between two enzymes for substrate removal in liver: Modulating effects of competitive pathways. J. Pharmacokinet. Biopharm. 15: 473—496, 1987.

75. K. S. Pang, H. Koster, I. C. M. Halsema. E. Scholtens, and G. J. Mulder. Aberrant pharmacokinetics of harmol in the perfused rat liver preparation: Sulfate and glucuronide conjugation. J. Pharmacol. Exp. Ther. 219: 134—140, 1981.

76. S. Hendrix-Tracy, S. M. Wallace, K. W. Hindmarsh, G. M. Wyant, and A. Danikewich. The effect of acetaminophen administration on its disposition and body stores of sulfate. Eur. J. Clin. Pharmacol. 30: 273—278, 1986.

77. L. Accatino and F. R. Simon. Identification and characterization of a bile acid receptor in isolated liver surface membranes. J. Clin. Invest. 57: 1280—1292, 1975.

78. B. F. Scharschmidt, J. G. Waggoner, and P. D. Berk. Hepatic organic anion uptake in the rat. J. Clin. Invest. 56: 1280—1292, 1975.

79. D. L. Eaton and C. D. Klaassen. Carrier-mediated transport of ouabain in isolated hepatocytes. J. Pharmacol. Exp. Ther. 205: 480–488, 1978.

80. K. Iwamoto, D. L. Eaton, and C. D. Klaassen. Uptake of morphine and nalorphine by isolated rat hepatocytes. J. Pharmacol. Exp. Ther. 206: 181–189, 1978.

81. M. Ookhtens, K. Hobdy, M. C. Corvasce, T. Y. Aw, and N. Kaplowitz. Sinusoidal efflux of glutathione in the perfused rat liver. Evidence for a carrier-mediated process. J. Clin. Invest. 75: 258–265, 1985.

82. K. S. Pang, W. F. Cherry, J. A. Terrell, and E. H. Ulm. Disposition of enalapril and its diacid metabolite, enalaprilat, in a perfused rat liver preparation. Presence of a diffusional barrier into hepatocytes. Drug Metab. Dispos. 12: 309–312, 1984.

83. J. R. Gillette and K. S. Pang. Theoretical aspects of pharmaco-kinetic drug interactions. Clin. Pharmacol. Ther. 22: 623–639, 1977.

84. R. Weisiger, J. Gollan, and R. Ockner. Receptor for albumin on the liver cell surface may mediate uptake of fatty acids and other albumin-bound substances. Science 211: 1048–1051, 1981.

85. E. L. Forker and B. A. Luxon. Albumin-mediated transport of rose bengal by perfused rat liver. Kinetics of the reaction at the cell surface. J. Clin. Invest. 72: 1764–1771, 1983.

86. M. Inoue, K. Okajima, S. Nagase, and Y. Morino. Plasma clearance of sulfobromophthalein and its interaction with hepatic binding proteins in normal and analbuminemic rats: Is plasma albumin essential for vectorial transport of organic anions in liver? Proc. Natl. Acad. Sci. USA 80: 7654–7658, 1983.

87. S. C. Tsao, Y. Sugiyama, Y. Sawada, S. Nagase, T. Iga, and M. Hanano. Effect of albumin on hepatic uptake of warfarin in normal and analbuminemic mutant rats: Analysis by multiple indicator dilution method. J. Pharmacokinet. Biopharm. 14: 51–65, 1986.

88. G. Levy and A. Yacobi. Effect of plasma protein binding on elimination of warfarin. 53: 805–806, 1974.

89. G. R. Wilkinson and D. G. Shand. Commentary. A physiological approach to hepatic drug clearance. Clin. Pharmacol. Ther. 18: 377–390, 1975.

90. K. S. Pang and M. Rowland. Hepatic clearance of drugs. I. Theoretical consideration of a "well-stirred" model and a "parallel tube" model. Influence of hepatic blood flow, plasma and blood cells binding, and the hepatocellular activity on hepatic drug clearance. J. Pharmacokinet. Biopharm. 5: 625–653, 1977.

91. U. Gartner, R. J. Stockert, W. G. Levine, and A. W. Wolkoff. Effect of nafenopin on the uptake of bilirubin and sulfobromo-phthalein by the isolated perfused rat liver. Gastroenterology 83: 1163–1169, 1982.

92. J. R. Gillette. Overview of drug-protein binding. Proc. Natl. Acad. Sci. USA 226: 6–17, 1973.

93. J. A. Jensen. Influence of plasma protein binding kinetics on hepatic clearance assessed from a "tube" model and a "well-stirred" model. J. Pharmacokinet. Biopharm. 9: 15–26, 1981.

94. J. D. Huang and S. Øie. Hepatic elimination of drugs with concentration-dependent binding. J. Pharmacokinet. Biopharm. 12: 67–81, 1984.

95. R. A. Weisiger. Dissociation from albumin. A potentially rate-limiting step in clearances of substances by the liver. Proc. Natl. Acad. Sci. USA 82: 1563–1567, 1985.

96. C. A. Goresky, G. G. Bach, and B. E. Nadeau. Red cell carriage of label. Its limiting effect on the exchange of materials in the liver. Circ. Res. 36: 328–351, 1975.

97. S. M. Wallace and S. Riegelman. Uptake of acetazolamide by human erythrocytes in vitro. J. Pharm. Sci. 66: 729–731, 1977.

98. M. Rowland, L. Z. Benet, and G. G. Graham. Clearance concepts in pharmacokinetics. J. Pharmacokinet. Biopharm. 1: 123–136, 1973.

99. G. M. Rubin and T. N. Tozer. Hepatic binding and Michaelis-Menten metabolism of drugs. J. Pharm. Sci. 75: 660–663, 1986.

100. K. S. Pang and M. Rowland. Hepatic clearance of drugs. II. Experimental evidence for acceptance of the "well-stirred" model over the "parallel tube" model using lidocaine in the perfused rat liver in situ preparation. J. Pharmacokinet. Biopharm. 5: 655–680, 1977.

101. C. A. Goresky. A linear method for determining liver sinusoidal and extravascular volumes. Am. J. Physiol. 204: 626–640, 1963.

102. D. G. Shand, D. M. Kornhauser, and G. R. Wilkinson. Effect of route of administration and blood flow on hepatic drug elimination. J. Pharmacol. Exp. Ther. 195: 424–432, 1975.

103. K. S. Pang and M. Rowland. Hepatic clearance of drugs. III. Additional experimental evidence supporting the "well-stirred" model, using metabolite (MEGX) generated from lidocaine under varying hepatic blood flow rates and linear conditions in the perfused rat liver in situ preparation. J. Pharmacokinet. Biopharm. 5: 681–699, 1977.

104. K. S. Pang, J. A. Terrell, S. D. Nelson, K. F. Feuer, M.-J. Clements, and L. Endrenyi. An enzyme-distributed system for lidocaine metabolism in the perfused rat liver preparation. J. Pharmacokinet. Biopharm. 14: 107–130, 1986.

105. M. T. Smith, N. Loveridge, E. R. Wills, and J. Chayen. The distribution of glutathione in the rat lobule. Biochem. J. 182: 103–108, 1979.

106. G. J. Mulder, and K. Keulemans. Metabolism of inorganic sulfate in the isolated perfused rat liver. Biochem. J. 176: 959–965, 1978.

107. R. L. Dills, and C. D. Klaassen. The effect of inhibitors of mitochondrial energy production on hepatic glutathione, UDP-glucuronic acid, and adenosine 3'-phosphate-5'-phosphosulfate concentrations. Drug Metab. Dispos 14: 190–196, 1986.

108. J. D. Adams, Jr., B. H. Lauterburg, and J. R. Mitchell. Plasma glutathione and glutathione disulfide in the rat: regulation and response to oxidative stress. J. Pharmacol. Exp. Ther. 227: 749–754, 1983.

109. K. R. Krijgsheld, E. Scholtens, and G. J. Mulder. An evaluation of methods to decrease the availability of inorganic sulfate for sulfate conjugation in the rat in vivo. Biochem. Pharmacol. 30: 1973–1979, 1981.

110. R. E. Galinsky, and G. Levy. Dose- and time-dependent elimination of acetaminophen in rats: Pharmacokinetic implications of cosubstrate depletion. J. Pharmacol. Exp. Ther. 210: 14–20, 1981.

111. J. J. Hjelle, G. A. Hazelton, and C. D. Klaassen. Acetaminophen decreases adenosine 3'-phosphate 5'-phosphosulfate and uridine diphosphoglucuronic acid in rat liver. Drug Metab. Dispos. 13: 35–41, 1985.

112. S. R. Howell, G. A. Hazelton and C. D. Klaassen. Depletion of hepatic UDP-glucuronic acid by drugs that are glucuronidated. J. Pharmacol. Exp. Ther. 236: 610–614, 1986.

113. H. Aune, H. Olsen, and J. Mørland. Diethyl ether influence on the metabolism of antipyrine, paracetamol and sulphanilamide in isolated rat hepatocytes. Br. J. Anaesth. 53: 621–626, 1981.

114. L. A. Reinke, S. A. Belinsky, R. K. Evans, F. C. Kauffman, and R. G. Thurman. Conjugation of p-nitrophenol in the perfused rat liver: the effect of substrate concentration and carbohydrate reserves. J. Pharmacol. Exp. Ther. 217: 863–870, 1981.

115. G. J. Mulder, T. J. M. Temmink, and H. J. Koster. The effect of fasting on sulfation and glucuronidation in the rat in vivo. Biochem. Pharmacol. 31: 1941–1944, 1982.

116. J. A. Hinson, J. B. Mays, and A. M. Cameron. Acetaminophen induced hepatic glycogen depletion and hyperglycemia in mice. Biochem. Pharmacol. 32: 1979–1988, 1983.

117. J. G. Conway, F. C. Kauffman, and R. G. Thurman. Effect of glucose on 7-hydroxycoumarin glucuronide production in periportal and pericentral regions of the liver lobule. Biochem. J. 226: 749—756, 1985.

118. B. H. Lauterburg, S. Davies, and J. R. Mitchell. Ethanol suppresses hepatic glutathione synthesis in rats in vivo. J. Pharmacol. Exp. Ther. 230: 7—11, 1984.

119. J. B. Watkins and C. D. Klaassen. Chemically-induced alteration of UDP-glucuronic acid concentration in rat liver. Drug Metab. Dispos. 11: 37—40, 1983.

120. V. F. Price and D. J. Jollow. Increased resistance of diabetic rats to acetaminophen induced hepatotoxicity. J. Pharmacol. Exp. Ther. 220: 504—513, 1982.

121. L. A. Reinke, F. C. Kauffman, and R. G. Thurman. Stimulation of p-nitroanisole 0-demethylation by ethanol in perfused livers from fasted rats. J. Pharmacol. Exp. Ther. 211: 133—139, 1979.

122. L. A. Reinke, F. C. Kauffman, S. A. Belinsky, and R. G. Thurman. Interactions between ethanol metabolism and mixed-function oxidation in perfused rat liver: Inhibition of p-nitroanisole 0-demethylation. J. Pharmacol. Exp. Ther. 213: 70—78, 1980.

123. T. Kashiwagi, S. Ji, J. J. Lemasters, and R. G. Thurman. Rates of alcohol dehydrogenase-dependent ethanol metabolism in periportal and pericentral regions of the perfused rat liver. Mol. Pharmacol. 21: 438—443, 1982.

124. L. A. Reinke, S. A. Belinksy, F. C. Kauffman, R. K. Evans, and R. G. Thurman. Regulation of NADPH-dependent mixed function oxidation in perfused livers. Comparative studies with sorbitol and ethanol. Biochem. Pharmacol. 31: 1621—1628, 1982.

125. O. Levenspiel. In Chemical Reaction Engineering, 2nd ed. John Wiley and Sons, New York, 1972, pp. 182—185.

126. S. Hwang, K. C. Kwan, and K. S. Albert. A linear model of reversible metabolism and its application to bioavailability assessment. J. Pharmacokinet. Biopharm. 9: 693—709, 1981.

127. J. G. Wagner, A. R. DiSanto, W. R. Gillespie, and K. S. Albert. Reversible metabolism and pharmacokinetics: Application to prednisone-prednisolone. Res. Commun. Chem. Pathol. Pharmacol. 32: 387—405, 1981.

128. J. Q. Rose, A. M. Yurchak, and W. J. Jusko. Dose dependent pharmacokinetics of prednisone and prednisolone in man. J. Pharmacokinet. Biopharm. 9: 189—417, 1981.

129. J. H. Lin, K. G. Yeh, and D. E. Duggan. Effect of uremia and anephric state on the pharmacokinetics of sulindac and its metabolites in rats. Drug Metab. Dispos. 13: 602—607, 1985.

130. W. F. Ebling and W. J. Jusko. The determination of essential clearance, volume, and residence time parameters of recirculating metabolic systems: The reversible metabolism of methylprednisolone and methylprednisone in rabbits. J. Pharmacokinet. Biopharm. 14: 557–599, 1986.

131. T. L. Ding and L. Z. Benet. The reversible biotransformation of N-acetylprocainamide in the rhesus monkey. Arzneimittelforsch. 28: 281–283, 1978.

132. S. A. Belinksy, F. C. Kauffman, P. M. Sokolove, T. Tsukuda, and R. G. Thurman. Calcium-mediated inhibition of glucuronide production by epinephrine in the perfused rat liver. J. Biol. Chem. 259: 7705–7711, 1984.

133. M. El Mouelhi and F. C. Kauffman. Sublobular distribution of transferases and hydrolases associated with glucuronide, sulfate, and glutathione conjugation in human liver. Hepatology 6: 450–456, 1986.

134. I. R. Anundi, F. C. Kauffman, M. El-Mouelhi, and R. G. Thurman. Hydrolysis of organic sulfates in periportal and pericentral regions of the liver lobule: Studies with 4-methylumbelliferyl sulfate in the perfused rat liver. Mol. Pharmacol. 29: 599–605, 1986.

135. L. I. Harrison and M. Gibaldi. Influence of cholestasis on drug elimination: Pharmacokinetics. J. Pharm. Sci. 65: 1346–1348, 1976.

136. J.-L. Steimer, Y. Plusquellec, A. Guillaume, and J.-F. Boisvieux. A time-lag model for pharmacokinetics of drugs subject to enterohepatic circulation. J. Pharm. Sci. 71: 297–302, 1982.

137. B. E. Dahlstrom and L. K. Paalzow. Pharmacokinetic interpretation of the enterohepatic recirculation and first-pass elimination of morphine in the rat. J. Pharmacokinet. Biopharm. 6: 505–519, 1978.

138. W. A. Colburn, P. C. Hirom, R. J. Parker, and P. Milburn. A pharmacokinetic model for enterohepatic recirculation in the rat: Phenolphthalein, a model drug. Drug Metab. Dispos. 7: 100–102, 1979.

139. K. C. Kwan, G. O. Breault, E. R. Umbenhauer, F. G. McMahon, and D. E. Duggan. Kinetics of indomethicin absorption, elimination, and enteroehepatic circulation in man. J. Pharmacokinet. Biopharm. 4: 255–280, 1976.

140. D. E. Duggan and K. C. Kwan. Enterohepatic circulation of drugs as a determinant of therapeutic ratio. Drug Metab. Rev. 9: 21–41, 1979.

141. F. L. S. Tse, F. Ballard, and J. Skinn. Estimating the fraction of reabsorbed in drugs undergoing enterohepatic circulation. J. Pharmacokinet. Biopharm. 10: 455–460, 1982.

142. T. A. Shepherd, D. J. Gannaway, and G. F. Lockwood. Accumulation and time to steady state for drugs subject to enterohepatic cycling: A simulation study. J. Pharm. Sci. 74: 1331–1333, 1985.

143. K. S. Pang and J. R. Gillette. A theoretical examination of the effects of gut wall metabolism, hepatic elimination, and enterohepatic recycling on estimates of bioavailability and hepatic blood flow. J. Pharmacokinet. Biopharm. 6: 355–370, 1978.

144. T. A. Shepherd, R. H. Reuning, and L. J. Aarons. Estimation of area under the curve for drugs subject to enterohepatic circulation. J. Pharmacokinet. Biopharm. 13: 589–608, 1985.

145. T. A. Shepherd, R. H. Reuning, and L. J. Aarons. Interpretation of area under the curve measurements for drugs subject to enterohepatic cycling. J. Pharm. Sci. 74: 227–228, 1985.

146. K. S. Pang. Metabolite pharmacokinetics: The area under the curve of metabolite and the fractional rate of metabolism of a drug after different routes of administration for renally and hepatically cleared drugs and metabolites. J. Pharmacokinet. Biopharm. 8: 477–487, 1981.

11

Recent Advances in Drug Metabolism Methodology

THOMAS F. WOOLF and TSUN CHANG *Parke-Davis Pharmaceutical Research, Warner-Lambert Company, Ann Arbor, Michigan*

I. INTRODUCTION

In the last two decades drug metabolism studies have expanded in
importance and scope in drug discovery and development processes.
Areas where major advances have occurred include (1) the discovery
of new and novel metabolic pathways, (2) increased mechanistic understanding of various metabolic processes, (3) a better understanding
of substrate specificities for metabolism, (4) a greater knowledge of
factors affecting drug metabolism, such as age, sex, genetics, disease
state, and environment (inducers and inhibitors of metabolism),
and (5) metabolic activation of drugs to toxic and reactive metabolites.
Contributing to these advances have been improvements in bioanalytical
techniques for metabolite isolation and formation as well as the development of highly sensitive and specific analytical instruments for detection
and identification of metabolites. This chapter describes some of
the more important developments in drug metabolism in terms of
metabolite formation, profiling (isolating), and identification.

II. IN VITRO METABOLISM METHODS

A. Microsomal Enzyme Systems

To help elucidate in vivo drug biotransformation processes, in vitro
drug metabolism studies are often carried out. The in vitro system
most often used for this purpose is the hepatic subcellular microsomal
fraction. Major metabolizing enzyme systems present in microsomes
include cytochrome P450 monooxygenases, flavin-containing monooxygenases, glycuronyltransferases, and glutathione transferases.
For a discussion on the preparation and properties of microsomes and
general conditions used to carry out oxidation reactions, see Eriksson
et al. (1).

A variety of factors can affect the activity of microsomal preparations, including species, tissue, sex, age, genetics, disease state,
and environment. Pretreatment of humans and other animals with such
agents as phenobarbital or ethanol can greatly affect the activities and
specificities of enzyme systems present in the microsomal fraction. In
addition, such agents as SKF-525A and cimetidine are known to inhibit
microsomal P450 oxidase systems (2).

In vitro microsomal incubations have provided a powerful tool
and approach for metabolic profiling and mechanistic studies. Perhaps
some of the more interesting applications have been in studying the
formation and reactivity of toxic metabolites (3,4).

A modification of classic microsomal enzyme incubation techniques
involves the use of immobilized microsomal enzymes on Sepharose
beads. These preparations, made by binding solubilized microsomal

enzymes to cyanogen bromide-activated Sepharose beads, have been shown to contain cytochrome P450, UDP-glucuronyltransferase, and glutathione transferase activities (5,6). For preparation of glucuronides this procedure offers the following advantages over other systems: (1) milligram quantities of reference glucuronides can be produced, (2) biosynthetic products can be readily isolated from the reaction mixture free from interfering substances, and (3) reaction temperature, pH, and time can be easily controlled.

A potential disadvantages of an immobilized microsomal enzyme system may involve alterations in enzyme substrate and product specificities.

Recently, immobilized phenobarbital-induced rabbit liver micro-somal enzymes have been used in studying nonsteroidal anti-inflam-matory drugs (NSAID), acyl glucuronide formation, and reactivity with respect to in vitro covalent binding (7). Future applications of immobilized enzyme systems as an aid in answering other metabolism and toxicology questions seems likely.

B. Cell Culture

The use of isolated hepatocytes represents an alternative to sub-cellular liver fractions, such as microsomes, that may produce arti-factural data not representative of the in vivo situation. Furthermore, the isolated hepatocyte cell system allows the study of sequential metabolism, that is, phase I metabolism followed by conjugation reactions, whereas in a microsomally based system specific cofactors are required for each step of the reaction sequence. A widely used technique for obtaining viable hepatocytes from rat liver envolves a two-step in situ collagenase perfusion followed by mechanical dispersion of the dissociated liver tissue into isolated hepatocytes. The isolated hepatocytes can be used in vitro either as a suspension or in primary culture (8–10). In general, the level of enzymatic activities in isolated hepatocytes without added cofactors is roughly equal to those found in microsomal preparations in the presence of appropriate cofactors, such as NADPH.

The major disadvantages of using isolated hepatocytes include the need of a sensitive analytical methodology to detect and quantitate the small amounts of metabolites produced, and short useful life span of the cells. However, the latst-mentioned problem has been partially overcome in recent years by improvement of isolation and preservation techniques. The use of hepatocyte cell cultures has been best illustrated in polyhydrocarbon metabolism studies and in the resultant toxicity of metabolites formed to the culture cells (11). With the availability of more sensitive analytical methods (i.e., MS/MS and

HPLC-RAM detection) and improvements in cell culture techniques, the use of cell cultures could provide a promising tool in the study of metabolism of drugs.

C. Microbial Systems

Isolation and identification of sufficient quantities of biotransformation products for structural characterization and biologic testing is often a formidable task in terms of efforts and expenses. Although chemical synthesis and biosynthesis are the most frequently used methods, a largely ignored alternative is the use of microorganisms that are capable of producing metabolites parallel to those in mammalian systems. This concept was first proposed in 1974 by Smith and Rosazza (12) as "microbial models of mammalian metabolism." Since then, considerable progress has been made in fermentation methodology as well as in defining the biochemical basis of microbial drug biotransformation.

Microbial cytochrome P450 systems characteristics similar to those of mammalian hepatic microsomes have been found in bacteria, fungi, and yeast. Detailed retrospective studies have shown that microorganisms are capable of producing biotransformation products similar to those obtained in mammalian systems. For laboratory-scale studies, the experimental technique typically entails preparation of an actively growing culture in a suitable sterile medium (e.g., soybean meal-glucose) by inoculating the medium with cultures maintained on agar. Following an incubation period of 3–4 days at 27°C, drug substrate is added and the mixture is further incubated for an additional 24–72 hr. The resulting biotransformation products are isolated and further purified for structural elucidation using conventional methodologies. The type of culture medium, pH, incubation temperature, and degree of oxygenation varies with the microorganism used (13). Typical phase I metabolic reactions found in microbial systems include hydroxylation and 0- and N-dealkylation as well as reductive and hydrolytic reactions (13).

Microbial drug hydroxylation reactions have been extensively studied with a variety of drugs and xenobiotics. Similar hydroxylation products in microbial and mammalian systems have been observed with a number of drugs, including coumarin (13), fenclozic acid (14), levodopa (15), and phencyclidine (16).

Microbial N- and 0-dealkylation reactions have been known to occur for a number of drugs, including griseofulvin (17), papaverine (18), clindamycin (19), N-(n-propyl)amphetamine (20), imipramine (21), and lergotrile (22).

Examples of microbial N-oxidation and S-oxidation of drugs are imipramine-N-oxide (16), spironolactone sulfoxide (23), and clindamycin (19).

Reduction of ketone groups is best exemplified by the recent work of Davis et al. on the microbial stereospecific reduction of pentoxifylline (24).

Hydrolysis of esters and amides by intestinal microorganisms has been known to occur for a number of drugs. Examples include the agents cyclomate and acetyldigitoxin (25).

These examples indicate that the microbial metabolism model approach is a very promising tool for the study of drug metabolism and the production of large quantities of metabolites for structural identification and pharmacological testing.

III. IN VIVO METABOLISM METHODS

In vivo drug disposition studies are generally more demanding and time consuming to perform than in vitro experiments. Factors complicating in vivo studies include inter- and intrasubject variability in absorption, distribution, metabolism, protein binding, first-pass effect, enterohepatic circulation, capacity-limited metabolism, and routes of excretion. Following the administration of a drug, biologic samples of plasma, urine, bile, and feces are collected for analysis of unchanged drug and metabolites. Methods used to profile and identify a drug and its metabolites from biologic fluids are described in Sections IV and V. The results obtained from such disposition studies can be used to help explain the pharmacological, toxicological, and pharmacokinetic properties of the drug. Protocols for performing in vivo studies can be designed in such a way as to ascertain information on specific aspects of a drug's disposition. For example, first-pass metabolism, enterohepatic circulation, and enzyme induction questions can be selectively addressed.

IV. QUANTITATIVE METABOLIC PROFILING

In order to understand the disposition of drugs, a detailed profile of the drug's metabolic fate is required. A variety of methods have been used, including high-performance liquid chromatography (HPLC), gas-liquid chromatograph (GLC), and thin-layer chromatograph (TLC). In the absence of radiolabeled drug, HPLC coupled with ultraviolet (UV), diode array, or electrochemical (EC) detection methods have been used, but complete accounting for drug disposition is questionable at best with these methods. TLC using a variety of methods (e.g., chemical reactivity and ultraviolet detection) for visualizing components of interest has been used extensively in metabolic identification

studies. Recent improvements in the performance and resolution of
TLC separations (HPTLC) coupled with the use of radioactivity detectors can provide a powerful technique for metabolite identification
and profiling studies.

A. HPLC Coupled to Radioactivity Detection

HPLC with on-line radioactivity detection (RAM) systems can provide
a direct method for metabolic profiling of radiolabeled drugs. In the
past, HPLC radioactivity profiling of drugs was carried out by
collecting HPLC eluates and counting them by liquid scintillation
spectrometry. The disadvantages of this technique include the small
volumes of eluate required and the inability to resolve closely related
radioactivity components and that the procedures are time consuming,
labor intensive, and expensive (26). HPLC-RAM overcomes some of
these disadvantages by monitoring eluate radioactivity in real time
by either homogeneous or heterogeneous radioactivity detectors.
Heterogeneous detectors, the first developed on-line radioactivity
detectors, had limited sensitivity and suffered from radioactive
contamination problems. Nevertheless this system does allow the recovery of radiolabeled metabolites following detection and homogeneous
systems do not. Homogeneous detectors differ from heterogeneous detectors in having the HPLC eluate mixed with a scintillation cocktail
prior to detection. The advantages of this system include increased
sensitivity and fewer problems with detector contamination. Recovery
of radiolabeled analytes from the scintillation cocktail mixture is
not possible; instead, if recovery of radiolabeled analyte is desired,
the HPLC eluate is split prior to the addition of the scintillation
cocktail.

Metabolic profiling by HPLC-RAM has been used to quantitate
radiolabeled metabolites in biologic fluids, such as urine and bile
for the diuretic etozolin, the α-blocker thymoxamine, and the non-
cardioselective β-blocker levobunolol (27).

B. Isotope Ratio Mass Spectrometry

Isotope ratio (IR) mass spectrometry has been explored as an alternative method in drug tracer and balance studies to the classic radio-
isotope techniques using liquid scintillation spectrometry (28). In
IR mass spectrometry, stable isotopes of hydrogen, carbon, and
nitrogen can be used with ratios of ^2H to ^1H, ^{13}C to ^{12}C, and ^{15}N
to ^{14}N determined in various tissues and body fluids by an IR
mass spectrometer. A major problem with the use of ^{13}C as a stable
isotope label is its high natural occurrence and natural variations
in $^{13}C/^{12}C$ isotope ratios in tissues and diets, which can lead to

systematic errors. This variability in natural isotope ratios generally results in limitations on sensitivity. Another problem is the requirement for stable isotopically label drugs. In spite of these drawbacks, examples of this technique applied to model compounds, such as antipyrine (28) and *N*-acetylprocainamide (29), have been reported.

V. METABOLITE IDENTIFICATION TECHNIQUES

A variety of methods have been developed for use in metabolite identification and characterization analyses. This section describes various mass spectrometric and nuclear magnetic resonance techniques used in drug disposition studies with an emphasis on new methodologies.

A. Mass Spectrometry

Mass spectrometry has historically been well suited to drug and xenobiotic metabolism studies mainly because of its ability to confirm the identity of drug metabolites by comparison to authentic reference materials, detection of metabolites in nanogram and lower quantities, and structural elucidation by information present in mass spectral data (30).

The use of mass spectrometry as a primary tool for metabolite identification has been facilitated by significant advances in ionization capabilities (i.e., liquid chromatography/mass spectrometry and fast-atom bombardment mass spectrometry), multiple ion detection techniques, instrument configuations (i.e., tandem mass spectrometry), and computer hardware and software capabilities (31). Of these advances, perhaps the most important has been in ionization techniques that allow direct analysis of intact polar metabolites. The ability to detect and identify intact polar metabolites, such as glucuronides, glutathione and mercapturic acid conjugates, amino acid and peptide conjugates, and carnitine and ornithine conjugates, has improved our understanding of drug metabolism processes and their implications in toxicity. This section briefly describes some of the more important advances in mass spectrometry with respect to drug metabolism applications.

1. Mass Spectrometer Instrumentation

Mass spectrometers can separate ions of different mass (m/z) by mass-charge ratios (quadrupole analyzer), momentum-charge ratios (magnetic analyzer), kinetic energy-charge ratios (electrostatic analyzer), time-of-flight (TOF), and ion cyclotron resonance (ICR). Magnetic and quadrupole analyzers are by far the most commonly used mass spectrometers for metabolite analysis. These instruments may have

mass ranges up to 2000 amu (atomic mass units). For higher mass
resolution studies, instruments combining magnetic and electrostatic
analyzers are used. Quadrupole mass analyzers use a combination
of direct-current voltage and radio-frequency to separate ions based
on mass. These instruments are particularly well suited for rapid
scanning of selected mass ranges or switching back and forth between
selected masses (multiple ion detection) as well as changing between
positive and negative ion detection capabilities. Advantages in cost
and instrument size have also contributed to the greater use of
quadrupole instruments. The increased use of magnetic analyzers in
drug metabolism studies is mainly a result of improvements in electromagnetic technology that has allowed faster scan rates, improved
signal-noise levels, and multiple ion detection capabilities. Improved
scan rates and signal-noise levels are necessary for applications to
gas chromatography/mass spectrometry (GC/MS), liquid chromato-
graph/mass spectrometry (LC/MS), secondary ionization mass spectrometry (SIMS), and tandem mass spectrometry (MS/MS).

Time-of-flight mass spectrometry (TOFMS), used extensively
in the late 1960s, has seen limited use in metabolic identification
applications in recent years. The limited use of TOF instruments
reflects developments and increased availability in quadrupole and
magnetic mass analyzers (32). TOF instruments have advantages
over sector instruments in being able to obtain complete mass spectra
of all ions generated in the source, absence of scan rate limitations,
simple instrument geometry (a hollow tube with high transmission
efficiency), and a wide mass range capability. At present, TOF is
mainly used in conjunction with laser desorption techniques for
ionization of polar compounds and metabolites, for which it is particular
well suited (33). A recent applications of Fourier transform technology
to TOFMS has been reported that should increase the possible uses
of TOF and may result in the development of GC/TOFMS instruments
(33). An application of TOF to form a hybrid MS/MS instrument
has also been reported involving coupling of a tandem quadrupole
instrument to a TOF instrument (33). Potential advantages over triple
quadrupole and magnetic sector/quadrupole MS/MS instruments
include increased speed, improved signal-noise levels, and greater
mass resolution capabilities.

Ion cyclotron resonance mass spectrometry (ICRMS) has found
increasing usefulness in identification of polar metabolites (34). This
technique involves trapping of ions, generated by a variety of
ionization techniques, inside a cubicle with magnetic fields and
electrical potentials followed by addition of sufficient energies to elicit
ion cyclotron resonance (35). Signals from the ion resonances are
recorded and converted by a Fourier transform into a frequency
domain signal and finally into the reported m/z mass spectrum. This

technique is also commonly described as Fourier transform MS (FTMS) (36). The advantages of this technique include mechanical simplicity, enhanced signal-noise ratios, high mass resolution capability, and high mass range. In theory, this system combined with collisional activated dissociation processes should provide spectral data similar to that of current MS/MS systems along with the possibility of higher mass resolution and greater sensitivity. Therefore, future applications of FTMS to metabolic profiling of drugs (see MS/MS discussion) can be expected as well as interfacing to GC and LC instruments.

2. Sample Ionization Methods

a. Desorption Ionization Techniques To aid in the detection of polar compounds and metabolites by mass spectrometry, alternative ionization techniques to classic direct electron impact and chemical ionization have been developed. Field desorption (FD) and secondary ionization mass spectrometry (SIMS) are two of the more important of these methods.

Field desorption mass spectrometry (FDMS) is a technique for ionizing and volatilizing of polar compounds without imparting excess thermal heat that could affect thermal stability. In general, polar compounds are desorbed from a polymeric acetonitrile wire emitter anode at a high potential with minimal excess thermal energy. The polymeric acetonitrile resembles whiskers growing on the emitter and is responsible for increased surface areas and intensities of electrostatic fields. This technique suffers from reproducibility and technical difficulties in preparing the emitters, thereby limiting its usefulness (37). In addition, this technique requires the use of relatively pure compounds to avoid high background peaks and complex intermolecular adduct formation.

Secondary ionization mass spectrometry (SIMS) involves the bombardment of a sample placed in a nonvolatile liquid matrix, such as glycerol, with a beam of energetic ions. A process described as high-energy sputter takes place whereby some sample and solvent molecules undergo direct collision and fragmentation with excess energy of momentum transferred throughout the matrix, generating ions and providing energy for desorption of ions for detection by the mass spectrometer (38). In fast-atom bombardment mass spectrometry (FABMS), a similar high-energy beam is used to effect desorption from the liquid matrix except it is comprised of neutral atoms. These techniques provide mainly molecular ions with little fragmentation as a result of the mild ionization procedure, thereby giving rise to the term "soft ionization" (35). The advanatages of this technique include the ability to ionize polar compounds to provide molecular ion data that may not be available by other techniques, such as electron impact or chemical ionization. A major problem with FABMS is getting useful information out of the generated mass spectrum. A typical FAB mass spectrum contains many ions formed from the matrix as well as quasi-molecular ions (e.g., $m+H^+$, $m+Na^+$, $m+k+$. and $m-H+Na_2^+$). Also present in most mass spectra are quasi-molecular ion polymers formed between the compound and liquid matrix. To aid in FAB mass spectrial interpretations, sample cleanup procedures, matrix manipulation, and covalent modifications have been used (39–41).

FABMS has found extensive use in identification of glucuronide conjugates, as with the antiallergy drug procaterol (42); NSAID, including indomethacine and zomepirac (43); and the quaternary ammonium-linked glucuronide of imipramine (44). In addition, this technique has been used to identify purified glutathionyl, cysteinyl, and mercapturic acid conjugates of acetaminophen (45). Perhaps the most exciting applications of FABMS is in coupling of this ionization technique to tandem MS/MS instruments, as is described later. Other forms of FABMS currently undergoing development include thermally assisted FAB, which does not require a liquid matrix, and early events FAB, which allows selected analysis of analytes over matrix background ions. A recent application of LC/FABMS has also been reported (46).

   b. *Gas Chromatography/Mass Spectrometry* GC/MS profiling of drug metabolites has improved tremendously by the development of capillary column gas chromatographs, in advancements in electromagnetic technology for magnetic sector instruments allowing faster scan rates over greater mass ranges, and in computer hardware for more rapid digitalization of data. Contributing to the increased use of capillary column GC has been the availability of fused silica capillary columns with a variety of bonded stationary phases (47,48). In general, capillary column GC allows higher sensitivity and selectivity than conventional packed column GC. In addition, lower flow rates for carrier gases into the mass spectrometer result in lower background noise levels to further enhance sensitivities (49).

GC/MS analysis of drug metabolites still suffers from the requirement that the metabolite be volatile and stable to heating. Therefore, a variety of more selective and specific derivatizing reagents have been developed to enhance the volatility of metabolites and unchanged drug (50). Nevertheless, volatility problems have limited the usefulness of GC/MS mainly to identification of classic phase I metabolites (oxidative, reductive, and hydrolytic products).

Further improvements in sensitivity and specificity in metabolite profiling for quantitative analysis have been made possible by multiple ion monitoring (SIM) (51,52). In multiple ion monitoring, the mass spectrometer is set up to monitor a small number of selected masses, usually diagnostic fragment ions. This technique has seen extensive use in stable isotope experiments (53). GC/MS-SIM coupled to a stable isotope-labeled chemical equivalent internal standard has been used to obtain accurate quantitation in the subnanogram range (54). For quantitation, care is required in selecting instrument parameters (i.e., ion monitoring position, window size for detection, dwell time, and peak width) and in avoiding hydrogen-transfer effects of isotope ratios, which is especially important if the internal standard stable isotope differs by only one or two mass units (55). Perhaps, the most exciting use of stable isotope methodology coupled to GC/MS-SIM is in monitoring the stereochemical disposition of individual enantiomers in drug racemates. This is accomplished by preparing pseudoracemates containing equimolar amounts of a stable isotopically labeled enantiomer with the opposite nonlabeled enantiomer. These studies generally require the placement of the stable label (i.e., ^{13}C, ^2H, and ^{15}N) in a location where little or no isotope effect would be expected (56). GC/MS-SIM has also been used successfully in mechanistic studies concerning metabolism of drugs, including valproic acid. A more detailed discussion of stable isotope methodology is beyond the scope of this chapter (see Refs. 51, 53, and 57 for reviews).

c. *Liquid Chromatography/Mass Spectrometry* Direct probe MS and GC/MS analysis of conjugates are confounded by the polar nature of metabolites and possible thermal instability problems. To analyze polar metabolites by these methods generally requires chemical derivatization or, if the metabolite is a conjugate, cleavage of the conjugate to a less polar product followed by chemical derivatization. These indirect methods have numerous disadvantages, including instability of conjugate cleavage products, instability of metabolite to derivatization conditions, formation of artifacts, and loss of direct structural information. The relatively new technique of LC/MS overcomes many of these difficulties by allowing the direct analysis of intact polar metabolites.

Until recently, the coupling or interfacing of HPLC to mass spectrometry has been difficult to achieve (58,59). These difficulties stem from the inherent differences in interfacing a system with high flow rates, relatively low temperatures, and high pressures to a system requiring high temperatures and vacuum pressures for operation. The two major approaches have been developed for HPLC interfacing are a moving belt technique in which the solvents are evaporated from the LC eluate prior to passing of the analyte into the mass spectrometer and a direct liquid introduciton technique (DLI) of which the eluate, or a portion of it, is injected directly into the mass spectrometer. Currently, the method of choice for DLI

is thermospray, developed by Blakley and Vestal (58). Thermospray
LC/MS has some of the following advantages over other DLI techniques:
(1) the ability to handle solvent flow rates of up to 2 ml/min, (2) a
preference for HPLC mobile phases with high percentages of water,
(3) a preference for volatile modifiers in the HPLC mobile phase,
and (4) provision of a relatively mild ionization technique (soft
ionization) for labile and polar analytes (59). In thermospray, the
LC eluate containing a volatile modifier, usually ammonium acetate
or formate, is passed through a heated capillary to form a super-
heated mist of charged and neutral droplets that are sprayed into
the ionization chamber of the mass spectrometer where they extrude
charged ions for transmission into the mass analyzer (58). The
nature of this soft ionization process may allow formation of molecular
ions for polar compounds that fail to give molecular ions by direct
probe electron impact or chemical ionization means. A variation of
thermospray whereby a filament-on-mode is used can result in ionization
by a chemical ionization method with the solvent acting as the reagent
gas. Ionization by thermospray results in the formation of positive
and negative ions in approximately equal amounts, making it possible
to obtain spectra in both the positive and negative ion modes with
close to equal intensity. Thermospray LC/MS instruments using
either quadrupole or magnetic sector analyzers are now commercially
available.

Negative ion thermospray LC/Ms has allowed the direct identification characterization, without the noeed for chemical derivatization,
of a 1-O-acyl glucuronide conjugate of the diuretic drug furosemide
(60). Typical of glucuronide conjugates in the negative ion mode is
the presence of a prominent $(m -1)^-$ ion and fragmentation of the
sugar moiety to give a characteristic sugar ion at m/z 175. Stability
and isomerization characteristics of the furosemide 1-O-acyl glucuronide
have also been studied using thermospray LC/MS detection (61). The
structure of the glutathione adduct of activated 3-methylindole was
determined using positive ion thermospray LC/MS in conjunction with
nuclear magnetic resonance (NMR) and UV analysis (62). Thermospray
LC/MS has also been used to identify the novel new class of metabolites,
quaternary acylcarnitines (63).

This technique has also been used for the detection of ornithine
conjugates of carboxylic acid containing drugs (Liberato, personal
communication). Quantification of choline and acetylcholine directly
by LC/MS has also been reported (64). Application of this technique
to the identification of polar N-oxide and sulfoxide metabolites of
phenothiazine tranquilizer drugs has been reported (59). These
metabolites are often not amenable to GC/MS analysis because of
thermal instability problems.

The disadvantages of thermospray LC/MS include (1) the lack of electron impact capability for structural elucidations owing to high ion-source pressures; (2) the need for volatile buffers to prevent the deposition of nonvolatile salts in the mass spectrometer; (3) the requirement that the LC mobile-phase conditions allow efficient proton-transfer reactions to take place for nonassisted thermospray (i.e., no discharge electrode); and (4) the compound must be stable to heating during thermospray volatilization (65,66).

Recently, thermospray LC/MS has been coupled to tandem mass spectrometry (LC/MS/MS), incorporating advantages of both systems in metabolite identification and profiling studies (67). Microbore LC/MS techniques have also been reported that allow direct coupling of LC to FABMS (46). The advantages of this technique are in the analysis of high-molecular-weight polar compounds not volatilized by thermospray techniques.

3. Tandem Mass Spectrometry

MS/MS is a relatively new form of mass spectrometry involving the combination of two or more mass spectrometers in series and offers significant advantages over other types of mass spectrometry, such as providing simultaneous information on several individual components present in a complex mixture without the need for extensive sample preparation and improved sensitivity to noise levels (35,68,69). In a typical MS/MS daughter ion experiment, the first mass spectrometer can be set up as a mass selector, selecting component ions at a particular m/z value, which can then be made to fragment by a collisional activated dissociation (CAD) process prior to analysis by the last mass spectrometer in series. The mass fragmentogram of this fragmented selected ion is termed the daughter ion spectrum. Using these conditions, the initial mass spectrometer can be made to act in a fashion similar to that of a GC or LC instrument. However, unlike LC/MS and GC/MS, MS/MS separations are carried out nearly instantaneously without the need for columns, heating, or mobile phases. Several variations besides the daughter ion experiments just described can be used to acquire data on the various components in a mixture, including parent ion and neutral loss experiments (70). The data obtained can be used to characterize the metabolic profile of drugs without the use of radiolabeled substrates. Application of MS/MS to drug metabolism studies of polar, potentially thermally labile, metabolites has been facilitated by developments in sample ionization methodologies, including coupling of SIMS and thermospray LC to MS/MS instruments (35).

The commercial availability of MS/MS instruments (triple quadrupole instruments) coupled with FAB (71) and thermospray ionization techniques can provide a powerful approach to metabolite profiling, as was shown by Perchalski et al. (70) with the antiepileptic drug primidone. This technique can also allow quantitative analyses when appropriate stable isotopically labeled internal standards are used.

B. Nuclear Magnetic Resonance

The use of nuclear magnetic resonance spectroscopy as a tool in drug metabolism has been generally limited to characterizations of isolated and purified metabolites. These applications are not covered in this chapter. Instead, recent uses of NMR as a tool for monitoring in vivo and in vitro metabolism are discussed. NMR offers several advantages over other methods of monitoring in vivo and in vitro drug metabolism, including (1) it provides a nonevasive method for monitoring drug metabolite formation; (2) it provides a method for simultaneous monitoring of normal endogenous compounds and metabolites in biologic systems; and (3) it can identify polar metabolites without the need for isolation and purification. A number of new advances have allowed the application of NMR to the study of biologic systems, including (1) the advent of wide-bore superconducting magnets, (2) developments in ^{13}C stable isotopically labeled NMR and other nuclei, and (3) improvements in pulse sequence and detection experiments for selectively editing the spectrum of resonances so that specific resonances of metabolites can be observed.

^{1}H-NMR spectroscopy has been used to monitor the urinary excretion of the analgesic drug acetaminophen and its metabolites in human subjects (72). In vitro metabolic studies with acetaminophen using intact hepatocytes allowed the detection of glucuronide and sulfate conjugates, thereby allowing direct determination of glucuronide-sulfate metabolite ratios (73). ^{1}H-NMR studies with the radiosensitizer metronidazole, using perfused rat liver, showed that glucuronidation is the major metabolic pathway (74). In addition, ^{1}H-NMR profiling of human urinary metabolites of metronidazole has resulted in identification and quantification of several oxidative metabolites along with glucuronidation products (75).

Disadvantages to the use of NMR include (1) the need to have authentic reference materials for accurate resonance assignments; (2) the need in most cases to have stable isotopically labeled drugs; (3) problems with the resolution of resonances due to excessive line broadening, which may be a particular problem with lipophilic drugs that are tightly bound or associated with protein or membranes; and (4) perhaps most importantly, the lack of adequate sensitivity for monitoring metabolites at physiological concentrations.

VI. CONCLUSION

Recent improvements in techniques for metabolite formation, isolation, and identification have greatly expanded our understanding of drug metabolism processes. Advances in methodologies in vitro have allowed exploration into specific metabolic reactions in isolated systems without the complications inherent in studies in vivo. Various oxidative reactions, such as N-dealkylations, O-dealkylations, hydroxylations, and epoxidations, have been studied extensively by use of in vitro systems, including subcellular, cellular, and microbial. Glucuronidation and gluthathione conjugation reactions have also been studied. Factors affecting drug biotransformation processes have been explored in these isolated systems (e.g., enzyme inducers, inhibitors, and substrate requirements). Mechanistic questions concerning the generation of reactive and potentially toxic metabolites have also been extensively studied with isolated in vitro systems.

The potential role of biotransformation processes in drug toxicity and pharmacological properties has made it necessary to more fully characterize a drug's disposition. Major improvements in analytical techniques for metabolic profiling and metabolite identification have been described in this chapter. These advances have been particularly significant in the area of sensitivity and the ability to identify intact polar metabolites. A result of these relatively new methodologies has been the identification of novel metabolic pathways, that is, carnitine conjugation. Other novel pathways of drug disposition may also be observed with future applications of new technologies. Another area, only recently being studied, is the stereochemical aspects of drug metabolism. This aspect of drug disposition has been greatly facilitated by the use of stable isotope methodologies coupled to mass spectrometric analysis.

REFERENCES

1. L. C. Eriksson, J. W. dePierre, and G. Dallner. Preparation and properties of microsomal fractions. In Hepatic Cytochrome P450 Monooxygenase System. Edited by J. B. Schenkman and D. Kupfer. Pergamon Press, New York, 1982, pp. 9—45.
2. J. C. Jensen and R. Gugler. Cimetidine interaction with liver microsomes in vitro and in vivo. Biochem. Pharmacol. 34: 2141—2146, 1985.
3. R. Sata and R. Kato. Microsomes, Drug Oxidations, and Drug Toxicity. Wiley-Interscience, New York, 1982.
4. M. W. Anders. Bioactivation of Foreign Compounds, Academic Press, New York, 1985.

5. J. P. Lehman, L. Ferrin, C. Feuselau, and G. S. Yost. Simultaneous immobilization of cytochrome P450 and glucuronyltransferase for synthesis of drug metabolites. Drug Metab. Dispos. 9: 15—18, 1981.

6. S. L. Pallante, K. C. A. Lise, D. M. Dulik, and C. Fenselau. Glutathione conjugates: Immobilized enzyme synthesis and characterization by fast atom bombardment mass spectrometry. Drug Metab. Dispos. 14: 313—318, 1986.

7. R. B. Van Breeman and C. Feuselau. Acylation of albumin by 1-0-acyl glucuronides. Drug Metab. Dispos. 13: 318—320, 1985.

8. M. N. Berry and D. S. Friend. High yield preparation of isolated rat liver parenchymal cells. J. Cell Biol. 43: 406—520, 1969.

9. P. O. Selgen. Preparation of isolated rats liver cells. Methods Cell Biol. 18: 29—83, 1976.

10. S. C. Strom, R. L. Jirtie, R. S. Jones, D. L. Novicki, M. R. Rosenberg, A. Novotny, G. Irone, J. R. McLain, and G. Michalopulos. Isolation, culture and transplantation of human hepatocyctes. JNCI 68: 771—778, 1982.

11. W. F. Benedict, J. E. Gielen, I. S. Owen, A. Niwa, and D. W. Mebert. Aryl hydrocarbon hydroxylase induction in mammalian liver cell culture. IV. Stimulation of the enzyme activity in established cell lines derived from rat or mouse hepatoma and from normal rat liver. Biochem. Pharmacol. 22: 2766—2769, 1973.

12. R. V. Smith and J. P. Rosazza. Microbial models of mammalian metabolism. Aromatic hydroxylation. Arch. Biochem. Biophys. 161: 551—558, 1974.

13. R. V. Smith and J. P. Rosazza. Microbial models of mammalian metabolism. J. Pharm. Sci. 64: 1737—1756, 1975.

14. R. Howe, R. H. Moore, H. S. Rao, and A. H. Wood. Metabolism of 2-(4-chlorophenyl)-thiazol-4-ylacetic acid (fenclozic acid) and related compounds by microorganisms. J. Med. Chem. 15: 1040—1045, 1972.

15. J. P. Rosazza, P. Foss, M. Lemberger, and C. J. Sih. Microbiological synthesis of L-dopa. J. Pharm. Sci. 63: 544—547, 1974.

16. C. D. Hufford, J. K. Baker, A. M. Clark. Metabolism of phenycyclidine by microorganisms. J. Pharm. Sci. 70: 155—158, 1981.

17. B. Boothroyd, J. Napier, and G. A. Somerfield. The demethylation of griseofulvin by fungi. Biochem. J. 80: 34—37, 1961.

18. J. P. Rosazza, M. Kammer, L. Youel, R. V. Smith, P. W. Erhardt, D. H. Troung, and S. W. Leslie. Microbial models of mammalian metabolism. O-Demethylation of papaverine. Xenobiotica 7: 133—143, 1977.

19. A. D. Argoudelis, J. H. Coats, D. J. Mason, and O. K. Sebek. Microbial transformation of antibiotics. III. Conversions of clindamycin and clindamycin sulfoxide by Streptomyces. J. Antibiot. 22: 309−314, 1969.

20. R. T. Coutus, B. C. Foster, G. R. Jones, and G. E. Myers. Metabolism of (+/−) *N*-(*n*-propyl)amphetamine by *Cumminghamelle echinulata*. Appl. Environ. Microbiol. 37: 429−432, 1979.

21. C. D. Hufford, G. A. Capiton, A. M. Clark, and J. K. Baker. Metabolism of imipramine by microorganism. J. Pharm. Sci. 70: 151−155, 1981.

22. P. J. Davis, J. C. Glade, K. Kerr, and R. V. Smith. N-demethylation of lergotrile by *Streptomyces platensis*. Appl. Environ. Microbiol. 38: 891−893, 1979.

23. W. J. Marsheck and A. Karim. Preparation of metabolites of spironolactone by microbial oxygenation. Appl. Microbiol. 25: 647−649, 1975.

24. P. J. Davis, S. K. Yang, and R. V. Smith. Microbial models of mammalian metabolism. Stereospecificity of ketone reduction with pentoxifylline. Xenobiotica 15: 1001−1010, 1985.

25. M. H. Bickel, B. Burkard, E. Meier-Strasser, and M. Van Den Broek-Boot. Entero-bacterial formation of cyclohexylamine in rats ingesting cyclamate. Xenobiotica 4: 425-439, 1974.

26. R. F. Roberts and M. J. Fields. Monitoring radioactive compounds in high-performance liquid chromatographic eluates: Fraction collection versus on-line detection. J. Chromatogr. 342: 25−33, 1985.

27. K. O. Vollmer, W. Klemisch, and A. von Hodenber. High performance liquid chromatography coupled with radioactivity detection: A powerful tool for determining drug metabolite profiles in biological fluids. Z. Naturforsch. 41-C; 115−125, 1986.

28. A. Nakagawa, A. Kitagawa, M. Asami, K. Nakamura, D. A. Schoeller, R. Slater, M. Minagawa, and I. R. Kaplan. Evaluation of isotope ratio (IR) mass spectrometry for the study of drug metabolism. Biomed. Mass. Spectrom. 12: 502−506, 1985.

29. J. M. Strong, J. S. Dutcher, W. K. Lee, and A. J. Atkinson. Absolute bioavailability in man of *N*-acetylprocainamide determined by a novel stable isotope method. Clin. Pharmacol. Ther. 18: 613−622, 1976.

30. C. E. Costello. Fundamentals of present-day mass spectrometry. J. Clin. Pharmacol. 26: 390−395, 1986.

31. P. B. Bowman and M. F. Grostic. Drug metabolism. In Biochemical Applications of Mass Spectrometry. Edited by G. R. Waller and O. C. Dermer, Wiley, New York, 1980, pp. 661−691.

32. F. J. Knorr, M. Ajami, and D. A. Chatfield. Fourier transform time-of-flight mass spectrometry. Anal. Chem. 58: 690–694, 1986.

33. G. L. Glish, D. E. Goeringer. Tandem quadrupole time-of-flight instrument for mass spectrometry/mass spectrometry. Anal. Chem. 56: 2292–2295, 1984.

34. M. L. Coates and C. L. Wilkins. Laser desorption/Fourier transform mass spectra of glycoalkaloids and steroid glycosides. Biomed. Environ. Mass Spectrom. 13: 199–204, 1986.

35. S. P. Markey. Mass spectrometry: Recent developments. J. Clin. Pharmacol. 26: 406–411, 1986.

36. M. L. Gross and D. L. Rempel. Fourier transform mass spectrometry. Science 226: 261–268, 1984.

37. A. M. Lawson. The scope of mass spectrometry in clinical chemistry. Clin. Chem. 21: 803–824, 1975.

38. C. Fenselau and B. S. Larsen. Fast atom bombardment and thermospray mass spectrometry. In Drug Metabolism: Molecular Approaches and Pharmacological Implications. Edited by G. Siest. Pergamon Press, New York, 1985, pp. 167–173.

39. B. D. Musselman, J. Allison, and J. T. Watson. Utility of silver ion attachment in fast atom bombardment mass spectrometry. Anal. Chem. 57: 2425–2427, 1985.

40. D. Renner and G. Spiteller. Mechanism of fragmentation reactions of [MH]$^+$ ions obtained from peptides by liquid secondary ion mass spectrometry. Biomed. Environ. Mass Spectrom. 13: 405–410, 1986.

41. W. T. Wang, N. C. LeDonne, B. J. Ackerman, and C. C. Sweeley. Structural characterization of oligosaccharides by high-performance liquid chromatography, fast atom bombardment-mass spectrometry and Exoglycosidase Digestion. Anal. Biochem. 141: 366–381, 1984.

42. T. F. Woolf and T. Chang. Biosynthetic preparation of racemic-erythro procaterol glucuronides using immobilized phenobarbital induced rabbit liver microsomal enzymes. Pharm. Res. 3: 159, 1986.

43. P. C. Smith and L. Z. Benet. Characterization of isomeric esters of zomepirac glucuronide by proton NMR. Drug Metab. Dispos. 14: 503–505, 1986.

44. J. P. Lehman and C. C. Fenselau. Synthesis of quaternary ammonium-linked glucuronides by rabbit hepatic microsomal UDP-glucuronyltransferase and analysis by fast-atom bombardment mass spectrometry. Drug Metab. Dispos. 10: 446–449, 1982.

45. B. L. Ackerman and J. T. Watson. Application of fast atom bombardment mass spectrometry to biological samples: Analysis of urinary metabolites of acetaminophen. Biomed. Mass Spectrom. 11: 502−511, 1984.

46. Y. Ito, T. Tadeuchi, D. Ishii, and M. Goto. Direct coupling of micro high-performance liquid chromatography with fast atom bombardment mass spectrometry. J. Chromatogr. 346: 161−166, 1985.

47. M. G. Horning, W. G. Stillwell, K. Lertrantanangkoon, and K. Halpaap-wood. Glass capillary chromatographic studies of the metabolism of drugs and environmental chemicals. In Glass Capillary Chromatographic Clin Med Pharmacol, Edited by H. Jaeger. Marcel Dekker, New York, 1985, pp. 473−495.

48. M. A. Kaiser and M. S. Klee. Current status of high resolution column technology for gas chromatography. J. Chromatogr. Sci. 24: 369−373, 1986.

49. A. G. De Boer, N. P. E. Vermeulen, and D. D. Breimer. Capillary GLC in pharmacokinetics and drug metabolism studies. IN Glass Capillary Chromatographic Clin Med Pharmacol, Edited by H. Jaeger. Marcel Dekker, New York, 1985, pp. 607−634.

50. D. R. Knapp. Handbook of Analytical Derivatization Reactions. Wiley, New York, 1979.

51. N. J. Haskins. The applications of stable isotopes in biomedical research. Biomed. Mass Spectrom. 9: 269−277, 1982.

52. W. A. Garland and M. L. Powell. Quantitative selected ion monitoring (QSIM) of drugs and/or drug metabolites in biological matrices. J. Chromatogr. Sci. 19: 392−434, 1981.

53. T. A. Baillie, A. W. Rettenmeier, L. A. Peterson, and N. Castagnoli. Stable isotopes in drug metabolism and disposition. Annu. Rep. Med. Chem. 19: 273−282, 1984.

54. W. F. Trager. Biotransformation and excretion: Quantitative studies. J. Clin. Pharmacol. 26: 443−447, 1986.

55. I. A. Low, R. H. Liu, S. A. Barker, F. Fish, R. L. Settine, E. G. Piotrowski, W. C. Damert, and J. Y. Liu. Selected ion monitoring mass spectrometry: Parameters affecting quantitative determination. Biomed. Mass. Spectrom. 12: 633−637, 1985.

56. E. D. Bush, L. K. Low, and W. F. Trager. A sensitive and specific stable isotope assay for warfarin and its metabolites. Biomed. Mass Spectrom. 10: 395−398, 1983.

57. T. A. Baillie and A. W. Rettenmeier. Recent advances in the use of stable isotopes in drug metabolism research. J. Clin. Pharmacol. 26: 481−484, 1986.

58. C. R. Blakley and M. L. Vestal. Thermospray interface for liquid chromatograph/mass spectrometry. Anal. Chem. 55: 750−754, 1983.

59. T. R. Covey, J. B. Crowther, E. A. Dewey, and J. D. Henion. Thermospray liquid chromatography/mass spectrometry determination of drugs and their metabolites in biological fluids. Anal. Chem. 57: 474—481, 1985.

60. A. Rachmel, G. A. Hazelton, A. L. Yergey, and D. J. Liberato. Furosemide 1-O-acyl glucuronide: In vitro biosynthesis and pH-dependent isomerization to β-glucuronidase-resistant forms. Drug Metab. Dispos. 13: 705—710, 1985.

61. D. J. Liberato and C. C. Fenselau. Characterization of glucuronides with a thermospray liquid chromatography/mass spectrometry interface. Anal. Chem. 55: 1741—1744, 1983.

62. M. R. Nocerini, G. S. Yost, J. R. Carlson, D. J. Liberato, and R. G. Breeze. Structure of the glutathione adduct of activated 3-methylindole indicates that an imine methide is the electrophilic intermediate. Drug Metab. Dispos. 13: 690—694, 1985.

63. A. L. Yergey, D. J. Liberato, and D. S. Millington. Thermospray liquid chromatography/mass spectrometry for the analysis of L-carnitine and its short-chain acyl derivatives. Anal. Biochem. 139: 278—288, 1984.

64. D. J. Liberato, A. L. Yergey, and S. T. Weintraub. Separation and quantification of choline and acetylcholine by thermospray liquid chromatography/mass spectrometry. Biomed. Environ. Mass Spectrom. 13: 171—174, 1986.

65. D. J. Liberato and A. L. Yergey. Solvent selection for thermospray liquid chromatography/mass spectrometry. Anal. Chem. 58: 6—9, 1986.

66. C. P. Tsai, A. Sahil, J. M. McGuire, B. L. Karger, and P. Vouros. High-performance liquid chromatographic/mass spectrometric determination of volatile carboxylic acids using ion-pair extraction and thermally induced alkylation. Anal. Chem. 58: 2—6, 1986.

67. R. D. Voyksner, J. T. Bursey, and J. W. Hines, and E. D. Pellizzari. A comparison of thermospray and direct liquid introduction high-performance liquid chromatography/mass spectrometry for the analysis of candidate antimalarials. Biomed. Mass Spectrom. 11: 616—621, 1984.

68. R. G. Cooks and G. L. Glish. Mass spectrometry. Chem. Eng. News November 30: 40—52, 1981.

69. K. L. Busch and G. C. Didonato. Expanded MS/MS applications through improved instrumentation. Am. Lab. August: 17—32, 1986.

70. R. J. Perchalski, M. S. Lee, and R. A. Yost. Biotransformation and excretion: Metabolite identification; other mass spectrometric methods. J. Clin. Pharmacol. 26: 435—442, 1986.

71. K. B. Tomer, N. J. Jensen, M. L. Gross, and J. Whitney. Fast-atom bombardment combined with tandem mass spectrometry for determination of bile salts and their conjugates. Biomed. Environ. Mass Spectrom. 13: 265–272, 1986.

72. J. R. Bales, J. K. Nicholson, P. J. Sadler, and J. A. Timbrell. Urinary excretion of acetaminophen and its metabolites as studied by proton NMR spectroscopy. Clin. Chem. 30: 1631–1636, 1984.

73. J. K. Nicholson, J. A. Timbrell, J. R. Bales, and P. J. Sadler. A high resolution proton nuclear magnetic resonance approach to the study of hepatocyte and drug metabolism: Application to acetaminophen. Mol. Pharmacol. 27: 634–643, 1985.

74. H. Allars, M. D. Coleman, and R. S. Norton. [1]H nuclear magnetic resonance study of metronidazole metabolism by perfused rat liver. Eur. J. Drug Metab. Pharmacokinet. 10: 253–260, 1985.

75. M. D. Coleman and R. S. Norton. Observation of drug metabolites and endogenous compounds in human urine by ^{1}H nuclear magnetic resonance spectroscopy. Xenobiotica 16: 69–77, 1986.

12

Saturable Kinetics and Bioavailability Determination

THOMAS N. TOZER and GERALD M. RUBIN* *University of California at San Francisco, San Francisco, California*

*Current affiliation: Drug Metabolism Department, Merrell Dow Research Institute, Cincinnati, Ohio.

In virtually all the theories and applications of pharmacokinetics, there
is an assumption of linearity. Linearity implies that, for a given route
and method of administration, the time course of drug in or eliminated
from the body, normalized to the dose administered, superimposes for
all doses. Thus, as shown in Figure 1, superposition is a primary test
for linearity. When, after appropriate corrections for variability, dose-
normalized curves do not superimpose, some form of nonlinearity is present. The term commonly applied here is "dose-dependent kinetics."

Most dose-dependent situations occur because one or more of the
processes involved in drug absorption, distribution, metabolism, or
excretion show *saturability*, a condition in which the rate of a given
process increases with the concentration driving it but approaches
a limiting value. Figure 2 is an example of saturable metabolism.

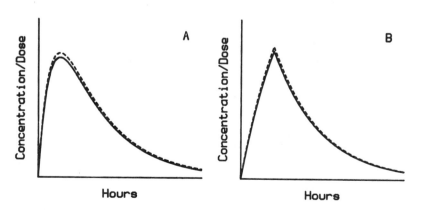

FIGURE 1 Following the oral administration (A) or intravenous infusion
(B) of a drug, one expects the plasma concentration following a high
dose to superimpose on that of a low dose when the concentration
is normalized to the dose given. A consistent deviation from this
condition is evidence of dose dependence in one or more of the input,
distribution, and elimination processes.

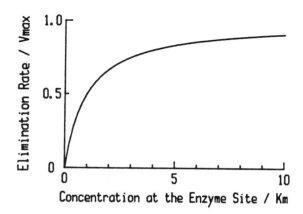

FIGURE 2 When the rate of metabolism approaches a limiting value as the drug concentration is increased, the metabolism is said to be *saturable*. In this example, the rate is expressed relative to the maximum rate V_{max} and the concentration is related to the Michaelis constant, K_m [see Eq. (1).]

TABLE 1 Selected Mechanisms and Examples of Drugs Showing Saturable Kinetic Behavior

Mechanism	Drug example
Absorption	
Saturable transport in gut wall	Riboflavin
Saturable metabolism during first pass	Propranolol
Distribution	
Saturable plasma protein binding	Disopyramide
Excretion	
Active tubular secretion	Penicillin
Active tubular reabsorption	Ascorbic acid
Metabolism	
Capacity-limited (saturable) metabolism	Phenytoin
Cofactor supply limitation	Salicylamide

TABLE 2 Additional Causes of Dose-Dependent Kinetics with Selected
Examples and Pharmacokinetic Parameter(s) Affected

Cause	Drug	Parameter affected
Physical property		
Low solubility	Griseofulvin	Bioavailability decreases with increased dose
Altered renal handling		
Diuresis	Theophylline	Renal clearance initially increased after single dose
Nephrotoxicity	Aminoglycosides (large chronic doses)	Renal clearance decreases with time
Altered hepatic handling		
Inhibition by end product	Lidocaine	Hepatic metabolic clearance decreased on repeated administration
Increased hepatic blood flow	Propranolol	Hepatic clearance increased
Hepatotoxicity	Acetaminophen (high doses)	Decreased hepatic clearance
Autoinduction	Carbamazepine	Hepatic clearance increases with time

Several saturable mechanisms are known to occur. Examples of such
mechanisms and of drugs exhibiting such kinetic behavior are shown
in Table 1. Other causes of dose-dependent kinetics and examples of
drugs with the corresponding kinetic behavior are given in Table 2.

This chapter examines problems associated with the determination
of the bioavailability of drugs that show saturable kinetics. The
primary focus is on drugs that exhibit saturable metabolism, a cause
of variable bioavailability as well as a problem for bioavailability
assessment.

After describing and defining saturable metabolism, several methods that have been applied to bioavailability assessment in the presence

of nonlinear kinetic mechanisms are reviewed. One of these methods, concurrent administration of a tracer dose with the oral dose, and the *conventional method* of giving *equally-sized* intravenous and oral doses on separate occasions are evaluated by computer simulation. The relationship between the accuracy of these methods (under one-compartment conditions) and various pharmacokinetic parameters, dose, and incomplete absorption are calculated, and the results for the two methods are compared. Modifications of the administration of the tracer dose to improve accuracy are also presented.

I. SATURABLE METABOLISM

When drug concentrations in blood or plasma are sufficiently high, the rate of metabolism appears to approach a limit (see Fig. 2). The Michaelis-Menten enzyme kinetics model is often applied in these circumstances. This model states that

$$\text{Rate of metabolism} = \frac{V_{max} \cdot C_s}{K_m + C_s} \tag{1}$$

where V_{max} is the maximum rate of metabolism, C_s is the drug concentration at the enzyme site, and K_m is the concentration at which the rate is one-half the maximum value. The K_m value is an index of the approximate concentration above which saturability becomes evident.

Phenytoin is an example of a drug for which the Michaelis-Menten model applies. The consequence of having a therapeutic concentration above K_m is shown for an individual patient in Figure 3. Only minor differences in the input rate cause large changes in the steady-state plasma concentration. For example, using the parameter values in Figure 3 and a daily dose of 400 mg, an increase in bioavailability from 0.8 to 1.0, a 25% change, increases the steady-state concentration from 7 to 16 mg/liter, an increase of more than 100%. Clearly, bioavailability is an important parameter of this drug to know and to control.

Drugs with saturable metabolism and a medium-to-high hepatic extraction ratio are expected to show an increase in bioavailability on increasing the dose or dosing rate. This phenomemon, called saturable first-pass metabolism, occurs because metabolism becomes capacity limited during the first pass through the liver. As reflected by data for propranolol (1), the combination of saturable first-pass metabolism (increased bioavailability) and saturable metabolism (decreased clearance) can lead to a markedly disproportionate increase in

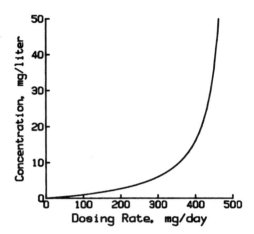

FIGURE 3 As a consequence of Michaelis-Menten kinetics, the steady-
state concentration of phenytoin increases disproportionately with
the dosing rate. Only minor changes in the dosing rate produce
large changes in the steady-state concentration. The usual therapeutic
range.is 10–20 mg/liter. In this example, V_{max} = 500 mg/day K_m = 4
mg/liter, V = 50 liters, and bioavailability = 1 [See Eq. (1) for definition
of symbols.]

the steady-state concentration with dosing rate. Similar dose-dependent behavior is reflected in single-dose data for lorcainide (2) and
alprenolol (3).

Therapeutically, saturable metabolism is important for two reasons.
First, the steady-state concentration increases disproportionately
with an increase in dosing rate. Second, the bioavailability should
become more variable as a consequence of the influence of absorption
rate on the fraction escaping first-pass metabolism at any point in
time. Thus, food, drugs, posture, and other factors that affect the
rate of absorption can influence the concentration entering the liver
and the corresponding degree of saturation.

II. BIOAVAILABILITY DETERMINATION

Ironically, for drugs like phenytoin, the conventional method for
determining bioavailability is less accurate than for drugs with linear
kinetics in spite of an even greater need for such information.

Bioavailability is defined as the fraction of a dose reaching the general circulation. It can be reduced by incomplete absorption into the portal vein or by metabolism during the first pass through the liver or gut. It is frequently determined by dividing the area under the concentration-time curve (AUC) of an oral dose by the AUC of a separate, equally-sized intravenous dose. This method is based on the premise that the overall clearance, defined as the amount of drug eliminated (not including first-pass elimination, if any) divided by AUC, is the same for both doses. When elimination of a drug follows Michaelis-Menten kinetics, as with phenytoin, this premise is violated (4), producing an error in the bioavailability estimate (4−6). Jusko et al. (6) have reported that, in the human, the conventional method underestimates the bioavailability of phenytoin (4.6 mg/kg) by about 10%. This problem has prompted various investigators to develop methods to determine the bioavailability of drugs with Michaelis-Menten elimination kinetics or others forms of nonlinear elimination. Both model-dependent and model-independent methods have been proposed.

III. BIOAVAILABILITY ESTIMATION FOR MICHAELIS-MENTEN DRUGS

A. Model-Dependent Methods

Martis and Levy (5) were the first to develop a method of bioavailability estimation for drugs with Michaelis-Menten elimination kinetics. Bioavailability is estimated with the following equation, which has a term for parallel first-order elimination:

$$F_{est} = \frac{1}{D_{po}} \int_0^\infty \left(\frac{V_{max} \cdot C}{K_m + C} + k \cdot V \cdot C \right) dt \qquad (2)$$

where F_{est} is the estimated value of bioavailability, D_{po} is the oral dose, C is the concentration of drug measured in the systemic circulation, k is the first-order elimination rate constant, and V is the volume of distribution.

For the simplest case of a one-compartment model drug, two potential sources of error result from the simplified pharmacokinetic model (5) used to derive Equation 2. First, the value of Km, which is determined from the systemic concentration-time profile after intravenous dosing, is based on the concentration entering the eliminating organ rather than the concentration at the enzyme site. Thus, Km is an apparent value. Assuming elimination occurs in the liver and if the fraction of drug which passes through the liver intact changes over a wide range during elimination, the apparent value of Km will vary widely. Because Km is thought to have a fixed value, variation in its apparent value may result in a poor fit of the Michaelis-Menten equation [Eq. (1)] to the concentration-time data. This potential problem can be solved by using a hepatic model that allows distinction between drug concentrations at the enzyme site and entering the liver. In practice, doing this may be difficult because it requries finding the appropriate hepatic model and determining hepatic blood flow.

The second, and probably more important source of error results from the assumption that the concentration entering the eliminating organ after oral dosing is equal to the systemic concentration. This assumption is not valid when elimination occurs in the liver. When oral absorption occurs, the concentration of drug entering the liver, C_{in}, is the sum of the systemic (recirculating) concentration, C, and that which is derived from oral absorption, C_{abs}:

$$C_{in} = C + C_{abs} \tag{3}$$

The concentration entering the liver is therefore underestimated. Because of Michaelis-Menten kinetics, this underestimation results in an overestimation of the rate of elimination and bioavailability. The method of Martis and Levy is thus potentially more suitable for drugs, such as nitrofurantoin (7), for which saturable elimination occurs in an organ other than the liver.

Simulation results (not given in text) demonstrate that the method of Martis and Levy, modified to handle differences between the concentrations entering the liver and at the enzyme site, tends to be accurate when elimination is slow relative to absorption, that is, for low extraction ratio, long half-life drugs such as phenytoin.

Keller and Scholle (8) presented another method for estimating the bioavailability of drugs showing Michaelis-Menten kinetics in the liver. Their method is based on the assumption that drug in the body does not recirculate to the liver, and thus is expected to be inaccurate for any drug for which the recirculating concentration substantially contributes to that entering the liver. The method of Keller and Scholle has the advantage, over that of Martis and Levy, of using an analytical equation to find bioavailability but has the disadvantage of requiring determination of the first-order absorption rate constant, a value that is difficult to estimate under Michaelis-Menten conditions. Furthermore, it assumes that the entire dose is absorbed. These authors (8) showed that their method gives a bioavailability for ethanol similar to that obtained by Wilkinson et al. (9) using the method of Martis and Levy.

Veng-Pederson (10) suggested that, when elimination is nonlinear, an empirical function describing the concentration dependence of elimination can be used for bioavailability estimation. When multiplied by the systemic drug concentration, this function gives the rate of elimination. Thus it can be considered a clearance function. Because its value tends to change with time, it can be defined as the instantaneous clearance and is denoted $CL(t)$. Accordingly, the bioabailability of the oral dose D_{po} is calculated as follows:

$$F_{est} = \frac{1}{D_{po}} \int_o^\infty CL(t) \cdot C \, dt \qquad (4)$$

Fundamentally, this approach is the same as that of Martis and Levy, except that it is more general and can be used for concentration-dependent nonlinearities other than Michaelis-Menten kinetics. As with the method of Martis and Levy, this method also neglects the effect that potentially high portal drug concentrations can have on the value of clearance during the absorption phase when hepatic elimination predominates. Furthermore, when elimination does in fact occur by Michaelis-Menten kinetics, an empirical function may not describe elimination as well as the Michaelis-Menten equation.

The method of Veng-Pederson does have the advantage of applying to other types of nonlinear disposition, such as saturable plasma protein binding, which occurs, for example, with disopyramide (11). There are many instances, however, in which concentration itself is not adequate to describe nonlinear elimination (12–14), and in such instances, the method of Veng-Pederson cannot be used unless some other variables or combination of variables are used to describe elimination.

The three approaches discussed so far require estimation of model parameters, and two of them assume one-compartment kinetics. These characteristics can make their practical use somewhat difficult and subject to error.

B. Model-Independent Methods

Another approach toward estimating the bioavailability of drugs with Michaelis-Menten (or other nonlinear) kinetics is to administer an intravenous reference dose as a labeled tracer at the time when the oral dose is given (14–16). Kornhauser et al. (15) suggested that this method could be used to "avoid [the effect of] known dose-dependent kinetics seen following oral administration of single doses," and thus enable accurate bioavailability estimation of drugs with dose-dependent kinetics. This suggestion implies that drug from both the intravenous and oral doses is subject to the same degree of saturation, resulting in equal values of clearance. This hypothesis is correct, however, only when the intravenous and oral concentration-time profiles are similar, that is, when absorption is much faster than elimination. The degree of error entailed in using this method under other conditions has not been determined.

Compared with the other methods discussed, concurrent dosing has the advantage of requiring few assumptions about the appropriate pharmacokinetic model. It also avoids the effect of changes in clearance that may occur between separate administrations of oral and intravenous doses, but has the potential disadvantage that kinetic isotope effect may cause a difference in the clearance of the two drug forms.

In a study of the dose-dependent first-pass metabolism of salicylamide in dogs, Waschek et al. (17) modified this method by delaying intravenous tracer dose administration for 4 min after the oral dose was given. This was done in an attempt to compensate for the slower oral input. Whether bioavailability estimation was improved here was not determined. It may be surmised, however, that better accuracy would result if the delay substantially increased the similarity of the concentration-time profiles.

Øie and Jung (18) have developed a method that is appropriate for drugs with nonlinear renal excretion. When nonlinear elimination is restricted to renal excretion and there is no renal metabolism, the amount of drug eliminated by the nonlinear route can be measured directly in urine. Thus, bioavailability can be calculated as

$$F_{est} = \frac{CL_{xr} \cdot AUC_{po} + A_{ex}}{D_{po}} \tag{5}$$

where CL_{xr} is the extrarenal clearance and A_{ex} is the amount of drug excreted in the urine. This method bypasses the problem of using clearance to estimate the amount of drug eliminated by the nonlinear pathway.

In the next section, the nonlinear model used for evaluating the conventional method and the concurrent administration of an intravenous tracer dose is presented. The sources of error and conditions resulting in reasonable accuracy for both methods are discussed. Finally, modifications of the time and method of administration of the tracer dose are explored as ways to improve the accuracy of the tracer method.

IV. SIMULATIONS

A. Model

The model used (19) is as simple as possible and yet includes the anatomic features necessary for testing the accuracy of each method of bioavailability estimation. The simulation model, Figure 4, meets

ORAL DOSE

$f \cdot D_{po}$

$\downarrow k_a$

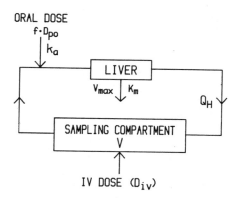

IV DOSE (D_{iv})

FIGURE 4 Simulation model for evalution of the error in oral bioavailability estimates when the oral dose is given: (1) on an occasion
separate from an equal intravenous dose and (2) concurrently with
a tracer intravenous dose. Elimination occurs in the liver according
to the venous equilibration model and follows Michaelis-Menten kinetics.
V_{max} is the maximum rate of metabolism, and K_m is the Michaelis-
constant. Hepatic blood flow is denoted Q_H. The liver is assumed to
have negligible volume; thus, the model has a single distribution
compartment and an apparent volume of distribution V equal to the
volume of the sampling compartment. Oral input occurs by a first-
order process, the rate constant for which is denoted k_a. The fraction
of the oral dose absorbed (reaching the portal circulation) is denoted f.

the requirement for simplicity by being limited to a single distribution
compartment (the hepatic volume is negligible), having elimination
occur only in the liver by a single metabolic pathway, and showing
no binding of drug to components in blood or liver. At the same
time, it includes the basic anatomic characteristics (lacking in a
true one-compartment model) necessary for simulating the oral absorption of drug into the blood entering the liver. Other important
features of the model include first-order absorption kinetics, Michaelis-
Menten elimination kinetics, and use of the venous-equilibration model
(20) to describe hepatic elimination.

The use of a single distribution compartment is based on the
assumption that equilibration of drug between the tissues and blood
is rapid relative to drug elimination. The disposition of a number
of drugs has been described with one distribution compartment, including the classic examples for Michaelis-Menten kinetics, phenytoin
(6) and ethanol (21). The assumption that the liver has a negligible
volume is made because the liver is small relative to the body and is

highly perfused so that drug equilibrates rapidly between the liver
and blood. Drugs that show a large distribution phase and/or a
large degree of hepatic binding, however, may require a more comprehensive model to evaluate the accuracy of their bioavailability estimation.

Oral absorption is modeled as a first-order process because
plasma concentration-time data can often be fit by assuming first-
order input. First-order kinetics have been shown to describe both
gastric emptying (22) and the absorption of drug through the
intestinal mucosa (23).

Orally absorbed drug passes directly into the blood entering the
liver. This process must be modeled to evaluate the accuracy of each
method of bioavailability estimation because direct input into the
blood entering the liver affects the clearance-time profile and thus
the overall clearance of the oral dose. The overall clearance is the
term that relates the area under the systemic concentration-time curve
to the amount of drug eliminated from the systemic circulation.

B. Parameter Values

Dose, V_{max}, first-order absorption rate constant, and volume of
distribution were varied one at a time in the simulations to determine
their relationships to error in bioavailability estimation. Dose, rather
than K_m, was varied to influence the degree of saturation of metabolism. The default values of the parameters used in the simulations
were: dose = 178 μmol, k_a = 0.02 min^{-1}, V = 50 liters, Q_H = 1.5
liters/min, V_{max} = 1.35 μmol/min, K_m = 0.1 μM, and f_u (the fraction
unbound in plasma) = 1. Unless otherwise specified, the default
values are used in all subsequent simulations. All parameters were
held constant during each simulation.

C. Bioavailability Calculations

Bioavailability determination is conventionally based on the following
principles: the amount of drug reaching the systemic circulation is
equal to the amount eliminated from the systemic circulation, which
in turn is equal to the product of the clearance CL_{po} and the area
under the systemic concentration-time curve AUC_{po} of the oral dose.
Thus,

$$F \cdot D_{po} = CL_{po} \cdot AUC_{po} \tag{6}$$

where F is bioavailability and D_{po} is the oral dose. Because CL_{op}
cannot be determined from the oral dose, an intravenous reference
dose is given, separately or concurrently, with the assumption that

its clerance CL_{iv} is equal to CL_{po}. Assuming tha the bioavailability of the intravenous dose is 1, its clearance is given as

$$CL_{iv} = \frac{D_{iv}}{AUC_{iv}} \tag{7}$$

where D_{iv} is the intravenous dose and AUC_{iv} is the area under the systemic concentration-time curve resulting from the intravenous dose. From Equations (6) and (7),

$$F = \frac{AUC_{po}}{AUC_{iv}} \cdot \frac{D_{iv}}{D_{po}} \cdot \frac{CL_{po}}{CL_{iv}} \tag{8}$$

and when the clearance are equal,

$$F = \frac{AUC_{po}}{AUC_{iv}} \cdot \frac{D_{iv}}{D_{po}} \tag{9}$$

When CL_{iv} and CL_{po} differ as a result of time-dependent or dose-dependent changes, erro results from using Equation (9).

D. Error Calculations

The error in bioavailability estimation is expressed as percentage error and is calculated from

$$\% \text{ Error} = 100 \cdot \frac{F_{est} - F_{true}}{F_{true}} \tag{10}$$

where F_{true} is the actual value of bioavailability. According to Equation (6), the calculated value of bioavailability is proportional to the value of CL_{iv} that is used to estimate CL_{po}. Hence, the percentage error can be described in terms of overall clearance:

$$\% \text{ Error} = 100 \cdot \frac{CL_{iv} - CL_{po}}{CL_{po}} \tag{11}$$

The magnitude of error is usually presented in absolute terms, that is, the sign of the error (which is negative when bioavailability is under-estimated) is disregarded. In the tables and figures, the sign of error is always given.

V. CONVENTIONAL METHOD

The conventional method of bioavailability estimation entails the
separate administration of intravenous and oral doses, usually of the
same size, and calculations based on Equation (9). Because of its
relative simplicity and common use in bioavailability studies, the
conventional method will likely continue to be used in studies of drugs
showing Michaelis-Menten elimination kinetics. For this reason, it
is useful to evaluate and predict the accuracy of this method over a
wide variety of pharmacokinetic conditions.

The conventional method serves as a standard against which the
accuracy of the concurrent dosing and other methods can be compared.
If the conventional method is predicted to be more accurate, then its
use would be indicated unless another reason can be given to support
using one of the alternative methods.

A. Overall Versus Instantaneous Clearance

The conventional dosing method is based on the assumption that the
overall clearances of the intravenous and oral doses are equal. With
Michaelis-Menten kinetics, however, the overall clearances tend to
differ. The reason for this tendency can be explained in terms of
the time courses of two variables, namely, instantaneous clearance
$CL(t)$ and the concentrations of drug C in the sampling compartment
(see simulation model, Fig. 4). The time courses of both variables
are influenced by the degree of saturation of elimination.

Instantaneous clearance is defined here as the proportionality
constant between the rate of elimination of drug from the sampling
compartment $Rate_{sys}$ and the concentration returning to the liver
from this compartment:

$$Rate_{sys} = CL(t) \cdot C \tag{12}$$

This definition is convenient for evaluating the methods of bioavailability estimation. Hereafter, instantaneous clearance is referred to
simply as clearance.

The relationships between instantaneous and overall clearances
for oral and intravenous doses are obtained by integrating Equation
(12) from time zero to infinity and substituting the result into the
equation

$$CL_{iv} = \frac{\text{Amount eliminated}}{AUC_{iv}} \tag{13}$$

for the intravenous dose and into an analogous equation for the oral dose. The resulting equations are

$$CL_{iv} = \int_0^\infty CL(t)_{iv} \cdot \frac{C_{iv}}{AUC_{iv}} \, dt \qquad (14)$$

$$CL_{po} = \int_0^\infty CL(t)_{po} \cdot \frac{C_{po}}{AUC_{po}} \, dt \qquad (15)$$

The built-up terms are the AUC-normalized concentrations in the sampling compartment. According to Equations (14) and (15), the overall clearances of the intravenous and oral doses can be thought of as the integrals of instantaneous clearance weighted to the AUC-normalized concentrations with respect to time. Equations (14) and (15) demonstrate that the overall clearance of the intravenous and oral doses may be unequal because of differences in either the AUC-normalized concentration-time or clearance-time profiles, or both (Fig. 5).

B. AUC-Normalized Concentration-Time Profiles

Differences in the AUC-normalized concentration-time profiles after equal intravenous and oral doses result from differences in the input rates of each. As a rule, the similarity of the profiles increases as oral absorption becomes faster relative to elimination, that is, when oral input becomes more like that of an intravenous bolus dose (Fig. 6).

Since the AUC-normalized concentration acts as a weighting factor for the instantaneous clearance [Equation (14) and (15)], the overall clearance of the intravenous dose is most influenced by clearance values that occur near the time of intravenous dosing; the overall clearance of the oral dose is most affected by values that occur near the peak concentration after oral dosing. Even if the clearance-time curves are the same for both doses, the weighting effect of the different profiles results in differing values of overall clearance for each dose and error in bioavailability estimation results.

C. Clearance-Time Profiles

Even when the same dose size is given, the clearance-time profiles usually differ after intravenous and oral dosing (bottom of Fig. 5) because differences in the input rate and input site influence the time course of the drug concentration entering the liver (Fig. 7).

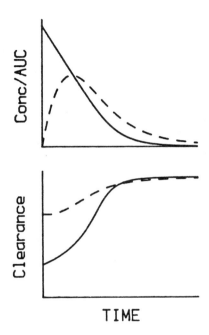

TIME

FIGURE 5 AUC-normalized concentration-time profiles (top) after
separate administration of equal intravenous (solid line) and oral
doses (dashed line). Corresponding clearance-time profiles (bottom)
after the intravenous (solid line) and oral (dashed line) doses are
shown. The potential for route-dependent differences in the profiles,
which cause differences in the overall clearances of the intravenous
and oral doses, is evident. In this case, the overall clearances were
0.65 and 1.13 liters/min, respectively, resulting in a 42% underestimation of bioavailability. The first-order absorption rate constant
was set to 0.01 min^{-1}.

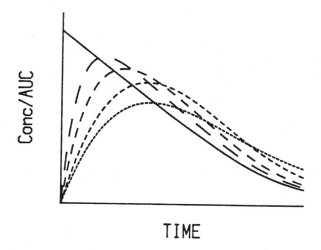

FIGURE 6 Effect of absorption rate constant on the degree of super-position of the AUC-normalized concentration-time profiles after single intravenous (solid line) and oral doses (various dashed lines) given on separate occasions. The values of k_a used were 0.1, 0.05, 0.02, and 0.01 min^{-1} (represented by successively shorter dashes).

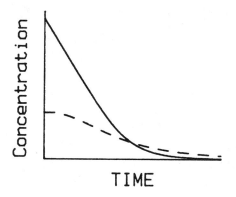

FIGURE 7 Concentrations of drug entering the liver after separate administrations of equal intravenous (solid line) and oral (dashed line) doses. The first-order absorption rate constant, volume of distribution, and hepatic blood flow were 0.01 min^{-1}, 50 liters, and 1.5 liters/min, respectively. The initial concentration entering the liver was three times greater after the intravenous dose than after the oral dose.

The tendency for this concentration to differ after each route of administration is most easily shown at the time of dosing. For the intravenous dose, the initial value of the concentration entering the liver is equal to the dose divided by the volume of distribution. The orally administered drug, which is absorbed by a first-order process and goes directly into the blood entering the liver, results in an initial concentration given by $k_a \cdot Dose/Q_H$ (24).

D. Simulation Results

1. Dose

The relationship between dose and percentage error in the bioavailability estimate is shown in Figure 8A. The results confirm that the coventional method is accurate when the dose is small enough to result in ap-

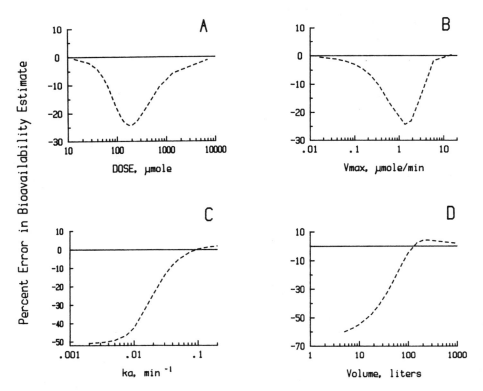

FIGURE 8 The relationship between percentage error in the bio-availability estimate and (A) Dose, (B) V_{max}, (C) k_a, and (D) V.

proximately first-order elimination (constant clearance) after both intravenous and oral doses. On increasing the dose, both routes lead to an increase in the degree of saturation of metabolism, especially early on, as evidenced by a tendency for the clearance values to drop. The degree of error increases because, up to a point, there tends to be a larger separation in the clearance-time profiles after intravenous and oral doses as the degree of saturation increases.

At doses above approximately 200 µmol, however, error decreases with further increases in dose. At these higher doses, there is a tendency for both the AUC-normalized concentration-time profiles and clearance-time profiles to be similar (superimpose) after intravenous and oral dosing (Fig. 9) and, thus, according to Equations (14) and (15), for equal values of overall clearance to occur. The increased

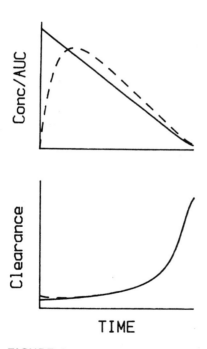

FIGURE 9 AUC-normalized concentration-time profiles (top) after separate administrations of equal (750 µmol) large intravenous (solid line) and oral doses (dashed line). Clearance-time profiles (bottom) after the same intravenous (solid line) and oral (dashed line) doses are also shown. This figure demonstrates the tendency of a highly saturating dose to result in AUC-normalized concentration and clearance-time profiles that superimpose.

superposition of both time-dependent variables is a result of a
reduction in the rate of elimination relative to absorption.

2. Maximum Rate of Metabolism

The relationship between V_{max} and percentage error in the bioavailability estimate is given in Figure 8B. For the conditions used in the
simulations, the lowest value of V_{max} tested results in a hepatic
extraction ratio of 0.1 when elimination is first order and much lower
extraction ratios when there is saturation of metabolism. A low extraction ratio tends to result in elimination being slow relative to
absorption. As seen in the simulations of high doses, slow elimination
results in a tendency for the AUC-normalized concentration-time
and clearance-time profiles to superimpose and for error in bioavailability estimates to be small.

Error becomes larger when V_{max} is increased because the rate
of elimination increases relative to the rate of absorption. When
V_{max} exceeds a value of about 1.35 μmol/min, however, error
decreases. At large values of V_{max}, the extraction ratio approaches 1
and clearance tends to remain constant (nearly equal to hepatic blood
flow), even when metabolism is partially saturated. Clearance also
tends to be constant at high values of V_{max} because, for a given
concentration entering the liver, higher values of V_{max} result in lower
concentrations of drug inside the liver and less saturation of metabolism. These results imply that high extraction ratio drugs which exhibit
saturable first pass metabolism, such as alprenolol (25), may be
amenable to accurate bioavailability determination by the conventional
method.

3. Absorption Rate Constant

The relationship between first-order absorption rate constant and
percentage error is shown in Figure 8C. At low values of k_a, the
relatively slow absorption of drug tends to result in little saturation
of the oral dose, but metabolism of the intravenously administration
drug is saturated to a large degree, especially at early times. Thus,
bioavailability is greatly underestimated when k_a is low.

As the first-order absorption rate constant is increased, the oral
dose saturates metabolism to a greater degree, resulting in a smaller
value of overall clearance and reduced error. At a certain value of
k_a (approximately 0.1 min^{-1} in the simulations done here), the overall clearances of both doses are equal and there is no error in bioavailability estimation [Eq. (11)]. At higher values of k_a, the oral
dose saturates metabolism to a greater degree than the intravenous
dose and bioavailability is overestimated. In this instance, direct
input of orally absorbed drug into the blood entering the liver is

rapid enough to more than compensate for the rapid intravenous bolus
input into the sampling compartment.

Even though the initial value of clearance after oral dosing can
be much lower than that of the intravenous dose when k_a is large,
error is never great here. This is true because, as k_a increases,
there is a shortening in the absorption period relative to the time
it takes for drug to be eliminated. Thus, the period in which large
differences in the clearance-time profiles occurs becomes shorter.
Error approaches zero as k_a approaches infinity.

4. Volume of Distribution

The relationship between volume of distribution and percentage error
in the bioavailability estimate is given in Fig. 8D. At low volumes of
distribution, the concentration-time profile for drug entering the
liver tends to be much lower for the oral dose than for the intravenous dose (Fig. 10). This is true because elimination, which tends
to be relatively fast at low volumes of distribution, occurs at the
same time that oral absorption is taking place. First-pass metabolism
also tends to lower the concentration of orally administered drug
entering the liver because it reduces the amount of drug reaching
the sampling compartment. Direct input of oral drug into the blood
entering the liver adds somewhat to the total concentration entering
the liver, but does not compensate for the concentration-lowering
effects of slower oral input and first-pass metabolism. As a result,
the overall clearance of the oral dose tends to be much higher than

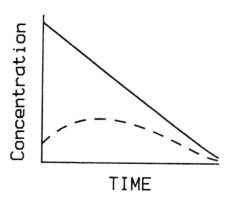

TIME

FIGURE 10 Typical concentration-time profiles of drug entering the
liver after separate administration of equal intravenous (solid line)
and oral (dashed line) doses when volume is low (10 liters).

that of the intravenous dose and bioavailability is underestimated
[Eq. (11)].

When the volume of distribution is increased, both doses result
in less saturation of metabolism. Because the concentration resulting
from the absorption of orally administered drug into the blood entering
the liver is not influenced by the volume of distribution, the degree
of saturation of the oral dose is less influenced by increases in
volume. Therefore, as volume is increased, the overall clearance
of the intravenous dose increases (relatively) more than that of
the oral dose and the error in bioavailability estimation declines
[Eq. (11)].

At a volume of distribution between 100 and 150 liters, the overall clearances of the intravenous and oral doses are nearly equal and
there is little error in bioavailability estimates. At higher volumes
of distribution, bioavailability is overestimated because elimination
of the intravenous drug becomes virtually first order. Oral administration, on the other hand, always results in saturable metabolism
during first pass (at the dose used in the simulation). Error is not
large in this circumstance because the half-life increases with the
volume of distribution; thus, the period in which oral absorption
occurs and clearance is reduced is relatively short compared with
the time it takes for the doses to be eliminated. Hence, only a small
fraction of the area under the systemic concentration-time curve
of the oral dose is associated with the low clearances that occur during
absorption. At volumes of distribution greater than 250 liters, the
error in bioavailability estimates declines when volume is increased.

There are a number of drugs with high volumes of distribution
that exhibit saturable elimination during absorption, but linear
elimination after absorption is complete (many drugs in Table 3 are
in this category). According to the preceding discussion, these
drugs may be adequately handled by the conventional method, but

TABLE 3 Drugs Exhibiting Saturable First-Pass Metabolism

Alprenolol	Phenacetin
5-Fluorouracil	Propoxyphene
Hydralazine	Propranolol
Lorcainide	Salicylamide
Methoxysalen	Thymidine
Metoprolol	

for any of them that show a substantial distribution phase, an appropriate distribution model may be required for estimation of accuracy.

5. Incomplete Absorption

Until now, all the simulations have been based on complete absorption of the oral dose into the portal system. Many drug products are characterized by incomplete absorption, a factor that reduces bioavailability both directly and potentially as a result of a reduction in the degree of saturation of first-pass metabolism. Because incomplete absorption reduces the saturation of the oral dose, it is expected to affect the accuracy of the bioavailability estimation by increasing the overall clearance of the oral dose relative to that of the intravenous dose. The effect on accuracy can be quite substantial, as is shown in Table 4.

TABLE 4 Relationship Between Selected Parameters and Error in the Conventional Method of Bioavailability Estimations Associated with Incomplete Drug Absorption

Parameter	Parameter Value	% Error Fraction of dose absorbed		
		1.0	0.9	0.5
Dose	27	-2.1	-2.3	-2.9
(μ mol)	66	-10.5	-11.5	-14.0
	178	-24.3	-29.9	-46.3
	255	-22.8	-30.2	-54.6
	1390	-5.7	-15.6	-55.0
V_{max}	0.017	-0.5	-10.0	-47.8
(μ mol/min)	0.15	-4.5	-13.9	-51.0
	1.35	-24.3	-29.9	-46.3
	2.85	-15.5	-17.0	-20.1
	14.9	0.2	0.2	0.2
k_a	0.005	-49.2	-49.7	-50.8
(min^{-1})	0.02	-24.3	-29.9	-46.3
	0.05	-5.3	-12.4	-36.9
	0.10	0.2	-7.3	-33.1
Volume	10	-54.7	-62.3	-84.8
(liters)	50	-24.3	-29.9	-46.3
	200	4.0	2.1	-4.1

Because the overall clearance of the oral dose is increased when absorption is incomplete, error tends to become less positive or more negative or become negative after being positive [Eq. (11)]. When the oral dose is eliminated under near first-order conditions, a reduction in the fraction absorbed will not materially change the overall clearance and bioavailability estimates remain relatively unaffected by reduction absorption. This occurs when dose or k_a is low or when V_{max} or volume of distribution is high, conditions that tend to result in first-order metabolism (Table 4). In all these cases, except that of low k_a, bioavailability tends to be accurate whether or not absorption is reduced.

When the pharmacokinetic parameters result in a high degree of saturation of the oral dose, incomplete absorption tends to result in substantial increases in overall clearance. This increases the error in bioavailability estimates whenever the overall clearance of the oral dose is normally greater than that of the intravenous dose, that is, when bioavailability is underestimated [Eq. (11)]. When error is normally small due to low extraction conditions (high dose or low V_{max}), reduced absorption causes a substantial increase in the error in bioavailability estimates (Table 4; $V_{max} = 0.017$ μmol/min and dose = 1390 μmol).

In summary, the conventional method is accurate for the estimation of bioavailability of Michaelis-Menten drugs when the clearance-time profiles of both doses are constant (low dose, high V_{max}, or large volume of distribution) and when the AUC-normalized concentration-time profiles and clearance-time profiles after intravenous and oral dosing superimpose (high dose, k_a, or volume of distribution; low V_{max}). Error tends to be large at low values of k_a and volume of distribution. In many instances, error is substantially increased when drug absorption is incomplete.

An important generalization that can be made for the conventional method is that, when absorption is complete and the clearance-time profile begins lower for the oral dose than for the intravenous dose, error tends to be moderate or low. This occurs at high values of k_a and volume of distribution. Simulations using other sets of values for k_a and volume of distribution have confirmed this observation. This characteristic may be used as a rough, but practical, guide for predicting whether the conventional method will be accurate.

VI. CONCURRENT DOSING METHOD

The basis for the concurrent dosing method is that, when there is no kinetic isotope effect, drug from both the tracer intravenous (labeled) and oral (unlabeled) doses should experience the same clearance values. Tracer quantities are given intravenously to avoid altering

the kinetics and the bioavailability of the oral dose. Before the concurrent dosing method is chosen in a given situation, it should first
be demonstrated to be more accurate than the conventional method.
This applies unless other characteristics make its use more favorable,
such as avoidance of between treatment changes in clearance.

In this section, the accuracy of the concurrent dosing method
is tested under the same conditions used to evaluate the conventional
method. The results for the two methods are compared, and ex-
planations are given for the relative accuracy of each.

Modification of intravenous dose input are investigated to determine
if the concurrent dosing method can be improved. These modifications
include delaying administration of the bolus and giving the intravenous
dose as a short-term constant-rate infusion. Finally, the effect of a
delay (lag time) in the absorption of drug from an oral dose is examined.

A. Error in Bioavailability

According to Equations (14) and (15), the overall clearances of the
oral and intravenous doses are equal when the AUC-normalized concentration-time profiles superimpose or when elimination is first order.
As with the conventional method, superpositioning is expected to
be approached with the concurrent dosing method when oral absorption
is fast relative to elimination, but exact superpositioning never
occurs. When oral absorption is slow relative to elimination, the
concentration-time profiles are very different. As the overall clearance
value of the intravenous dose is most influenced by the clearance
values near the time of dosing and that of the oral dose is most
affected by the values occurring near the time of the peak concentration, there may be substantial error in the bioavailability estimate.

B. Simulation Results

1. Dose

The relationship between error in the bioavailability estimate and the
size of the oral dose is shown in Figure 11A. The results of the
conventional method are shown for comparison. As with the conventional
method, when the dose is small enough to result in a relatively constant value of clearance, error tends to be small. As dose is increased,
clearance varies over a wider range and the difference between
clearance values at the time of dosing and the peak time becomes
larger. This results in an increased tendency to underestimate bioavailability because the overall clearance of the intravenous dose,
which peaks when clearance is lowest, declines relative to that of
the oral dose [Eq. (11)]. In this series of simulations, error reaches
a maximum of approximately 15% between doses of 150 and 300 μmol.

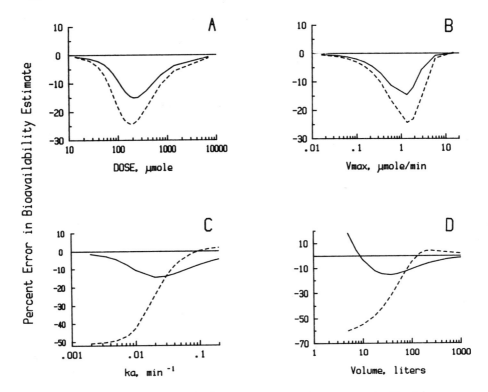

FIGURE 11 The relationship between percentage error in the bioavailability estimate and (A) dose, (B) V_{max}, (C) k_a, and (D) V.
The solid and dashed lines connect the values determined for the
concurrent dosing and conventional methods of bioavailability estimation,
respectively.

When dose is further increased, the increased degree of superpositioning of the AUC-normalized concentration-time profiles becomes
the most important factor influencing error, which thus becomes
smaller. As with the conventional method, increased superpositioning
occurs because increased saturation of elimination increases the length
of the elimination phase of the oral dose relative to its absorption
phase.

Bioavailability is underestimated at all the oral doses tested. This
is explained as follows. When drug absorption is first order and
the rate constant is large enough, the concentration of drug entering

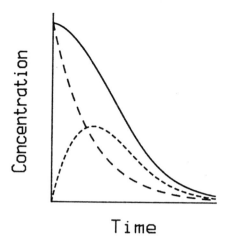

FIGURE 12 Typical concentration-time profile for drug entering the liver (solid line). This concentration is the sum of the concentrations from first-order (oral) input into the blood entering the liver (large dashes) and returning to the liver from the sampling compartment (small dashes). The concentration entering the liver declines at the outset because the concentration from oral input initially declines more rapidly than the concentration in the sampling compartment rises.

the liver tends to fall with time (Fig. 12) because of the continuous decrease in the amount of drug at the absorption site and a corresponding reduction in absorption rate. In response, clearance, which changes inversely with concentration, tends to rise with time, as shown at the top of Figure 13. Because the intravenous input is not prolonged in a manner similar to oral input (bottom of Fig. 13), the overall clearance value determined for the intravenous tracer dose reflects earlier and lower values of instantaneous clearance. The overall clearance of the intravenous dose is therefore smaller than that of the oral dose and bioavailability is underestimated [Eq. (11)].

2. Maximum Rate of Metabolism

The relationship between error in the bioavailability estimate and V_{max} is shown in Figure 11B and is compared to the same relationship determined for the conventional method. At low values of V_{max}, which result in low hepatic extraction ratios, elimination tends to be slow relative to absorption and the AUC-normalized intravenous and oral

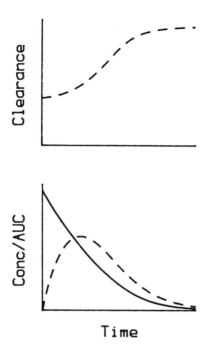

FIGURE 13 Typical clearance-time (top) and AUC-normalized concentration-time profiles (bottom) after concurrent intravenous (solid line) and oral (dashed line) dosing.

concentration-time profiles tend to superimpose. This results in relatively small error. As V_{max} is increased, elimination becomes faster and the tendency toward superpositioning is reduced and hence error becomes larger.

As V_{max} exceeds a value of about 1.35 μmol/min, error tends to decrease. The explanation for this is the same as given for the conventional method; that is, when the extraction ratio is high, there is a tendency for clearance to remain constant even when metabolism is partially saturated.

Comparing the results for both dose and V_{max}, the concurrent dosing method is, in all cases, more accurate than the conventional method. For any given value of dose or V_{max}, the degree of superpositioning of the intravenous and oral AUC-normalized concentration-time profiles is similar for both methods, and hence the differences in accuracy can be primarily ascribed to the clearance-time profiles.

Error is higher with the conventional method because the clearance-
time profile of the intravenous dose is lower than that of the oral
dose, adding to the error resulting from the lack of superpositioning.
It should be noted that the difference in clearance profiles is a function
of k_a, V, and Q_H as well as dose and V_{max}. Thus when the accuracy
of the two methods is compared by changing the value of a single
parameter, the results of the comparison may be different from those
using a different combination of fixed parameter values.

It might be predicted that if the clearance-time profiles were
reversed, that is, the oral dose resulted in a lower clearance-time
profile, the conventional method would be more accurate than the
concurrent dosing method. This prediction is tested in the following
sections on first-order absorption rate constant and volume of distribution where a reversal in the order of the clearance-time profiles
is observed.

3. Absorption Rate Constant

The relationship between error and the first-order absorption rate constant is shown in Figure 11C and is compared to the results obtained
with the conventional method. At low values of k_a, the concentration
that enters the liver from the oral dose tends to be small and there
is little reduction of clearance from its first-order value. Drug from
the concurrently administered intravenous tracer dose follows the
same clearance-time profile; consequently, the error in bioavailability
estimation is small. With the conventional method, when equal doses
are administered separately, the intravenous dose produces a much
lower clearance-time profile, resulting in error that is much greater
than that observed with the concurrent dosing method.

As the first-order absorption rate constant is increased, drug
from oral dose exhibits an increased degree of saturation and clearance
varies more during elimination. The error in bioavailability estimation
by the concurrent dosing method thus increases, reaching a maximum
of about 15% at a k_a value of 0.02 min^{-1}. For the conventional method,
on the other hand, bioavailability estimates improve with increasing
values of the absorption rate constant because the overall clearance
of the intravenous dose is unaffected but that of the oral dose
decreases toward the value for the intravenous dose.

When the absorption rate constant is large, oral input becomes
kinetically similar to intravenous input. This results in AUC-normalized
concentration-time profiles that tend to superimpose, thus giving
a high degree of accuracy. The conventional method, however, is
even more accurate than the concurrent dosing method when the
absorption rate constant is large ($k_a > 0.03$ min^{-1}). This is true,
as was predicted, because at high values of k_a, the clearance-time
profile of the oral dose tends to be lower than that of the intravenous

dose, compensating for the differences in the AUC-normalized concentration-time profiles.

4. *Volume of Distribution*

The relationship between error in the bioavailability estimate and
volume of distribution is shown in Figure 11D. When the volume of
distribution is low, clearance tends to be lowest near the oral dose
peak time, as shown in Figure 14. Because the intravenous tracer
input is complete at the time of dosing when clearance is higher,
the overall clearance of the intravenous dose tends to be higher than
that of the oral dose and bioavailability is overestimated. The decrease

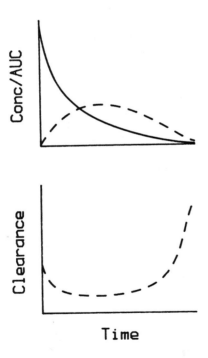

FIGURE 14 Typical AUC-normalized concentration-time profiles
(top) resulting from concurrent intravenous (solid line) and oral
(dashed line) doses when the volume of distribution is low (7.5
liters). The clearance-time profile (bottom) results from the total
concentration entering the liver from the oral dose.

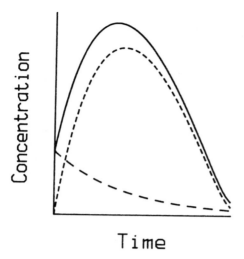

FIGURE 15 Concentration-time course of drug entering the liver (solid line), which is the sum of the concentrations from first-order input into the blood entering the liver (large dashes) and returning to the liver from the sampling compartment (small dashes). The curves are typical for a drug with a small volume of distribution (7.5 liters). The concentration entering the liver rises at the outset because the concentration in the sampling compartment rises faster than the concentration from direct oral input declines.

in clearance at early times is a result of the relatively fast buildup of concentrations in the sampling compartment, which occurs at low volumes of distribution. More specifically, the initial rate of increase in drug concentration in the sampling compartment is faster than the initial rate of decline in the concentration derived from the absorption site (Fig. 15). Because the concentration of drug entering the liver is the sum of the two, its value initially increases with time.

When the volume of distribution is equal to about 10 liters, the error in bioavailability estimates changes from positive to negative (Fig. 11D). This happens because the rate of increase in the concentration in the sampling compartment is reduced enough so that the concentration entering the liver tends to fall with time, resulting in little or no decrease in clearance from its initial value after oral dosing. The natural tendency for clearance to rise with time as drug is removed from the absorption site and eliminated from the body causes of the overall clearance of the later-peaking oral dose to be higher than that of the intravenous dose, and bioavailability is under-estimated [Eq (11)]. The accuracy of the bioavailability estimate in-creases at volumes of greater than 40 liters because the difference in intravenous and oral input periods becomes small in relation in the in-creasingly long half-life, resulting in an increased superpositioning of the curves.

Up to a volume of distribution of approximately 75 liters, the concurrent dosing method tends to be more accurate than the con-ventional method. Between volumes of about 75 and 400 liters, the conventional method is more accurate because the clearance-time profile of the oral dose tends to be lower than that of the separately administered intravenous dose. Above a volume of 400 liters, both methods are accurate, with the concurrent dosing method the more accurate of the two.

5. Incomplete Absorption

The relationship between the bioavailability estimate and the fraction of the oral dose that is absorbed is given in Table 5. Changes in er-ror as absorption is decreased tend to be relatively small, especially when the fraction of the dose absorbed drops from 1.0 to 0.9.

Table 5 shows that error can either increase or decrease as the fraction absorbed is reduced, depending on the pharmacokinetic conditions evaluated. When there is a high degree of saturation and a resultant high degree of superpositioning of the AUC-normalized concentration-time profiles (high dose or low V_{max}), incomplete absorption results in less saturation and therefore increased error. When the degree of saturation is low and error is small because clearance is almost constant (low dose or k_a; high V_{max} or V), reduced absorption causes an increase in accuracy. In the situation in which error tends to be large because neither of the conditions for accuracy is approached, error may either increase or decrease when the extent of absorption is decreased, depending on whether the effect of reduced superpositioning (increased error) or the effect of a more constant clearance-time profile (reduced error) predominates.

Compared with the conventional method, the concurrent dosing method is generally more accurate when there is incomplete absorption. With the conventional method, reduced absorption almost always makes error worse, and the increases in error are often large (Table 4).

Summarizing the simulations to this point, the concurrent dosing method tends to be more than the conventional method under conditions in which the clearance-time profile of the intravenous dose is lower than that of the oral dose, that is, when the first-order absorption rate constant is less than 0.03 min^{-1} or the volume of distribution is

TABLE 5 Relationship Between Selected Parameters and Error in the Concurrent Dosing Method of Bioavailability Estimation Associated with Incomplete Drug Absorption

Parameter	Parameter Value	% Error Fraction of dose absorbed		
		1.0	0.9	0.5
Oral dose	27	-1.3	-1.2	-0.6
(μmol)	66	-4.8	-4.0	-1.7
	178	-14.6	-14.0	-7.6
	255	-14.9	-15.1	-11.8
	1390	-3.8	-4.3	-7.6
V_{max}	0.017	-0.3	-0.4	-0.6
(μmol/min)	0.15	-3.0	-3.3	-5.4
	1.35	-14.6	-14.0	-7.6
	2.85	-5.8	-4.7	-1.5
	14.9	-0.1	-0.1	-0.0
k_a	0.005	-4.4	-3.8	-1.6
(min^{-1})	0.02	-14.6	-14.0	-7.6
	0.05	-11.6	-11.9	-10.5
	0.10	-7.6	-8.0	-8.6
Volume	10	-2.9	-4.4	-6.4
(liters)	50	-14.6	-14.0	-7.6
	200	-6.3	-5.7	-2.7

less than 75 liters. Although the concurrent dosing method is not always more accurate than the conventional method, it is more robust because its error is almost always less than 15%; with the conventional method, error is greater than 50% at low values of k_a and volume of distribution. Furthermore, with the concurrent dosing method, the degree of error is less sensitive to differences in parameter values and hence is more predictable in individuals for whom the parameter values are uncertain.

C. Delay in the Intravenous Dose

An approach for improving the concurrent dosing method is to delay the intravenous bolus dose to increase the degree of superpositioning of the AUC-normalized concentration-time profiles. For the pharmacokinetic conditions studied, the most accurate bioavailability estimation generally occurs when the intravenous dose is delayed for a period

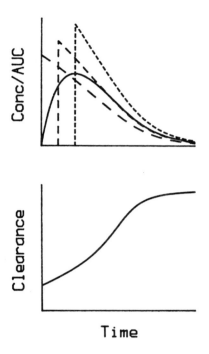

Time

FIGURE 16 Typical relationship between delay in intravenous dosing and the tendency of the AUC-normalized concentration-time profiles (top) resulting from intravenous (dashed lines) and oral (solid line) doses to superimpose. Intravenous doses were given at 0, 50, and 100% of the oral dose peak time. The initial concentration appears to be increased when the dose is delayed because of its normalization to AUC. The clearance-time profile is given in the lower graph.

that results in its AUC-normalized concentration-time profile over-lapping that of the oral dose after the peak is reached (top of Fig. 16, dose given at one-half peak time). This observation tends to confirm the hypothesis that the delay improves accuracy by increasing the degree of superpositioning of the AUC-normalized concentration-time curves. Delaying the intravenous dose, however, never results in perfect superpositioning because the normalized concentration-time profiles cannot superimpose during the absorption phase. Because clearance changes with time during this period, the overall clearances of the intravenous and oral doses are different even if the terminal portions of the normalized concentration profiles overlap.

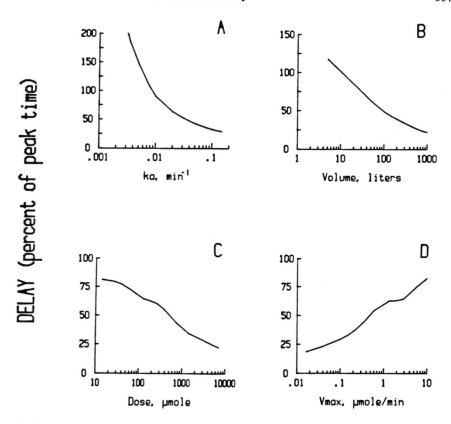

FIGURE 17 The delay (as a percentage of the oral dose peak time) in the intravenous bolus input that results in no error in the bioavailability estimate. The relationship between best delay time and k_a, (A), V (B), dose (C), and V_{max} (D) is shown. Using the errors calculated for delays of 0, 25, 50, 75, and 100% of peak time, the best delay was estimated by interpolation. The results are presented as lines that connect the calculated values of best delay. When the best delay was greater than the peak time, it was calculated by extrapolating the results for delays of 75 and 100% of peak time.

The time delay that results in no error is therefore not the one that produces perfect overlapping, although it should be close.

A summary of the best delay times (reported as percentage of peak time) for each pharmacokinetic parameter studied in the simulations is given in Figure 17. Shorter delays are required as the first-order absorption rate constant, volume of distribution, or dose becomes larger and as V_{max} becomes smaller. From this observation it appears that pharmacokinetic conditions that tend to result in a high degree of superpositioning when there is no delay in the intravenous dose also tend to require shorter delays for best accuracy. Although the optimum delay varies, in most cases a delay of 50% of peak time results in a sizable improvement over the accuracy seen with no delay (Table 6).

D. Short-Term Constant-Rate Infusion

Another approach to improving bioavailability estimation is to administer the reference dose as a short-term constant-rate infusion. The results, summarized in Table 6, show that in most cases infusion until peak time is much more accurate than bolus dosing with no delay. Interestingly, similar results are obtained either when the infusion is continued until the peak time or when the intravenous bolus dose is delayed by 50% of peak time. In both cases, the mean delay in input time is the same.

Error persists when infusion is used because the AUC-normalized intravenous and oral concentration-time profiles never perfectly superimpose; the input rate of drug from the oral dose (into the sampling compartment) is a function of first-order absorption and time-dependent changes in hepatic extraction; intravenous input is a zero-order process, however. Furthermore, a certain fraction of the oral dose, which can be large, remains to be absorbed when the intravenous infusion is finished at the peak time.

When either the first-order absorption rate constant or the volume of distribution is small, elimination tends to be fast relative to absorption and the peak concentration is reached early with respect to the time it takes to absorb the entire dose. Because of this, the fraction of the oral dose that remains to be absorbed when the infusion is finished at the peak time tends to be large, and poor superpositioning results. To improve accuracy in this situation, the infusion rate must be slowed and the infusion continued past the peak time. For example, when k_a is less than 0.02 min^{-1} or volume of distribution is less than 50 liters, accuracy is improved when the infusion is continued until 150% of the peak time (Table 6).

At the highest values of k_a, volume of distribution, or dose shown in Table 6, on the other hand, infusions of only 50% of the peak time are more accurate than infusions continued until the peak time. High values of k_a, V, and dose result in a high degree of superpositioning of the AUC-normalized concentration-time profiles when intravenous dosing is not modified. It is probably for this reason that less change is needed in the intravenous input (in this case, shorter infusions) to produce the optimal degree of superpositioning.

TABLE 6 Relationship Between Selected Parameters and Error in the Concurrent Dosing Method of Bioavailability Estimation as a Function of Delay in Intravenous Bolus Dosing or Infusion Period

Parameter	Parameter value	% Error				
		Delay in bolus (% of peak time)		Infusion period (% of peak time)		
		0	50	50	100	100
Oral dose (μ mole)	27	-1.3	-0.4	-0.7	-0.4	-0.1
	66	-4.8	-1.2	-2.6	-1.4	-0.2
	178	-14.6	-3.6	-8.7	-3.5	3.5
	739	-7.2	1.3	-3.4	1.6	7.5
	6960	-0.8	1.2	0.1	1.2	2.4
V_{max} (μ mole/min)	0.017	-0.3	0.7	1.6	0.7	1.8
	0.15	-3.0	2.0	-0.8	2.1	5.4
	1.35	-14.6	-3.6	-8.7	-3.5	3.5
	2.85	-5.8	-1.0	-3.3	-1.4	0.1
	14.9	-0.1	-0.0	0.5	0.0	0.2
$k_a(min^{-1})$	0.005	-4.4	-3.1	-3.5	-3.1	-2.2
	0.01	-10.7	-5.3	-7.9	-5.2	-2.1
	0.02	-14.6	-3.6	-8.7	-3.5	3.5
	0.05	-11.6	2.2	-4.6	1.7	8.9
	0.10	-7.6	4.3	-1.8	3.7	9.0
Volume (L)	5	18.1	-17.3	-10.8	-12.0	-6.1
	10	-2.9	-14.4	-12.8	-10.9	-3.9
	25	-14.7	-8.7	-12.4	-7.5	0.4
	50	-14.6	-3.6	-8.7	-3.5	3.5
	100	-10.5	0.3	-4.5	-0.3	4.3
	500	-2.7	1.6	-0.2	1.2	2.0

TABLE 7 Relationship Between Selected Parameters and Error in the Concurrent Dosing Method of Bioavailability Estimation as a Function of Lag Time in Absorption of an Oral Dose

	Parameter value	% Error lag time (min)			
Parameter		0	15	30	60
Oral dose	66	-5	-1	1	4
(μ mol)	178	-15	1	15	35
	739	-7	30	78	201
	6960	-1	48	119	374
V_{max}	0.017	0	4	9	18
(μ mol/min)	0.15	-3	18	43	106
	1.35	-15	1	15	35
	2.85	-6	-2	1	5
k_a	0.01	-11	-2	4	12
(min^{-1})	0.02	-15	1	15	35
	0.05	-12	8	27	58
	0.10	-8	13	34	67
Volume	10	-3	188	289	310
(liters)	25	-15	30	68	108
	50	-15	1	15	35
	100	-10	-5	1	8

E. Lag Time in Oral Absorption

Some dosage forms are characterized by a lag time before oral absorption begins. When this occurs, the estimate of bioavailability is increased, sometimes resulting in a great degree of overestimation (Table 7). This happens because a fraction of the intravenous tracer dose is eliminated under first-order conditions (maximum clearance) before oral absorption, and hence saturation of metabolism, begins. In some instances, however, our results show that a relatively short lag time can result in improved estimates of bioavailability. Overestimating bioavailability due to lag time in oral absorption is expected to be a problem when a large fraction of the intravenous dose is eliminated before oral absorption begins, that is, when the elimination half-life is short relative to the lag time. This is confirmed by the strong tendency for large positive error when the volume of distribution is small and results in a short half-life.

The tendency to overestimate bioavailability is also expected to be increased by factors that reduce clearance during elimination of the oral dose, making clearance differences larger before and after the start of absorption. The results demonstrate this to be true; greater overestimation of bioavailability occurs with increases in the dose and first-order absorption rate constant and decreases in the volume of distribution, all of which reduce the clearance-time profile of the oral dose. With respect to V_{max}, the tendency for positive error is small both at low values (long half-life) and high values (small reduction in clearance) of this parameter. To compensate for the effect of lag time, the estimated lag time should be added to the time of intravenous dosing estimated to be optimal when there is no delay in oral absorption. Because of the potential for a very large error, it is important to adjust input appropriately.

VII. CONCLUSION

The concurrent dosing method of bioavailability determination is accurate for drugs eliminated by Michaelis-Menten kinetics when either the clearance-time profile is constant)low dose or k_a; high V_{max} or V) or the AUC-normalized concentration-time profiles superimpose (high dose or V; low V_{max}). Bioavailability is underestimated except at low volumes of distribution, and error is rarely greater than 15%. The accuracy of this method generally compares favorable to the conventional method and can be further improved by modification of the time or duration of the intravenous dose input. However, a lag time in absorption of drug following an oral dose can be a serious limitation to the method.

In principle, the conventional and concurrent dosing methods can be used for other conditions, for example other sets of parameter values or models of drug distribution and nonlinear elimination. Before doing so, however, error analysis, similar to that performed here, can be helpful in estimating the error potentially involved for any specific set of conditions.

ACKNOWLEDGMENTS

This chapter was extracted, in part, from the Ph.D. dissertation, Bioavailability Determination of Drugs with Michaelis-Menten Elimination Kinetics by Gerald M. Rubin, University of California, San Francisco. The dissertation is available through University Microfilms International. Support (GM) from grant GM 26556 and training grant GM 07175 of the National Institutes of Health is gratefully ackowledged. We also wish to acknowledge Plenum Press for giving permission to use selected text and figures from our manuscript (Ref. 19).

REFERENCES

1. B. Silber, N. Holford, and S. Riegelman. Dose-dependent elimination of propranolol and its major metabolites in humans, J. Pharm. Sci. 72: 725–732, 1983.
2. E. Jähnchen, H. Bechtold, W. Kasper, F. Kersting, H. Just, J. Heykants, and T. Meinertz. Lorcainide. I. Saturable presystemic elimination. Clin. Pharmacol. Ther. 26: 187–195, 1979.
3. B. Ablad, M. Ervik, J. Hallgren, G. Johnsson, and L. Sölvell. Pharmacological effects and serum levels of orally administered alprenolol in man. Eur. J. Clin. Pharmacol. 5: 44–52, 1972.
4. G. Rubin and T. Tozer. Theoretical considerations in the calculation of bioavailability of drugs exhibiting Michaelis-Menten elimination kinetics. J. Pharmacokinet. Biopharm. 12: 437–450, 1984.
5. L. Martis and R. Levy. Bioavailability calculations for drugs showing simultaneous first-order and capacity-limited elimination kinetics. J. Pharmacokinet. Biopharm. 1: 283–294, 1973.
6. W. Jusko, J. Koup, and G. Alván. Nonlinear assessment of phenytoin bioavailability. J. Pharmacokinet. Biopharm. 4: 327–336, 1976.
7. N. Watari, T. Funaki, K. Aizawa, and N. Kaneniwa. Nonlinear assessment of nitrofurantoin bioavailability in rabbits. J. Pharmacokinet. Biopharm. 11: 529–545, 1983.
8. F. Keller and J. Scholle. First-pass effect: Nonlinear concept comprising an explicit solution of integrated Michaelis-Menten equation. J. Pharm. Sci. 70: 195–198, 1981.
9. P. Wilkinson, A. Sedman, E. Sakamar, D. Kay, and J. Wagner. Pharmacokinetics of ethanol after oral administration in the fasting state. J. Pharmacokinet. Biopharm. 5: 207–224, 1977.
10. P. Veng-Pederson. Novel method of calculating absolute bioavailability in nonlinear pharmacokinetics. J. Pharm. Sci. 74: 90–93, 1985.
11. P. Meffin, R. Edward, R. Winkle, S. Harapat, F. Peters, and D. Harrison. Role of concentration-dependent plasma protein binding in disopyramide disposition. J. Pharmacokinet. Biopharm. 7: 29–47, 1979.
12. R. Galinsky and G. Levy. Dose- and time-dependent elimination of acetaminophen in rats: Pharmacokinetic implications of co-substrate depletion. J. Pharmacol. Exp. Ther. 219: 14–20, 1981.
13. P. Dayton and J. Sanders. Dose-dependent pharmacokinetics. Emphasis on phase I metabolism. Drug Metab. Rev. 14: 347–405, 1983.
14. J. Waschek, R. Fielding, S. Pond, G. Rubin, D. Effeney, and T. Tozer. Dose-dependent sulfoconjugation of salicylamide in

dogs: Effect of sulfate depletion or administration. J. Pharmacol. Exp. Ther. 234: 431–434, 1985.

15. D. Kornhauser, A. Wood, R. Vestal, G. Wilkinson, R. Branch, and D. Shand. Biological determinants of propranolol disposition in man. Clin. Pharmacol. Ther. 23: 165–174, 1978.

16. Y. Kasuya, K. Mamada, S. Baba, and M. Matsukura. Stable-isotope methodology for the bioavailability study of phenytoin during multiple-dosing regimens. J. Pharm. Sci. 74: 503–507, 1985.

17. J. Waschek, G. Rubin, T. Tozer, R. Fielding, W. Couet, D. Effeney, and S. Pond. Dose-dependent bioavailability and metabolism of salicylamide in dogs. J. Pharmacol. Exp. Ther. 230: 89–93, 1984.

18. S. Øie and D. Jung. Bioavailability under variable renal clearance conditions. J. Pharm. Sci. 68: 128–129, 1979.

19. G. Rubin, J. Waschek, S. Pond, D. Effeney, and T. Tozer. Concurrent intravenous administration of a labeled tracer to determine the oral bioavailability of a drug exhibiting Michaelis-Menten metabolism. J. Pharmacokinet. Biopharm. 15: 615–631, 1987.

20. K. Pang and M. Rowland. Hepatic clearance of drugs. I. Theoretical considerations of a "well-stirred" model and a "parallel-tube" model. Influence of hepatic blood flow, plasma and blood cell binding and the hepatocellular enzymatic activity on hepatic drug clearance. J. Pharmacokinet. Biopharm. 5: 625–653, 1977.

21. P. Wilkinson, A. Sedman, E. Sakamar, R. Earhart, D. Weidler, and J. Wagner. Blood ethanol concentrations during and following constant-rate intravenous infusion of alcohol. Clin. Pharmacol. Ther. 19: 213–223, 1976.

22. D. Stubbs. Models of gastric emptying. Gut. 18: 202–207, 1977.

23. K. Yorgey, J. Pritchard, N. Renzi, and B. Dvorchik. Evaluation of drug absorption and presystemic metabolism using an in situ intestinal preparation. J. Pharm. Sci. 75: 869–872, 1986.

24. S. Pond and T. Tozer. First-pass elimination: Basic concepts and clinical consequences. Clin. Pharmacokinet. 9: 1–25, 1984.

25. G. Alván, M. Lind, B. Mellström, and C. von Bahr. Importance of "first-pass elimination" for interindividual differences in steady-state concentrations of the adrenergic β-receptor antagonist alprenolol. J. Pharmacokinet. Biopharm. 5: 193–205, 1977.

13

Time-Dependent Pharmacokinetics: Recent Developments

RENE H. LEVY and C. R. BANFIELD *University of Washington, Seattle, Washington*

I. INTRODUCTION

Time-dependent pharmacokinetics belong among nonlinear phenomena in pharmacokinetics. In the first review on this subject (1), time-dependent phenomena were classified in two categories: physiologically induced, such as chronopharmacokinetics, and chemically induced, such as auto- and heteroinduction. This classification is still valid and is followed in this chapter. Comprehensive compilations of chronopharmacokinetic studies can be found in the reviews of Reinberg and Smolensky (2) and Labrecque and Bélanger (3). Mechanistic aspects of time-dependent phenomena were recently considered (4). This chapter constitutes an update and emphasizes new developments not covered in earlier reviews.

II. CHRONOPHARMACOKINETICS

A. Prevalence and Manifestation of the Phenomenon

1. Theophylline

Theophylline plays an important role in the treatment of asthma. In light of its pharmacokinetic characteristics (short half-life and narrow therapeutic range) and because the disease is worse at night in most patients, controlled-release dosage forms were developed.

After introduction of sustained-release formulations, a number of reports indicated diurnal differences in plasma steady-state levels (5-7). These observations raised the question of a diurnal cycle in systematic clearance of this drug, and this issue was addressed in several studies. Although four studies found no diurnal change in intravenous clearance (8-11), two reports support the existence of a diurnal phenomenon (12,13).

A number of recent studies continued to examine circadian effects associated with oral theophylline. Watanabe et al. (9) reported that in 16 volunteers administered aminophylline in a powder form at 9 a.m. or at 9 p.m., the time to peak was shorter and peak plasma concentration was higher in the morning than in the evening. No difference in $t_{1/2}$ or area under the concentration-time curve (AUC) was observed.

In subjects administered either a compressed or sustained-release tablet, a longer time to reach peak concentration was observed after administration at 8 p.m. than at 8 a.m. (10). The chronopharmaco-kinetic behavior of theophylline was studied in eight patients with obstructive airway disease during regular 12-hr dosing at 9 a.m. and 9 p.m. (sustained-release formulation with pH-independent dissolution) (14). On day 4, the plasma concentrations for the first 5 hr after the morning dose were significantly higher than after the evening dose. However, the areas under the drug concentration-time curve were not significantly different. Therefore, although the rate of absorption appeared to be delayed in the evening, the extent of absorption was not impaired. In contrast, nine nocturnal asthmatics dosed with a sustained-release formulation of theophylline at either 8 a.m. or 8 p.m. for 5 days showed a statistically significantly smaller mean AUC when administered at 8 p.m. (15).

In a recent study conducted by Uematsu et al. (11), data were obtained from patients with an acute exacerbation of asthma or chronic obstructive lung disease. Aminophylline was infused for at least 30 hr followed by oral administration of a slow-release preparation (Xantivent) at 2 p.m., 10 p.m., and 6 a.m. Following oral dosing, the mean AUC after daytime administration (2—10 p.m.) was significantly larger ($p < 0.01$) than that following night administration (10 p.m. to 6 a.m.). In the six patients the AUC difference between morning and evening ranged from no change in two subjects to a 32% increase.

2. Indomethacin

In an early study in which indomethacin and its odemethyl metabolite were measured following administration of a sustained-release preparation at 8 a.m., 12 noon, and 8 p.m., it was found that demethylation was higher at night (8 p.m.) compared with either 8 or 12 a.m. (16). In contrast, administration of an indomethacin suppository (100 mg) to 12 healthy males at 9 a.m. and 9 p.m. failed to show any diurnal variation in C_{max}, t_{max}, $t_{1/2}$, AUC, or 24 hr urinary elimination (17).

3. Lithium

In a recent study, Olesen et al. (18) examined the diurnal disposition of lithium in rats. Li clearance was statistically significantly higher in the dark period than during the light period. The increase in clearance was 50% in a low-Li group and 80% in a high-Li group. However, no diurnal variation in serum Li was observed. In parallel, the mean Na and K clearances and mean urine flow showed the same diurnal variation. Urine flow was 200% larger during the dark period. Li is reabsorbed in the proximal tubule to the same extent as Na and water but is not reabsorbed in the loop of Henle, the distal tubules, or collecting ducts. The authors concluded that Li clearance is equal to the volume of fluid delivered from the proximal tubules to the loop of Henle. Therefore, the increase Li clearance following high doses of Li was due to an increase in the volume of fluid delivered from the proximal tubules.

4. Heparin

Heparin is the most widely used drug in the initial treatment and prevention of venous thrombosis. During continuous infusion with heparin over a 2-day period, a circadian variation in anticoagulant effect was observed using either activated partial thromboplastin time, thrombin time, or factor Xa inhibition assays (19). Maximum

anticoagulation was observed at night (4 a.m.) and minimum effect
in the morning (8 a.m.). The mean differences were 50% in activated
partial thromboplastin time, 60% in thrombin time, and 40% in factor
Xa inhibition assay. These findings suggested that a circadian rhythm
in the pharmacokinetics of heparin may exist and contribute to the
observed differences.

The time dependency of the pharmacokinetics of $^{99}Tc^m$-labeled
heparin was studied in six healthy volunteers who received the drug
as an intravenous bolus (160 IU) at four different times: 8 a.m.,
2 p.m., 8 p.m., and 2 a.m. (20). A 7-day interval was allowed between
consecutive injections. Cosinor analysis and the Gauss-Marquardt
method showed no significant circadian rhythm for the apparent
volume of distribution V, plasma clearance CL, or extrarenal metabolic
clearance (ERMC) expressed as the mean of the raw values. However,
a circadian rhythm in CL was apparent when data were expressed as
a percentage of the individual 24 hr mean (p < 0.04). For V, CL,
and ERMC, significant variations were observed between 8 a.m. and
2 p.m. (p < 0.01) and between 2 and 8 p.m. (p < 0.05). The magnitude
of peak-trough difference over 24 hr varied from subject to subject.
The largest differences were 110% for V, 87% for CL, and 120% for
ERMC. Although circadian rhythms in the pharmacokinetic parameters
were observed, the maximum clearance value at 2 p.m. did not correspond to minimum anticoagulant effect (8 a.m.). Similarly, the
lowest clearance (at 8 p.m.) did not correspond to maximum anticoagulant effect (4 a.m.). Thus the temporal variation in pharmacokinetics does not explain the circadian variation in anticoagulant
effect.

5. Cyclosporin

Major success in organ grafting has been attributed to the use of
cyclosporin as an immunosuppressant. Diurnal variations in cyclosporin kinetics were investigated as a possible explanation for marked
variations in cyclosprin trough levels seen within patients (21).

Th maintenance dose (140—150 mg) as an infusion (1 hr) in the
morning and at night was administered to two patients who underwent
orthotopic liver transplant. The trough concentration following administration at night was lower than that obtained after morning
dosing. The difference was 42% in one patient.

The differences in blood clearance between night and day were
39 and 42% in the patients under study. During re-evaluation of one
patient a third time, the clearance and trough concentrations showed
the same trends as previously described. The authors attributed
the time of day phenomenon to circadian variations in hepatic drug
metabolizing enzymes or diurnal changes in plasma lipoprotein profiles,
the primary transport agent for cyclosporin.

6. Cis-diamine Dichloroplatinum (Cisplatin)

Cisplatin is an important anticancer agent that binds irreversibly to plasma proteins and is eliminated by renal excretion. Severe irreversible renal damage, predominantly tubular, is associated with cisplatin therapy. Reports suggest that the degree of nephrotoxicity is related to the urinary concentration of free platinum. Since there are circadian rhythms in renal function (22), some investigations focused on correlating renal damage and time of administration. Hrushesky et al. (23) tested that hypothesis in 11 patients who had advanced malignancies. Of the 11 patients, 5 had one kidney. Patients were randomly assigned to one of two treatment protocols. Schedule A consisted of 60 mg/m^2 doxorubicin (D) given at 6 a.m. followed 12 hr later (at 6 p.m.) by 60 mg/m^2 cisplatin (C); in schedule B the same dose of D was given at 6 p.m. followed 12 hr later by the identical dose of C. Each drug was administered as an intravenous infusion over 30 min. Patients were alternated monthly between the two schedules.

Regardless of kidney number, the average diuresis over 4.5 hr after cisplatin infusion was greater when the drug was given at 6 p.m. than when given at 6 a.m. (1140 and 900 ml, respectively) (21%). The urine volume (at each 30-min collection) was always greater following evening than morning administration (except at 3.5 hr) resulting in a lower concentration of free platinum. Patients receiving the drug at 6 p.m. had a mean peak urinary concentration (29.6 ± 1.7 μg/ml) approximately 50% lower than that achieved (43.8 ± 2 μg/ml) by the same subjects after 6 a.m. administration. The more rapid urinary clearance in cisplatin following evening administration resulted in a significant reduction (71%) in the area under the urinary concentration-time curve for free platinum over the 4.5 hr period.

Hecquet et al. (24), in a series of in vitro experiments, investigated the circadian variation of cisplatin binding to plasma proteins by evaluating the rate of binding in plasma from nine patients at several different times of the day. Cisplatin was incubated in vitro at 37°C with each sample of plasma. A plot of log concentration versus incubation time was linear, and its slope was the rate of binding k. Plasma samples from the same subject corresponding to different times yielded different binding values (k). Cosinor analysis of k showed a significant circadian rhythm with the acrophase at 4.1 p.m. (range 1—7.2 p.m.).

Cisplatin binding and plasma protein content were evaluated in nine other subjects in plasma collected at 4 a.m. and at 4 p.m. The protein concentration and the value of k were always higher at 4 p.m. than at 4 a.m.

In four patients prehydrated for 6 hr prior to blood sampling at

9 a.m. or at 3 p.m., the value of k was always greater at 3 p.m. than
at 9 a.m. The authors suggest that the level of unbound cisplatin
must be lower in the afternoon. This effect may thus partly explain
the decrease in toxicity observed when cisplatin is administered in
that part of the activity span (25—27).

B. Mechanistic Aspects

Diurnal variation in cytochrome P_{450}-mediated drug-metabolizing
activity has been previously reported (28—31). Temporal variations
in enzyme systems that control the rates of formation and degradation
of glucuronide and sulfate conjugates were studied by Bélanger et al.
(32). Male albino Sprague-Dawley rates were maintained on a 12-hr
light dark cycle (7 a.m. to 7 p.m.). Rats were sacrificed at 9 a.m. or
9 p.m., and the 10,000 g supernatant fraction, soluble fraction,
and microsomal pellets obtained from their livers were examined. The
regulation of these systems by food intake was also investigated by
using a freely fed group and a fasted group (deprived of food and
water 12—16 hr before sacrifice). UDP-glucuronosyltransferase and
β-glucuronidase activities were determined in the microsomal and
10,000 g fractions, respectively, whereas sulfotransferase and sulfatase
activities were measured in the soluble fraction.

In freely fed rats there was a significant increase (57%) in V_{max}
of UDP-glucuronosyltransferase at 9 p.m. compared with the activity
at 9 a.m. The microsomal protein, however, showed a significant
decrease ($p < 0.05$) at 9 p.m. No diurnal variation in the apparent
K_m value was observed. Fasting was associated with an increase
in the values of V_{max} at both diurnal periods, reaching significance
at 9 a.m. However the diurnal variation in V_{max} was not present in
the fasted group. There was no time dependency for microsomal
protein or K_m in fasted animals.

The sulfotransferase V_{max} exhibited diurnal variation in freely
fed rats with a significant reduction (54%) at 9 p.m. In the fasted
group no diurnal variation was observed. In freely fed rats, K_m
was 4.5 times greater at 9 a.m. than at 9 p.m. However, there was
no diurnal variation in the K_m in the fasted group. No diurnal variation
was observed for the soluble fraction protein either in freely fed
or fasted animals.

The activities of β-glucuronidase and sulfatase and the 10,000 g
supernatant protein content showed no diurnal variation in freely
fed animals. However, in the fasted group there was appreciable
(two- to threefold) diurnal variation in both V_{max} of K_m of sulfatase
activity.

III. CHEMICALLY INDUCED TIME DEPENDENCY

A. Autoinduction in Metabolic Clearance

Using antipyrine autoinduction in the rat, Chang et al. (33) tested the monoexponential kinetic model of induction proposed by Levy et al. (34). This model assumes that the time course of the increase in drug clearance is controlled by the turnover half-life of the induced enzyme(s). As predicted by this kinetic model, the increase in antipyrine clearance as a function of time was well defined by a monoexponential equation. In four of the five rats studied, the half-life for induction varied between 30 and 36 hr. These values were found to be comparable to in vitro estimates for the half-life of induced cytochrome P_{450} enzymes in this species.

B. Heteroinduction

Bai and Abramson (35) examined the time course of induction of α_1-acid glycoprotein by phenobarbital in dogs and its impact of the protein binding of propanolol. They observed that after discontinuation of phenobarbital, the washout of the stimulation of propanolol plasma protein binding was delayed. In order to account for this lag time, they invoked an induction model in which the kinetics of the inducer may be rate limiting. Abramson (36) examined the relationship between the kinetics of the inducer and those of the induced substance (enzyme or precursor). When the elimination rate constant of the inducer is much larger (i.e., five times or more) than the turnover rate constant of the induced substance, the kinetics of the induction phase and deinduction phase are both governed by the turnover rate constant of the induced substance.

When the elimination rate constant of the induced substance is not much larger (i.e., equal to or smaller) than the turnover rate constant of the induced substance, the extent of induction achieved by the concentration of the inducer must be considered. If the concentration of the inducer is sufficiently high such that the production rate of the induced substance is maximal, the induction and deinduction phases are not symmetrical. The induction phase is controlled by the turnover rate constant of the induced substance (i.e., the kinetics of accumulation of the inducer are unimportant). However, in the deinduction phase, the return to baseline conditions is much slower than predicted by the turnover rate constant of the induced substance. Indeed, the stimulation of induction persists after withdrawal of the inducer and is controlled by the elimination rate constant of the inducer. If the concentration of the inducer is much smaller than the concentration associated with maximum induction (or production rate of induced substance), the extent of induction increases slowly as the concentration of inducer rises. After withdrawal of the inducer, the extent of induction decreases slowly and is governed by the elimination rate constant of the inducer. In both phases of induction and deinduction, the turnover rate constant of the induced substance does not play a role.

In a second paper, Abramson (37) examined the alternative mechanism for induction, a decrease in the turnover rate constant of the enzyme [or precursor(s)]. When the elimination rate constant of the inducer is larger than the original (noninhibited) turnover rate constant of the induced substance, the time course of induction during the induction phase is governed by the inhibited turnover rate constant of the induced substance. After withdrawal of the inducer, the time course of deinduction is rapid and is controlled by the noninhibited turnover rate constant of the induced substance.

When the elimination rate constant of the inducer is rate limiting (smaller than the baseline value of the turnover rate constant of the induced substance), both the induction and deinduction phases are governed by the elimination rate constant of the inducer. Similar behavior is obtained when the inducer inhibits the turnover rate constant of a precursor of the induced substance.

IV. CONCLUSIONS

This literature review, which covers the period between 1983 and 1987, shows that diurnal phenomena in drug disposition were pursued for several drugs with narrow therapeutic ranges. For theophylline, the increased use of controlled-release formulations was a motivating factor. Also of interest is that attempts were made to understand the mechanisms underlying the changes in drug clearance. For chemically induced time dependencies, most advances were made in model testing and model development. The monoexponential model of induction of clearance was validated with antipyrine autoinduction in the rat. In the induction of α_1-acid glycoprotein by phenobarbital in the dog, the induction model was expanded to consider the kinetics of the inducer.

REFERENCES

1. R. H. Levy. Time-dependent pharmacokinetics. Pharmacol. Ther. 7: 383–397, 1982.
2. A. Reinberg and M. H. Smolensky. Circadian changes in drug disposition in man. Clin. Pharmacokinet. 7: 401–420, 1982.

3. G. Labrecque and P. M. Bélanger. In Topics in Pharmaceutical Sciences 1985. Edited by D. D. Briemer and P. Speiser. Elsevier, New York, 1985, pp. 167–178.

4. R. H. Levy. In Topics in Pharmaceutical Sciences 1985. Edited by D. D. Briemer and P. Speiser. Elsevier, New York, 1985, pp. 161–166.

5. L. J. Lesko, D. Brousseau, A. T. Canada, and G. Eastwood. Temporal variation in trough serum theophylline concentrations of steady state. J. Pharm. Sci. 69(3): 358–359, 1980.

6. P. H. Scott, E. Tabachnik, S. MacLeod, J. Carreia, C. Newth, and H. Levison. Sustained-release theophylline for childhood asthmaL Evidence for circadian variation of theophylline pharmacokinetics. J. Pediatr. 99(3): 476–479, 1981.

7. W. Primrose. Asthma at night. Lacet 927, April 23, 1983.

8. K. P. Coulthard, D. J. Birkett, D. R. Lines, N. Grgurinovich, and J. J. Grygiel. Bioavailability and diurnal variation in absorption of sustained release theophylline in asthmatic children. Eur. J. Clin. Pharmacol. 25: 667–672, 1983.

9. H. Watanabe, S. Nakano, K. Nagai, and N. Ogawa. Time-dependent absorption of theophylline. J. Clin. Pharmacol. 24: 509–514, 1984.

10. M. St.-Pierre, M. Spino, A. Isles, A. Tesoro, and S. M. MacLeod. Circadian variation in theophylline disposition. Clin. Pharmacol. Ther. IV-A: 278, 1984.

11. T. Uematsu, F. Follath, and S. Vozeh. Circadian changes in the absorption and elimination of theophylline in patients with bronchial obstruction. Eur. J. Clin. Pharmacol. 30: 309–312, 1986.

12. J. H. G. Jonkman, W. J. V. van der Boon, L. P. Balant, R. Schoenmaker, and A. Holtkamp. Chronopharmacokinetics of theophylline after sustained release and intravenous administration to adults. Eur. J. Clin. Pharmacol. 26: 215–222, 1984.

13. B. L. Chauhan, B. S. Doshi, and R. D. Kulkarni. Diurnal variation in the pharmacokinetics of intravenous theophylline and etophylline in healthy subjects. Eur. J. Clin. Pharmacol. 30: 635–636, 1986.

14. D. R. Taylor, D. Duffin, C. D. Kinney, and D. G. McDevitt. Circadian variation in plasma theophylline concentrations during maintenance therapy with a sustained-release preparation in patients with obstructive airway disease. Br. J. Clin. Pharmacol. 18: 27–30, 1984.

15. H. Neuenkirchen, J. H. Wilkens, M. Oellerich, and G. W. Sybrecht. Nocturnal astham: Effect of a once per evening dose of sustained release theophylline. Eur. J. Respir. Dis. 66: 196–204, 1985.

16. P. Guissou, G. Cuisinaud, G. Llorca, E. Lejeune, and J. Sassard. Chronopharmacokinetic study of a prolonged release form of indomethacin. Eur. J. Clin. Pharmacol. 24: 667—670, 1983.

17. A. J. Taggart, J. C. McElnay, B. Kerr, and P. Passmore. The chronopharmacokinetics of indomethacin suppositories in healthy volunteers. Eur. J. Clin. Pharmacol. 31: 617—619, 1987.

18. O. V. Olesen and K. Thomsen. Diurnal variation in serum lithium and renal lithium clearance in rats given lithium as a single small dose or as multiple high doses. Acta Pharmacol. Toxicol. 57: 171—175, 1985.

19. H. A. Decousus, M. Croze, F. A. Levi, J. G. Jaubert, B. M. Perpoint, J. F. De Bonadona, A. Reinberg, and P. M. Queneau. Circadian changes in anticoagulant effect of heparin infused at a constant rate. Br. Med. J. 290: 341—344, February 2, 1985.

20. M. Decousus, E. Gremillet, H. Decousus, A. Champailler, C. Houzard, B. Perpoint, and J. Jaubert. Nyctothermeral variations of $^{99}Tc^m$-labelled heparin pharmacokinetic parameters. Nucl. Med. Commun. 6: 633—640, 1985.

21. R. Venkataramanan, S. Yang, G. J. Burckart, R. J. Ptachcinski, D. H. Van Thiel, and T. E. Starzl. Diurnal variation in cyclosporine kinetics. Ther. Drug Monit. 8: 380—381, 1986.

22. J. H. Sirota, D. A. Balwin, and H. Villarreal. Diurnal variations of renal function in man. J. Clin. Invest. 29: 187—192, 1950.

23. W. J. M. Hrushesky, R. Borch, and F. Levi. Circadian time dependence of cisplatin urinary kinetics. Clin. Pharmacol. Ther. 32(3): 330—339, 1982.

24. B. Hecquet, J. Meynadier, J. Bonnetree, L. Adenis, and A. Demaille. Time dependency in plasmatic protein binding of cisplatin. Cancer Treat. Rep. 69(1): 79—83, 1985.

25. W. J. M. Hrushesky, F. A. Levi, and F. Halberg. Circadian stage dependence of cis-diammine-dichloroplatinum lethal toxicity in rats. Cancer Res. 42: 945—949, 1982.

26. F. A. Levi, W. J. M. Hrushesky, and F. Halberg. Lethal nephrotoxicity and hematologic toxicity of cis-diamine-dichloroplatinum ameliorated by optimal circadian timing and hydration. Eur. J. Cancer Clin. Oncol. 18: 471—477, 1982.

27. F. A. Levi, W. J. M. Hrushesky, and R. F. Borch. Cisplatin urinary pharmacokinetics and nephrotoxicity: A common circadian mechanism. Cancer Treat. Rep. 66: 1933—1938, 1982.

28. F. M. Radzialowski and W. F. Bousquet. Daily rhythmic variation in hepatic drug metabolism in the rat and mouse. J. Pharmacol. Exp. Ther. 163(1): 229—238, 1968.

29. A. Colas, D. Gregonis, and N. Moir. Daily rhythms in the hydroxylation of 3-β-hydroxyandrost-5-en-17-one by rat liver microsomes. Endocrinology 84: 165—167, 1969.

30. A. Jori, E. DiSalle, and V. Santini. Daily rhythmic variation and drug metabolism in rats. Biochem. Pharmacol. 20: 2965−2969, 1971.

31. T. L. Holcslaw, T. S. Miya, and W. S. Bousquet. Circadian rhythms in drug action and drug metabolism in the mouse. J. Pharmacol. Exp. Ther. 195(2): 320−332, 1975.

32. P. M. Bélanger, M. Lalande, G. Labrecque, and F. M. Dore. Diurnal variation in the transferases and hydrolases involved in glucuronide and sulfate conjugation of rat liver. Drug Metab. Dispos. 13(3): 386−388, 1985.

33. S.-L. Chang, K. Emmick, and P. Wedlund. Characterization of antipyrine autoinduction in the rat utilizing a new micro-sampling technique for serial blood sample collection. J. Pharm. Sci. 75(5): 456−458, 1986.

34. R. H. Levy, A. A. Lai, and M. S. Dumain. Time-dependent kinetics. IV. Pharmacokinetic theory of enzyme induction. J. Pharm. Sci. 68(3): 398−399, 1979.

35. S. A. Bai and F. P. Abramson. Interaction of phenobarbital with propranolol in the dog. 1. Plasma protein binding. J. Pharmacol. Exp. Ther. 222(3): 589−594, 1982.

36. F. P. Abramson. Kinetic models of induction. 1. Persistence of the inducing substance. J. Pharm. Sci. 75(3): 223−228, 1986.

37. F. P. Abramson. Kinetic models of induction. 2. Decreased turnover of a product or its precursor. J. Pharm. Sci. 75(3): 229−232, 1986.

Index